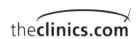

ENDOCRINOLOGY AND METABOLISM CLINICS

OF NORTH AMERICA

Andrology

GUEST EDITOR
Ronald Tamler, MD, PhD, MBA

CONSULTING EDITOR
Derek LeRoith, MD, PhD

June 2007 • Volume 36 • Number 2

SAUNDERS

An Imprint of Elsevier, Inc.
PHILADELPHIA   LONDON   TORONTO   MONTREAL   SYDNEY   TOKYO

W.B. SAUNDERS COMPANY
A Division of Elsevier Inc.

1600 John F. Kennedy Boulevard • Suite 1800 • Philadelphia, Pennsylvania 19103-2899

http://www.theclinics.com

ENDOCRINOLOGY AND METABOLISM	Volume 36, Number 2
CLINICS OF NORTH AMERICA	ISSN 0889-8529
June 2007	ISBN-13: 978-1-4160-4309-6
Editor: Rachel Glover	ISBN-10: 1-4160-4309-8

The ideas and opinions expressed in *Endocrinology and Metabolism Clinics of North America* do not necessarily reflect those of the Publisher. The Publisher does not assume any responsibility for any injury and/or damage to persons or property arising out of or related to any use of the material contained in this periodical. The reader is advised to check the appropriate medical literature and the product information currently provided by the manufacturer of each drug to be administered to verify the dosage, the method and duration of administration, or contraindications. It is the responsibility of the treating physician or other health care professional, relying on independent experience and knowledge of the patient, to determine drug dosages and the best treatment for the patient. Mention of any product in this issue should not be construed as endorsement by the contributors, editors, or the Publisher of the product or manufacturers' claims.

Endocrinology and Metabolism Clinics of North America (ISSN 0889-8529) is published quarterly by Elsevier Inc., 360 Park Avenue South, New York, NY 10010-1710. Months of publication are March, June, September, and December. Business and editorial offices: 1600 John F. Kennedy Boulevard, Suite 1800, Philadelphia, PA 19103-2899. Customer Service Office: 6277 Sea Harbor Drive, Orlando, FL 32887-4800. Periodicals postage paid at New York, NY and additional mailing offices. Subscription prices are USD 193 per year for US individuals, USD 319 per year for US institutions, USD 99 per year for US students and residents, USD 242 per year for Canadian individuals, USD 383 per year for Canadian institutions, USD 264 per year for international individuals, USD 383 per year for international institutions and USD 138 per year for Canadian and foreign students/residents. To receive student/resident rate, orders must be accompanied by name of affiliated institution, date of term, and the *signature* of program/residency coordinator on institution letterhead. Orders will be billed at individual rate until proof of status is received. Foreign air speed delivery is included in all *Clinics* subscription prices. All prices are subject to change without notice. POSTMASTER: Send address changes to *Endocrinology and Metabolism Clinics of North America*, Elsevier Periodicals Customer Service, 6277 Sea Harbor Drive, Orlando, FL 32887-4800. **Customer Service: (+1) 800-654-2452 (US). From outside of the US, call (+1) 407-345-4000; e-mail: hhspcs@harcourt.com.**

Reprints. For copies of 100 or more, of articles in this publication, please contact the Commercial Rights Department, Elsevier Inc., 360 Park Avenue South, New York, NY 10010-1710; phone: (+1) 212-633-3813; fax: (+1) 212-462-1935; e-mail: reprints@elsevier.com.

Endocrinology and Metabolism Clinics of North America is covered in *Index Medicus, EMBASE/Excerpta Medica, Current Contents/Clinical Medicine, Current Contents/Life Sciences, Science Citation Index, ISI/BIOMED, BIO-SIS, and Chemical Abstracts.*

Printed in the United States of America.

CONSULTING EDITOR

DEREK LᴇROITH, MD, PhD, Chief, Division of Endocrinology, Metabolism, and Bone Diseases, Mount Sinai School of Medicine, New York, New York

GUEST EDITOR

RONALD TAMLER, MD, PhD, MBA, CNSP, Co-Director, The Mount Sinai Program for Men's Wellness; and Instructor of Medicine, Division of Endocrinology, Diabetes, and Bone Disease, Mount Sinai School of Medicine, New York, New York

CONTRIBUTORS

NATAN BAR-CHAMA, MD, Associate Professor of Urology, Obstetrics/Gynecology and Reproductive Medicine, Mount Sinai School of Medicine, Mount Sinai Medical Center, New York, New York

ANTHONY J. BELLA, MD, Clinical Instructor and American Urological Association Robert J. Krane Scholar, Department of Urology, University of California, San Francisco, California

JOHN P. BILEZIKIAN, MD, Department of Medicine; Department of Pharmacology, Division of Endocrinology, College of Physicians and Surgeons, Columbia University, New York, New York

WILLIAM O. BRANT, MD, Assistant Clinical Professor of Surgery, University of Colorado School of Medicine, Denver, Colorado

HAROLD E. CARLSON, MD, Professor of Medicine and Head, Division of Endocrinology, Diabetes, and Metabolism, Health Sciences Center, Stony Brook University, Stony Brook, New York

PAUL C. CARPENTER, MD, FACE, Associate Professor of Medicine and Consultant, Divisions of Endocrinology-Metabolism and Bioinformatics Research, Mayo Clinic College of Medicine, Mayo Clinic, Rochester, Minnesota

IAN D. CATERSON, MBBS, FRACP, PhD, Boden Professor of Human Nutrition, Royal Prince Alfred Hospital, Human Nutrition Unit, University of Sydney, Sydney, Australia

BRIAN G. CHOI, MD, MBA, Cardiology Fellow, The Zena and Michael A. Wiener Cardiovascular Institute, Mount Sinai School of Medicine, New York, New York

ADRIAN S. DOBS, MD, MHS, Professor of Medicine and Oncology, Division of Endocrinology and Metabolism, Johns Hopkins School of Medicine; and Department of Medicine, Johns Hopkins School of Medicine, Baltimore, Maryland

ANDREAS M. FINNER, MD, Fourth-Year Resident in Dermatology, Department of Dermatology, University Clinic, Magdeburg, Germany

SRAVANYA GAVINI, BS, Medical Student, Division of Endocrinology and Metabolism, Johns Hopkins School of Medicine, Baltimore, Maryland

LUIGI GENNARI, MD, Department of Internal Medicine, Endocrine-Metabolic Sciences, and Biochemistry, University of Siena, Siena, Italy

IRWIN GOLDSTEIN, MD, Director, Sexual Medicine, Alvarado Hospital, San Diego, California; Editor-in-Chief, The Journal of Sexual Medicine, Milton, Massachusetts

RONALD R. GRUNSTEIN, MBBS, FRACP, PhD, Professor of Medicine and Head, Sleep and Circadian Group, Royal Prince Alfred Hospital, Woolcock Institute, University of Sydney, Sydney, Australia

ANDRÉ T. GUAY, MD, FACP, FACE, Director, Center for Sexual Function/ Endocrinology, Lahey Clinic Northshore, Peabody; Clinical Assistant Professor of Medicine (Endocrinology), Harvard Medical School, Boston, Massachusetts

SIMON J. HALL, MD, Chair, Department of Urology; and Director, Deane Prostate Health and Research Center, Mount Sinai School of Medicine, New York, New York

DAVID J. HANDELSMAN, MBBS, FRACP, PhD, Professor of Reproductive Endocrinology and Andrology, and Director, ANZAC Research Institute, Concord Hospital, University of Sydney, Sydney, Australia

NIGEL HUNT, PhD, Associate Professor in Health Psychology, Institute of Work, Health, and Organisations, University of Nottingham, Nottingham, United Kingdom

CHRISTOPHER IP, MD, Chief Resident, Department of Urology, Mount Sinai School of Medicine, New York, New York

JONATHAN P. JAROW, MD, Professor of Urology, Pathology, Radiology, and Biochemistry and Molecular Biology, Johns Hopkins University, Baltimore, Maryland

RITA R. KALYANI, MD, Fellow, Division of Endocrinology and Metabolism, Johns Hopkins School of Medicine, Baltimore, Maryland

LAWRENCE C. LAYMAN, MD, Professor and Chief, Section of Reproductive Endocrinology, Infertility, and Genetics, Department of Obstetrics and Gynecology; and Director, Program in Reproductive Medicine, Developmental Neurobiology Program, Institute of Molecular Medicine and Genetics, Medical College of Georgia, Augusta, Georgia

PETER Y. LIU, MBBS, FRACP, PhD, Associate Professor, Department of Andrology, ANZAC Research Institute, Concord Hospital, University of Sydney, Sydney, Australia

TOM F. LUE, MD, Professor and Vice-Chairman of Urology, Department of Urology, University of California, San Francisco, California

SUE McHALE, PhD, Senior Lecturer in Biopsychology, Psychology Group, Sheffield Hallam University, Sheffield, United Kingdom

MARY ANN McLAUGHLIN, MD, MPH, Assistant Professor of Cardiology, The Zena and Michael A. Wiener Cardiovascular Institute, Mount Sinai School of Medicine, New York, New York

JEFFREY I. MECHANICK, MD, FACP, FACE, FACN, Director, Metabolic Support; and Associate Clinical Professor of Medicine, Division of Endocrinology, Diabetes, and Bone Disease, Mount Sinai School of Medicine, New York, New York

HARMEET SINGH NARULA, MD, Assistant Professor of Clinical Medicine, Division of Endocrinology, Diabetes, and Metabolism, Health Sciences Center, Stony Brook University, Stony Brook, New York

NINA OTBERG, MD, Clinical Hair Fellow/Research Fellow, Hair Research and Treatment Centre, Department of Dermatology and Skin Science, University of British Columbia, Vancouver, British Columbia, Canada

MICHELLE L. RAMÍREZ, BA, Medical Student, Male Reproductive Medicine and Surgery, Mount Sinai School of Medicine, Mount Sinai Medical Center, New York, New York

JONATHAN D. SCHIFF, MD, Assistant Clinical Professor of Urology, Mount Sinai School of Medicine, Mount Sinai Medical Center, New York, New York

JERRY SHAPIRO, MD, FRCPC, Clinical Professor and Director, Hair Research and Treatment Centre, Department of Dermatology and Skin Science, University of British Columbia, Vancouver, British Columbia, Canada

RONALD TAMLER, MD, PhD, MBA, CNSP, Co-Director, The Mount Sinai Program for Men's Wellness; and Instructor of Medicine, Division of Endocrinology, Diabetes, and Bone Disease, Mount Sinai School of Medicine, New York, New York

CONTENTS

> Gonadotropin-releasing hormone (GnRH) and olfactory neurons migrate together from the olfactory placode, and GnRH neurons eventually reside in the hypothalamus. Hypogonadism in male infants may be diagnosed in the first 6 months of life but cannot be diagnosed during childhood until puberty occurs. Patients with low serum testosterone and low serum gonadotropin levels have idiopathic hypogonadotropic hypogonadism (IHH). Mutations in three genes (KAL1, FGFR1, and GNRHR) comprise most of the known genetic causes of IHH. Treatment with testosterone is indicated if fertility is not desired, whereas GnRH or gonadotropin treatment induces spermatogenesis and fertility.

> There are several objectives to be achieved during the diagnostic evaluation of a male partner of an infertile partnership. The first is to identify whether or not there is a male factor present and, if so, whether this is attributable to an underlying medical illness. The second is to identify the cause of reduced male fertility and whether or not it is amenable to therapeutic intervention.

alone or in conjunction with standard therapies, the controversies of timing of therapy, and the completeness of ablation and its use on an intermittent basis are reviewed.

Androgen insufficiency and erectile dysfunction are highly prevalent medical disorders in aging men who have associated multiple risk factors. Good clinical practice requires the use of appropriate strategies for patient- and goal-directed diagnosis and treatment. This article focuses on a rational, evidence based clinical management paradigm that combines diagnosis and treatment of men who have androgen insufficiency and erectile dysfunction.

Erectile dysfunction (ED) is a common condition in men, and increases with age. Cardiovascular disease (CVD) is the leading cause of death in men and also increases in prevalence with advancing years. The common link between the two conditions is endothelial dysfunction that leads to vascular insufficiency of the coronary and penile arteries. Because the penile arteries are smaller, symptoms of ED may precede those of CVD by several years. It is logical, therefore, that a patient complaining of ED should alert the physician to look for cardiovascular risk factors. Early treatment of these risk factors may help to prevent or retard symptoms of vascular insufficiency.

A wide variety of medications, devices, and surgical interventions are available to patients who have ED. These range from first-line oral agents to second-line therapy with injections or vacuum devices to third-line options, such as penile prosthesis implantation. In this article, we cover available treatments for erectile dysfunction, ranging from first-line to third-line therapies.

This discussion reviews the concept and history of ergogenic aides, the penetration of use in society, some benefit/risk information, drug sources in our society, detection and regulation of these agents, and provides a look to the future. It also examines the role of the clinician/endocrinologist for these patients and uses some cases as examples of drug use among adolescents/teens.

FORTHCOMING ISSUES

RECENT ISSUES

THE CLINICS ARE NOW AVAILABLE ONLINE!

Access your subscription at:
http://www.theclinics.com

Endocrinol Metab Clin N Am
36 (2007) xiii–xvi

ENDOCRINOLOGY
AND METABOLISM
CLINICS
OF NORTH AMERICA

Foreword

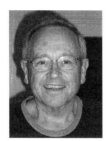

Derek LeRoith, MD, PhD
Consulting Editor

Ronald Tamler has developed an issue dealing with Andrology that is comprehensive in scope but is also of value to the reader, having many practical aspects to each topic. The authors are obviously experts in their fields but have presented their knowledge in a very down-to-earth manner and are to be complimented for their efforts.

In the first article, Lawrence Layman describes the normal development of the hypothalamic–pituitary axis and physiologic changes occurring in puberty. This is followed by a review of hypogonadism and delayed puberty in boys and a description of the syndrome of hypogonadotropic hypogonadism, which is diagnosed by the presence of low circulating testosterone and gonadotopin levels. There are a few genetic mutations that cause this abnormality, namely mutations in KAL1, FGFR1, and GNRHR genes. Hypothalamic–pituitary destruction can have the same result. The disorder can be treated either with testosterone if fertility is not desired, or GHRH or gonadotropins if spermatogenesis is also to be induced.

Evaluation of the infertile male has become an important topic given the extent to which the practice of in vitro fertilization has evolved. Low sperm counts warrant an extensive and complete evaluation of the male partner. In his article, Jonathan Jarow describes in detail the physical, genetic, and hormonal studies that are required to determine whether a treatable cause can be discovered. Jonathan Schiff, Michelle Ramírez, and Natan Bar-Chama complete the picture in their article by discussing the surgical and medical treatments of the infertile male. They present a comprehensive, practical

doi:10.1016/j.ecl.2007.03.016

algorithm for management of male infertility that, they suggest, is adaptable and should be individualized and used as a guideline for the male partner of an infertile couple.

Systemic disease can be associated with hypogonadism and low serum testosterone. This effect may explain loss of lean body mass, loss of bone mineral, changes in mood, lack of energy, and, of course, sexual dysfunction. A similar effect is seen with the normal aging process. Rita Kalyani, Sravanya Gavini, and Adrian Dobs describe in their article several chronic disorders associated with low testosterone and propose that replacement therapy may be warranted on an individual basis to improve patients' well-being, though careful monitoring is very important.

Liu, Caterson, Grunstein, and Handelsman present an interesting hypothesis to explain the relationship between obesity, hypogonadism, and obstructive sleep apnea in men. They propose that low serum testosterone is the central feature. Obesity leads to a reduction in circulating testosterone, which is also associated with erectile dysfunction. Weight loss reverses this effect. Low testosterone in turn may lead to worsening of obesity and exacerbate the sleep apnea that is characteristic of obesity. As they point out, more controlled trials will be needed to confirm these interesting interrelationships and perhaps support potential therapeutic options.

Coronary artery disease (CAD) is more common in males than females, until women are postmenopausal. This had led to the suggestion that sex steroids play an important role. Indeed, Brian Choi and Mary McLaughlin describe in their article the effect of testosterone on many of the risk factors that are involved in CAD. A subset of studies in the literature even show a positive effect of testosterone replacement on cardiac function. The studies they present appear quite convincing, but they do caution that more studies are required to evaluate this effect.

Androgenic alopecia, otherwise known as male pattern hair loss, has a strong genetic component. As described by Nina Otberg, Andreas Finner, and Jerry Shapiro, although it is not completely preventable or reversible, progression of the disorder can be attenuated using minoxidil and finasteride. Alternatively, hair restoration surgery is always an option.

Gennari and John P. Bilezikian discuss male osteoporosis, an increasing disorder that is commonly thought to be unique to postmenopausal women. The loss of bone mineral density (BMD) occurs later in men; therefore, BMD measurements may be determined in men over the age of 70 years. Earlier investigations are warranted if there are specific indications. Loss of bone is often related to hormonal changes in men. Treatment of men with osteoporosis is similar to females; bisphosphonates are the mainstay, but parathyroid hormone can be considered. Some recent studies suggest testosterone supplementation in hypogonadism or selective estrogen receptor modulators if the circulating estrogen levels are low.

Ip and Hall describe in their article the dilemmas surrounding the diagnosis and treatment of prostate cancer, a very common and sometimes fatal disorder. Androgens do affect prostate-specific antigen (PSA) levels, but the effect is less relevant than the proportional increase with recent enlargements of the prostate. PSA is useful in screening for prostate cancer, with the definitive diagnosis being histologic. Therapy for the primary tumor has generally involved surgery, although it has been replaced in some cases by radiation ablation. Prostate cancer with metastases involves antiandrogen therapy, because the tumors are commonly androgen-responsive. Orchiectomy, GnRH agonists, and antiandrogens have all been used to reduce or treat cancer recurrence, though the authors point out their appropriate use still requires more appropriate trials.

Hypoandrogenism and erectile dysfunction are conditions that occur commonly in men, more often when they age, and are often undiagnosed because the health care provider is not attentive to these conditions. They are often interrelated, and Irwin Goldstein presents in his article an algorithm for the diagnosis and treatment of these conditions. History, physcial examination, and blood chemistry are the mainstay of diagnosis. Therapy often addresses a condition that secondarily causes the disorder and is treatable. On the other hand, various hormonal replacements or pharmacologic therapies are required, as outlined. The importance lies in an awareness of how common these conditions are in men and that successful outcomes are often achievable.

The relationship of erectile dysfunction and endothelial dysfunction is discussed by Andre Guay. Endothelium in the coronary arteries is similar to that seen in penile arteries; indeed, erectile dysfunction may be caused by the same factors that predispose to coronary events and in fact often precede CHD. Not surprisingly, therefore, phosphodiesterase-5 inhibitors have been shown to improve both erectile and endothelial dysfunction. Brant, Bella, and Lue present a more in-depth and balanced discussion on the treatment of erectile dysfunction that covers all the available medications and surgical treatments.

A major concern of the medical community is the use of performance enhancers in sport. In a case-based article, Paul Carpenter describes the use and abuse of these agents, discussing the harmful side effects that eventuate and emphasizing the role of physicians and supervisory boards in educating athletes to avoid these harmful drugs.

Enlargement of the breast is commonly seen in adolescent boys, probably due to an imbalance between testosterone and androgens during that phase of development. It generally resolves spontaneously. On the other hand, it may be secondary to several disorders and warrants investigation, especially in postadolescent individuals. Narula and Carlson describe in detail the causes of gynecomastia, the process of investigating an underlying cause and the available treatments, both hormonal and nonhormonal.

Nigel Hunt and Susan McHale tackle an important though less-recognized problem that arises with various andrologic disorders, namely the psychological consequences. As they describe, treatment for these conditions should not focus entirely on the medical aspects but simultaneously on overcoming the serious concomitant psychologic problems.

In the last article, Ronald Tamler and Jeffrey Mechanick discuss the increasing use of nutraceuticals in treating erectile dysfunction, decreased libido, and related conditions, and strongly supports further rigorous testing before their use in these conditions can be recommended. On the other hand, certain antioxidants such as lycopene have been tested and may play a role in preventing prostate cancer.

Derek LeRoith, MD, PhD
Division of Endocrinology
Metabolism, and Bone Diseases
Mount Sinai School of Medicine
One Gustave L. Levy Place
Box 1055, New York
NY 10029, USA

E-mail address: derek.leroith@mssm.edu

ELSEVIER
SAUNDERS

Endocrinol Metab Clin N Am
36 (2007) xvii–xviii

ENDOCRINOLOGY
AND METABOLISM
CLINICS
OF NORTH AMERICA

Preface

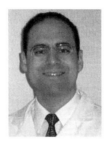

Ronald Tamler, MD, PhD, MBA, CNSP
Guest Editor

Are men the weaker sex? With higher rates of cancer, cardiovascular disease, and poor use of health care resources, all leading to an average life expectancy about 6 years less than in women, it may seem so. However, the last andrology issue of *Endocrinology and Metabolism Clinics of North America* dates back as far as 1998 and mainly concerns itself with fertility. Since then, significant developments have happened: We have become more aware of diagnoses such as hypogonadism and erectile dysfunction and have become more adept at diagnosing and treating them. Certainly, great strides have been made in fertility medicine. However, the contemporary practice of andrology, which, according to Webster's dictionary, is "a branch of medicine concerned with male diseases and especially with those affecting the male reproductive system," covers more than just reproduction. This demand in complete care for the entire man is mirrored in the creation of centers specializing in the care of men across the world, and the newly founded Mount Sinai Men's Wellness Program in New York is no exception. To mirror this comprehensive approach, we have assembled specialists from the realms of endocrinology, cardiology, dermatology, urology, sleep medicine, and psychology to give a wide-ranging interdisciplinary overview of physiologically interesting and clinically useful information. I sincerely hope that this issue will provide you with up-to-date yet durable knowledge on matters as diverse as prostate health, male fertility, gynecomastia, male psychology, hypogonadism in a variety of conditions, erectile dysfunction, alopecia, nutritional supplements, and the vastly underdiagnosed osteoporosis in men. May it be as stimulating for the reader as it was for me as a guest editor.

Ronald Tamler, MD, PhD, MBA, CNSP
Division of Endocrinology, Diabetes and Bone Disease
Mount Sinai School of Medicine
1 Gustave L Levy Pl, Box 1055
New York, NY 10029, USA

E-mail address: ronald.tamler@mssm.edu

ELSEVIER
SAUNDERS

Endocrinol Metab Clin N Am
36 (2007) 283–296

ENDOCRINOLOGY
AND METABOLISM
CLINICS
OF NORTH AMERICA

Hypogonadotropic Hypogonadism

Lawrence C. Layman, MD[a,b,*]

[a]*Section of Reproductive Endocrinology, Infertility, and Genetics, Department of Obstetrics and Gynecology, Medical College of Georgia, 1120 15th Street, Augusta, GA 30912, USA*
[b]*Program in Reproductive Medicine, Developmental Neurobiology Program, Institute of Molecular Medicine and Genetics, Medical College of Georgia, 1120 15th Street, Augusta, GA 30912, USA*

Maturation of the hypothalamic-pituitary-gonadal axis

Somatic changes

Normal puberty is usually a progression of events, and once puberty is initiated, it is generally completed in 3 to 4 years. Adrenarche is the result of adrenal androgen stimulation (androstenedione, dehydroepiandrosterone [DHEA], and dehydroepiandrosterone sulfate [DHEAS], and it begins at approximately 6 to 8 years of age and continues through the middle teens in boys and girls. In boys, the initial pubertal event is testicular growth, which usually begins at approximately 10.5 years of age. When the testes exceed 2.5 cm in any dimension, puberty is beginning. Pubarche frequently starts simultaneously with testicular development. Axillary hair growth occurs at approximately the time of peak height velocity, which occurs at approximately 14 years of age in boys.

Endocrinology of childhood and puberty

In the embryo, gonadotropin-releasing hormone (GnRH) neurons migrate with olfactory neurons from the olfactory placode to their normal position in the hypothalamus [1]. This embryologic event illustrates the close interaction of the reproductive and olfactory systems, the disruption of which may result in pathologic change. The GnRH pulse generator is the principal regulator of puberty through its control of pituitary gonadotropins and is active even in fetal life. As a result, gonadotropin levels change during

Research in hypogonadotropic hypogonadism is supported by National Institutes of Health grants HD33004 and HD040287.

* Section of Reproductive Endocrinology, Infertility, and Genetics, Department of Obstetrics and Gynecology, Medical College of Georgia, 1120 15th Street, Augusta, GA 30912.

E-mail address: llayman@mcg.edu

0889-8529/07/$ - see front matter © 2007 Published by Elsevier Inc.
doi:10.1016/j.ecl.2007.03.010

fetal development, childhood, puberty, and adulthood. In the embryo, gonadotropins begin to rise at 10 weeks of gestation, peak at midgestation, and decline at term because of the negative feedback from placental steroids [2]. At birth, when there is a withdrawal of gestational steroids, follicle-stimulating hormone (FSH) and luteinizing hormone (LH) rise, with a subsequent decline that is gender specific. Girls tend to have a higher FSH-to-LH ratio at all times compared with boys, and their gonadotropin levels decline by 2 to 4 years of age. Within the first 6 months of life, gonadotropin stimulation of the testes may result in testosterone production in male infants. During this "window period," gonadal function may be assessed clinically in male infants; however, unfortunately, this is rarely accomplished [2]. After 6 months of age in male infants, serum gonadotropins drop and the diagnosis of hyper- and hypogonadotropic hypogonadism is no longer possible until puberty. During childhood, gonadotropins remain low in both genders, with an LH/FSH ratio less than 1 until puberty.

Other hormones in the neonatal period reflect testicular function and are useful clinically [2]. These consist of two Sertoli cell proteins: inhibin B and anti-müllerian hormone (AMH)/müllerian inhibiting substance (MIS). Inhibin B (male humans have essentially no inhibin A) increases soon after birth, peaks at 4 to 12 months of age, declines to low levels at 3 to 9 years of age, and then increases again with the onset of puberty (however, at lower levels than in the neonate). AMH/MIS is evident in the first month of life and peaks at approximately 6 months of age, drops during childhood, and becomes extremely low with puberty, probably secondary to increased testosterone inhibition. These hormones are also useful markers of testicular function in early childhood.

The exact central inhibitor of GnRH (and gonadotropin levels) until the initiation of puberty remains unknown [2]. From identified gene mutations in patients with idiopathic hypogonadotropic hypogonadism (IHH), it has become apparent that leptin and kisspeptin signaling is important in normal puberty. Gonadotropins begin to rise by the age of approximately 9 years—first FSH and then LH. These increases reflect the increase in pulse frequency of the GnRH pulse generator. Slower GnRH pulses lead to the preferential secretion of FSH, whereas more rapid pulses favor LH secretion. Initially, LH pulses are nocturnal but then become apparent throughout the 24-hour day, which stimulate gonadal steroid production. In male adults, LH pulses occur roughly every 2 hours, resulting in testosterone stimulation [3]. There is evidence in younger male adults of a diurnal rhythm of testosterone secretion, with morning levels being higher than at other times during the day.

Delayed puberty

Diagnosis of hypogonadism and associated anomalies

Delayed puberty in boys is usually defined as the absence of signs of puberty by the age of 14 years that is 2.5 SDs greater than the mean for North

American boys [4]. A careful history and physical examination of the patient with delayed puberty are extremely important. It is important to ascertain if there were any initial signs of a voice change, axillary and pubic hair growth, and a growth spurt. Obtaining all pediatric records provides extremely useful information, because height and weight can be plotted to evaluate growth velocity. A complete lack of growth velocity indicates an absence of sex steroid–induced growth, which is more likely to portend serious pathologic change. Symptoms of thyroid disease (weight changes, constipation/diarrhea, sleep disturbances, and skin dryness/sweatiness) and hyperprolactinemia (headache, visual disturbances, and impotence) should be ascertained.

A history of anomalies in the patient and family should be discussed, because hypergonadotropic hypogonadism may be associated with Turner stigmata (shield chest, short fourth metacarpal, and webbed neck), short stature, cardiac anomalies, renal anomalies, and cryptorchidism (45,X/46,XY cell line) as well as with testicular fibrosis, mental deficiency, and behavior problems (47,XXY cell line) [5]. A variety of anomalies are also associated with hypogonadotropic hypogonadism, such as anosmia/hyposmia, cleft palate, dental agenesis, visual abnormalities, deafness, mental retardation, renal agenesis, pes cavus, and neurologic abnormalities (eg, cerebellar dysfunction, synkinesia). It must also be remembered that hypogonadism, hypergonadotropic and hypogonadotropic, may be associated with a variety of chromosomal abnormalities as well as with autosomal dominant and recessive syndromes. At the time of this writing, there are 32 entries in the Online Mendelian Inheritance in Man for hypergonadotropic hypogonadism and 55 for hypogonadotropic hypogonadism. It must also recognized that a variety of chronic medical diseases cause hypogonadotropic hypogonadism (Box 1).

A thorough general physical examination should be performed, with particular attention to height, weight, body mass index (BMI), and a search for the previously mentioned anomalies. Special emphasis should be placed on an ophthalmologic examination for papilledema, thyroid disease, a breast examination for gynecomastia, pattern of axillary and pubic hair, penis size, and testicular size. Tanner staging of pubic hair and testicular growth should be performed (with Tanner 1 being prepubertal and Tanner 5 being full adult development). Testicular size may be measured in centimeters of length and width or by a Prader orchidometer, with 15 to 25 mL usually being considered normal.

Etiology of delayed puberty

Delayed puberty usually indicates a hypogonadal state, or at least a disruption in the tempo of puberty (it is further complicated in girls, because outflow obstruction of the genital tract can occur with normal sex steroid production). An algorithm for the evaluation of delayed puberty in boys

---

Box 1. Medical conditions associated with hypogonadotropic hypogonadism

Disorders
Central nervous system (CNS) developmental abnormalities
Parasitic diseases
Head trauma
Crohn's disease
β-thalassemia/hemoglobinopathies
Metabolic disorders, such as amino acidopathies and
    carbohydrate, lipid metabolism, or lysosomal storage disease
Hemochromatosis
Malignancy
Pituitary tumors
Autoimmune diseases
Granulomatous disease
HIV
Lymphocytic hypophysitis

---

is shown in Fig. 1. All patients who present with delayed puberty should have a thyrotropin, total thyroxine (T_4; more robust assay than the potentially problematic free T_4 assay), and prolactin assessment and a detailed psychosocial history [4]. Hypothyroidism (which may be central in origin rather than primary hypothyroidism), hyperprolactinemia, and eating disorders/stress/exercise may occur in these patients, although eating disorders are more common in girls [5]. Serum FSH, LH, and testosterone levels should be obtained, which permits the localization of the defect as of hypothalamic-pituitary or gonadal origin; the two have quite different prognoses for fertility.

Classification of hypogonadism

If the serum testosterone level is low (usually < 100 ng/dL, with a normal range of 300–1100 ng/dL) and FSH and LH are elevated, the defect encompasses the endocrine and exocrine functions of the testis and hypergonadotropic hypogonadism is present. It is wise to repeat the studies once for confirmation because of the pulsatile nature of gonadotropin secretion. A karyotype should be performed in all boys with elevated gonadotropins to rule out a chromosomal abnormality, such as 47,XXY; 46,XX; or 45,X/46,XY, which may occur in 10% to 15% of such boys. In some infertile male patients, FSH may be elevated but LH and testosterone are normal; thus, these patients have spermatogenic failure.

If testosterone is < 100 ng/dL and gonadotropins are low or normal, the patient has hypogonadotropic hypogonadism attributable to hypothalamic

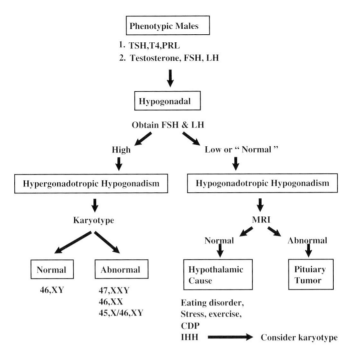

Fig. 1. An algorithm for the evaluation of delayed puberty in a phenotypic male patient is shown.

or pituitary disease. Again, repeating the laboratory studies for confirmation of the diagnosis is wise. Because sex steroids are necessary for growth, performing a bone age measurement should be considered in all hypogonadal patients, who may have delayed bone age compared with chronologic age (the bone age does not usually progress beyond 11–12 years). In cases of short stature and a markedly delayed bone age, growth hormone (GH) deficiency, hypothyroidism, and combined pituitary hormone deficiency should be strongly considered.

Hypogonadotropic hypogonadism

Phenotype

If the testosterone level is low and serum gonadotropins are low or normal ("normal" is inappropriate, given the hypogonadism), hypogonadotropic hypogonadism is present. MRI of the brain is necessary to exclude a pituitary tumor, a prolactinoma or craniopharyngioma most commonly [4]. If a prolactinoma is present, it is usually treated medically with a dopamine agonist, but surgery may be required for a craniopharyngioma, which may be malignant [5]. In the absence of a tumor, the cause is generally thought to be hypothalamic by exclusion. Although it is possible to perform a triple test (insulin-induced hypoglycemia, GnRH, and thyrotropin-releasing hormone (TRH) stimulation and checking baseline and stimulated levels every 15 minutes for 1–2 hours: thyrotropin, prolactin, cortisol, LH, FSH, and GH), the cost is great and the yield is low except in patients who have extreme short stature, suggesting pituitary failure. If the patient has a height less than the fifth percentile, especially with a family history of pituitary failure, the diagnosis of combined pituitary hormone deficiency (CPHD) should be entertained. Genetic counseling and testing for mutations in genes, such as PROP1, HESX1, or LHX3, should be considered [6].

In the absence of a tumor, strong consideration must be given to the history and physical examination, with particular attention to BMI, eating and exercise patterns, and stress. Eating disorders, such as anorexia nervosa or bulimia, are much more common in girls but should be excluded because of the significant morbidity and mortality. Morning cortisol levels may be elevated in patients with eating disorders as well as reverse triiodothyronine (rT_3) levels because of a preferential conversion of T_4 to rT_3 instead of the more active T_3. Correction of the underlying problem with an increase in weight, exercise reduction, or stress relief should restore eugonadism.

Associated medical disease usually presents with disease-specific symptoms (see Box 1); however, hemochromatosis is an exception. This disorder of iron overload may be quite insidious without specific symptoms other than fatigue and hypogonadism until significant liver disease is present. Hemochromatosis is an autosomal recessive disorder caused most commonly by mutations in the HFE gene, although the phenotype may not be adequately predicted by the genotype. Diagnosis can be obtained by performing transferrin saturation, ferritin, and total iron studies, and treatment is by phlebotomy.

For male patients with hypogonadotropic hypogonadism who have no pituitary tumor and are of normal weight, two diagnoses must be considered. Constitutional delay of puberty (CDP) is often diagnosed in retrospect if boys initiate puberty spontaneously before the age of 18 years and is more common in boys than in girls. If hypogonadotropic hypogonadism is present at 18 years of age or older, the diagnosis is IHH or isolated hypogonadotropic hypogonadism. The history should be reviewed for anosmia/hyposmia; midline facial defects; associated neurologic deficits, such as synkinesia (eg, mirror movements tested by raising both arms when asked to raise one arm [corticospinal tract abnormality]), hearing loss, or visual abnormalities. When IHH is combined with anosmia/hyposmia, the patient has Kallmann syndrome. IHH, which is most commonly recognized as being irreversible (although exceptions are becoming increasingly reported), is usually defined as pubertal delay at 18 years of age or older, testosterone levels less than 100 ng/dL, and low/normal serum FSH and LH levels [3]. A presumptive diagnosis of IHH may be made in male patients aged 14 to 18 years if they fit IHH criteria but should not be considered definitive until they are 18 years of age or older (because CDP is more common in boys).

Gonadotropin responses to exogenous GnRH in patients with IHH may be quite variable, ranging anywhere from completely absent LH pulses to normal LH pulses [3]. More prolonged GnRH therapy typically results in normal sex steroid levels and gonadotropin levels. When serial measurements of gonadotropins are performed over 12 hours, however, four different patterns of LH emerge (FSH does not display these changes); the most common is an apulsatile pattern, but nocturnal LH pulses similar to those during puberty, decreased frequency of LH pulses, and decreased amplitude of LH pulses are also registered (Fig. 2) [3]. These findings help to explain the tremendous variability in response to exogenous GnRH administration.

IHH may be classified according to the severity of the pubertal defect. If there is no evidence of puberty, it is referred to as complete IHH; if there is any evidence of puberty, the patient has incomplete IHH [7,8]. A clear dichotomy between the two types is not always possible. Male patients with testes less than 4 cm have complete IHH, whereas those with testes 4 cm or greater (15–25 cm is normal) have incomplete IHH. Testes 4 cm or greater have had some prior exposure to gonadotropins, as found during pubertal development. This subclassification has been suggested to be superior to endocrinologic values, because gonadotropins and testosterone values do not differentiate complete and incomplete forms of IHH [7].

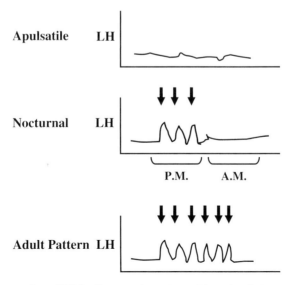

Fig. 2. Shown are pulses of LH for the normal man (every 2 hours) and abnormal LH pulses in IHH (apulsatile and nocturnal, nocturnal LH pulses; pulses that are decreased in frequency or amplitude are not shown).

Molecular basis of idiopathic hypogonadotropic hypogonadism

Chromosome abnormalities

It has generally been suggested that a karyotype is usually not necessary in men with IHH unless multiple congenital anomalies are present or there is suspicion for Prader-Willi syndrome (deletion 15q11–q13) [9]. Although some chromosomal translocations have been reported in patients with IHH, no systematic study was performed until recently, when the author's group found that 3 (4%) of 76 patients with IHH had chromosomal abnormalities [8]. Of 76 patients with IHH who were karyotyped, 73 were normal (19 are 46,XX and 54 are 46,XY). Three (4.1%) male patients without any family history of IHH had karyotypic abnormalities, however: 46,XY,t(10;12)(q26.3;q13.1); 46,XY/46,X,inv(Y)(p11.2q11.2); and mos46, XY,t(3;12)(p13;p13)[18]/46,XY[3]. The male patient with the 10;12 translocation had complete IHH and hyposmia, whereas the male patient with the pericentric inversion had incomplete IHH and a normal sense of smell.

The male with mosaicism for a 3;12 translocation had complete IHH, normosmia, and cerebellar ataxia. Balanced translocations may or may not cause the disorder but could provide some evidence of the location of newly etiologic genes for IHH.

Mendelian forms of idiopathic hypogonadotropic hypogonadism

Mutations in three genes—KAL1, GNRHR, and FGFR1—account for most of the known cases of IHH, and clinical testing may be reasonable. Although initial studies suggested that the etiology of IHH might be different for anosmic/hyposmic patients versus those with a normal sense of smell, it has become clear that mutations in at least one gene—fibroblast growth factor receptor-1 (FGFR1)—may cause IHH with anosmia (Kallmann syndrome) or normosmic IHH [10,11]. To date, mutations in KAL1 have been exclusively identified in Kallmann syndrome [12,13], whereas GNRHR mutations have been found only in normosmic patients with IHH [14].

KAL1

Mutations in the KAL1 gene on the X chromosome encoding the neural cell adhesion molecule anosmin-1 were first described in male patients with X-linked recessive Kallmann syndrome [15–18]. Initially, this was thought to be the most common etiologic mechanism of Kallmann syndrome, but several investigations (including that of the author's group) have shown that KAL1 mutations probably only comprise approximately 10% to 15% of the cases of anosmic male patients [19] in apparent sporadic cases but may comprise 30% to 60% of familial cases. KAL1 mutations have not been described in normosmic male patients or in female patients. As stated previously, patients with Kallmann syndrome may display a variety of non-reproductive anomalies, including midfacial clefting, renal agenesis, and neurologic abnormalities (eg, synkinesia [mirror movements], cerebellar dysfunction, deafness, mental retardation, eye abnormalities). Interestingly, these phenotypic findings correlate nicely with the expression patterns in chick and human embryos [20,21], providing an excellent example whereby understanding the molecular basis of a disease aids in the clinical management. A careful search for midfacial and brain defects, along with documenting the presence of two kidneys by ultrasound, now becomes important in taking care of these patients. Interestingly, the mouse ortholog has not yet been cloned, although human anosmin-1 antibodies recognize its existence in the lateral olfactory tract and olfactory cortex in mice [22].

FGFR1

Mutations in the FGFR1 (KAL2) gene occur in approximately 7% to 10% of patients (male and female) with autosomal dominant IHH, anosmic/hyposmic or normosmic [10,11]. These patients may also have neurologic abnormalities and midfacial defects, similar to those with X-linked Kallmann syndrome and in contrast to those with normosmia. A remarkable complicating feature among families with these inactivating FGFR1 mutations is reduced penetrance and variable expressivity [10,11]. Although approximately 7% to 10% of probands with Kallmann syndrome have been reported to have FGFR1 mutations, less than half of these are nonsense, frameshift deletion/insertions, or splice mutations, whereas the remainder seem to be missense mutations that await confirmation by in vitro functional studies [10,11]. Recently, some mutations have been shown to impair fibroblast growth factor (FGF) signaling in vitro [23]. A potential connection between the FGFR1 and KAL1 (anosmin-1) pathways has been suggested, because there is similar developmental expression and both use heparan sulfate proteoglycans for their function [10]. KAL1 and FGFR1 have been implicated in GnRH neuron migration, which explains the defects in olfactory and GnRH neuronal deficits in these patients. This has led to the speculation that anosmin-1 might be a ligand for FGFR1. Although most FGFR1 mutations have been reported in anosmic patients with IHH, mutations in this gene have been identified in normosmic patients [11], which is typical of autosomal dominant modes of inheritance with variable expressivity.

GNRHR

For patients with normosmia, mutations in the GNRHR gene seem to be the most common etiology, yet they comprise only approximately 5% of the cases and are inherited in an autosomal recessive fashion. Mutations in the GNRHR gene, a G-protein coupled transmembrane receptor, may affect ligand binding or signal transduction. Recently, the author's group (Bhagavath and colleagues [14]) published a series of 185 patients with IHH screened for GNRHR mutations. A total of 3 (1.6%) patients with IHH demonstrated compound heterozygous GNRHR mutations, but all 3 were identified from a cohort of 85 normosmic patients (3.5%), whereas none were identified in hyposmic or anosmic patients with IHH. GNRHR mutations were identified in 1 (6.7%) of 15 families with at least two affected siblings and in 2 (11.1%) of 18 normosmic female patients. None were found in presumably autosomal dominant families. The finding that GNRHR mutations account for approximately 3.5% of all normosmic IHH and 7% to 11% of presumed autosomal recessive IHH suggests that additional genes play an important role in normal puberty [14].

Other genes

Although mutations in other genes have been reported, they are currently thought to be rare. These include mutations in the leptin (LEP) and leptin receptor (LEPR), which have been detected in a minority of obese patients with IHH. Mutations in the GPR54 gene have been found in a few families with normosmic IHH, which have led to the importance of kisspeptin (the ligand for GPR54) signaling in normal puberty. Mutations in genes, such as LHX3 [24], HESX1 [25], and PROP1 [26], cause combined pituitary deficiency syndromes that may include hypogonadotropic hypogonadism, but these are rare in isolated IHH.

Testing for deletions of KAL1 may be performed commercially by fluorescent in situ hybridization (FISH), but this does not detect point mutations. If the results of FISH testing are negative, KAL1 testing may be performed in research laboratories, as can be done for FGFR1 and GNRHR genes.

Treatment for hypogonadotropic hypogonadism

Treatment for patients with hypogonadotropic hypogonadism depends on the desire for fertility. GnRH or gonadotropin treatment results in fertility for a substantial number of male patients, even though final sperm parameters may be subnormal. This approach is discussed in greater detail in the article by Schiff and colleagues elsewhere in this issue [27–37].

Once men with IHH have successfully fathered children or do not desire fertility, testosterone therapy may be instituted, as may be used for hypogonadism in general. It is wise to make sure that a complete metabolic panel and complete blood cell count (CBC) are normal and that there is no unexplained elevation of prostate-specific antigen (PSA). Reasonable choices of administration include intramuscular testosterone enanthate or cypionate (100 mg/wk or 200 mg every 2 weeks), a scrotal patch (6 mg/d), nongenital patches (5–10 mg/d), testosterone gel (5–10 g containing 50–100 mg/d), or buccal bioadhesive testosterone tablets (30 mg twice daily) [38]. Follow-up in 3 months should be done, with efforts to keep the serum total testosterone in the normal midrange. As outlined in the Endocrine Society's Clinical Guidelines (evidence-based), adverse events associated with testosterone treatment include erythrocytosis, acne/oily skin, detection of subclinical prostate cancer, growth of metastatic prostate cancer, and reduced sperm production and fertility [38]. Uncommon adverse events more weakly associated with testosterone consist of gynecomastia, male pattern balding, worsening of benign prostatic hypertrophy symptoms, growth of breast cancer, and induction or worsening of obstructive sleep apnea.

Adult-onset hypogonadotropic hypogonadism

Hypogonadism may also occur after puberty, commonly in couples experiencing infertility. If a man has several semen analyses with oligospermia (concentration <20 million sperm per mL), which is often accompanied by asthenospermia (<50% motility), with or without teratospermia (<30% normal forms by the World Health Organization [WHO] classification or <14% by strict Kruger morphology), an evaluation is indicated. In the normal aging man, there may be a loss of diurnal testosterone; if severe, testosterone becomes low. The hypogonadism that occurs with age in men is not as clearly abrupt and completely attributable to gonadal failure as in women, but it is probably a combination of hypothalamic-pituitary and gonadal dysfunction. Androgen deficiency of the aging man is discussed in greater detail in the article by Goldstein elsewhere in this issue.

Men may also present with hypogonadism in adulthood, commonly in the setting of infertility [39]. This adult-onset form of IHH has been defined as signs and symptoms of testosterone deficiency (infertility or sexual dysfunction [eg, decreased libido, impotence]), low serum testosterone levels (<100 ng/dL), low serum gonadotropin levels, and apulsatile LH secretion in men who completed puberty by the age of 18 years. Similar to those with the congenital form discussed previously, other known causes must be excluded. These men have a larger mean testes size (18 versus 3 cm) and a greater response to GnRH than men with the congenital form of IHH. In one study, spermatogenesis was evident earlier than in men with congenital IHH and semen parameters averaged 55 million sperm per milliliter after 8 months. Because GnRH is not available any longer, gonadotropin treatment with human chorionic gonadotropin (hCG) alone may be sufficient, because testes are typically larger.

Summary

During embryologic development, GnRH and olfactory neurons migrate from the olfactory placode, and GnRH neurons eventually reside in the hypothalamus. Hypogonadism in male infants may be diagnosed in the first 6 months of life with low serum testosterone and elevated gonadotropins (hypergonadotropic hypogonadism) or low/normal (hypogonadotropic hypogonadism) but cannot be diagnosed during childhood until puberty occurs. In male patients older than 14 years of age, hypogonadotropic hypogonadism is diagnosed with low serum testosterone and low serum gonadotropin levels. Imaging of the brain is necessary to exclude a pituitary tumor.

If a eugonadal state returns, the patient has CDP. If hypogonadism occurs at the age of 18 years or older, however, the diagnosis is IHH. Mutations in three genes—KAL1 (X-linked recessive), FGFR1 (autosomal dominant), and GNRHR (autosomal recessive)—comprise most of the known genetic causes of IHH and approximately 25% of all cases. Treatment of male patients with IHH with testosterone is indicated if fertility is not desired, whereas GnRH or gonadotropin treatment induces spermatogenesis and fertility. An adult-onset form of IHH has also been described and responds well to treatment.

References

[1] Wierman ME, Pawlowski JE, Allen MP, et al. Molecular mechanisms of gonadotropin-releasing hormone neuronal migration. Trends Endocrinol Metab 2004;15(3):96–102.

[2] Grumbach MM. A window of opportunity: the diagnosis of gonadotropin deficiency in the male infant. J Clin Endocrinol Metab 2005;90(5):3122–7.

[3] Crowley W Jr, Filicori M, Spratt D, et al. The physiology of gonadotropin-releasing hormone (GnRH) secretion in men and women. Recent Prog Horm Res 1985;41:473–531.

[4] Layman LC, Reindollar RH. The diagnosis and treatment of pubertal disorders. Adolescent Medicine: State of the Art Reviews 1994;5:37–55.

[5] Reindollar RH, Byrd JR, McDonough PG. Delayed sexual development: study of 252 patients. Am J Obstet Gynecol 1981;140:371–80.

[6] Wit JM, Vulsma T, de Vijlder JJ. [From gene to disease; POU1F1- and PROP1-mutations in pituitary hormone deficiency]. Ned Tijdschr Geneeskd 2001;145(50):2425–7 [in Dutch].

[7] Burris AS, Rodbard HW, Winters SJ, et al. Gonadotropin therapy in men with isolated hypogonadotropic hypogonadism: the response to human chorionic gonadotropin is predicted by initial testicular size. J Clin Endocrinol Metab 1988;66:1144–51.

[8] Bhagavath B, Podolsky RH, Ozata M, et al. Clinical and molecular characterization of a large sample of patients with hypogonadotropic hypogonadism. Fertil Steril 2006;85(3): 706–13.

[9] Layman LC. Human gene mutations causing infertility. J Med Genet 2002;39(3):153–61.

[10] Dode C, Levilliers J, Dupont JM, et al. Loss-of-function mutations in FGFR1 cause autosomal dominant Kallmann syndrome. Nat Genet 2003;33(4):463–5.

[11] Pitteloud N, Acierno JS Jr, Meysing A, et al. Mutations in fibroblast growth factor receptor 1 cause both Kallmann syndrome and normosmic idiopathic hypogonadotropic hypogonadism. Proc Natl Acad Sci U S A 2006;103(16):6281–6.

[12] Sato N, Katsumata N, Kagami M, et al. Clinical assessment and mutation analysis of Kallmann syndrome 1 (KAL1) and fibroblast growth factor receptor 1 (FGFR1, or KAL2) in five families and 18 sporadic patients. J Clin Endocrinol Metab 2004;89(3):1079–88.

[13] Albuisson J, Pecheux C, Carel JC, et al. Kallmann syndrome: 14 novel mutations in KAL1 and FGFR1 (KAL2). Hum Mutat 2005;25(1):98–9.

[14] Bhagavath B, Ozata M, Ozdemir IC, et al. The prevalence of gonadotropin-releasing hormone receptor mutations in a large cohort of patients with hypogonadotropic hypogonadism. Fertil Steril 2005;84(4):951–7.

[15] Franco B, Guioli S, Pragliola A, et al. A gene deleted in Kallmann's syndrome shares homology with neural cell adhesion and axonal path-finding molecules. Nature 1991;353: 529–36.

[16] Legouis R, Hardelin J, Levilliers J, et al. The candidate gene for the X-linked Kallmann syndrome encodes a protein related to adhesion molecules. Cell 1991;67:423–35.

[17] Hardelin JP, Levilliers J, Blanchard S, et al. Heterogeneity in the mutations responsible for X chromosome-linked Kallmann syndrome. Hum Mol Genet 1993;2(4):373–7.

[18] Bick D, Franco B, Sherins RS, et al. Intragenic deletion of the KALIG-1 gene in Kallmann's syndrome. N Engl J Med 1992;326:1752–5.

[19] Georgopoulos NA, Pralong FP, Seidman CE, et al. Genetic heterogeneity evidenced by low incidence of KAL-1 gene mutations in sporadic cases of gonadotropin-releasing hormone deficiency. J Clin Endocrinol Metab 1997;82(1):213–7.

[20] Rugarli E, Ballabio A. Kallmann syndrome from genetics to neurobiology. JAMA 1993;270: 2713–6.

[21] Lutz B, Karatani S, Rugarli EI, et al. Expression of the Kallmann syndrome gene in human fetal brain and in the manipulated chick embryo. Hum Mol Genet 1994;3(10):1717–23.

[22] Soussi-Yanicostas N, de Castro F, Julliard AK, et al. Anosmin-1, defective in the X-linked form of Kallmann syndrome, promotes axonal branch formation from olfactory bulb output neurons. Cell 2002;109(2):217–28.

[23] Pitteloud N, Meysing A, Quinton R, et al. Mutations in fibroblast growth factor receptor 1 cause Kallmann syndrome with a wide spectrum of reproductive phenotypes. Mol Cell Endocrinol 2006;254–5, 60–9.

[24] Howard PW, Maurer RA. A point mutation in the LIM domain of Lhx3 reduces activation of the glycoprotein hormone alpha-subunit promoter. J Biol Chem 2001;276(22):19020–6.

[25] Dattani MT, Martinez-Barbera J-P, Thomas PQ, et al. Mutations in the homeobox gene HESX1/Hesx1 associated with septo-optic dysplasia in human and mouse. Nat Genet 1998;19:125–33.

[26] Wu W, Cogan JD, Pfaffle RW, et al. Mutations in PROP1 cause familial combined pituitary hormone deficiency. Nat Genet 1998;18:147–9.

[27] Pitteloud N, Hayes FJ, Boepple PA, et al. The role of prior pubertal development, biochemical markers of testicular maturation, and genetics in elucidating the phenotypic heterogeneity of idiopathic hypogonadotropic hypogonadism. J Clin Endocrinol Metab 2002;87(1): 152–60.

[28] Barrio R, de Luis D, Alonso M, et al. Induction of puberty with human chorionic gonadotropin and follicle-stimulating hormone in adolescent males with hypogonadotropic hypogonadism. Fertil Steril 1999;71(2):244–8.

[29] Burgues S, Calderon MD. Subcutaneous self-administration of highly purified follicle stimulating hormone and human chorionic gonadotrophin for the treatment of male hypogonadotrophic hypogonadism. Spanish Collaborative Group on Male Hypogonadotropic Hypogonadism. Hum Reprod 1997;12(5):980–6.

[30] D'Agata R, Heindel JJ, Vicari E, et al. hCG-induced maturation of the seminiferous epithelium in hypogonadotropic men. Horm Res 1984;19(1):23–32.

[31] Jones TH, Darne JF. Self-administered subcutaneous human menopausal gonadotrophin for the stimulation of testicular growth and the initiation of spermatogenesis in hypogonadotrophic hypogonadism. Clin Endocrinol (Oxf) 1993;38(2):203–8.

[32] Kliesch S, Behre HM, Nieschlag E. Recombinant human follicle-stimulating hormone and human chorionic gonadotropin for induction of spermatogenesis in a hypogonadotropic male. Fertil Steril 1995;63(6):1326–8.

[33] Ley SB, Leonard JM. Male hypogonadotropic hypogonadism: factors influencing response to human chorionic gonadotropin and human menopausal gonadotropin, including prior exogenous androgens. J Clin Endocrinol Metab 1985;61(4):746–52.

[34] Liu L, Banks SM, Barnes KM, et al. Two-year comparison of testicular responses to pulsatile gonadotropin-releasing hormone and exogenous gonadotropins from the inception of therapy in men with isolated hypogonadotropic hypogonadism. J Clin Endocrinol Metab 1988; 67(6):1140–5.

[35] Schopohl J. Pulsatile gonadotrophin releasing hormone versus gonadotrophin treatment of hypothalamic hypogonadism in males. Hum Reprod 1993;8(Suppl 2):175–9.

[36] Schopohl J, Mehltretter G, von Zumbusch R, et al. Comparison of gonadotropin-releasing hormone and gonadotropin therapy in male patients with idiopathic hypothalamic hypogonadism. Fertil Steril 1991;56(6):1143–50.

[37] Weinstein RL, Reitz RE. Pituitary-testicular responsiveness in male hypogonadotropic hypogonadism. J Clin Invest 1974;53(2):408–15.

[38] Bhasin S, Cunningham GR, Hayes FJ, et al. Testosterone therapy in adult men with androgen deficiency syndromes: an Endocrine Society clinical practice guideline. J Clin Endocrinol Metab 2006;91(6):1995–2010.

[39] Nachtigall LB, Boepple PA, Pralong FP, et al. Adult-onset idiopathic hypogonadotropic hypogonadism—a treatable form of male infertility. N Engl J Med 1997;336(6):410–5.

ELSEVIER
SAUNDERS

Endocrinol Metab Clin N Am
36 (2007) 297–311

ENDOCRINOLOGY
AND METABOLISM
CLINICS
OF NORTH AMERICA

Diagnostic Approach to the Infertile Male Patient

Jonathan P. Jarow, MD

*Johns Hopkins University, 601 North Caroline Street, Room 4068,
Baltimore, MD 21287, USA*

Approximately 15% of couples have difficulty in conceiving, and of these, at least half have a male factor as the underlying cause [1]. Couples experiencing difficulty in conceiving are typically first seen by the wife's medical doctor unless the husband has a known risk factor for infertility. Subfertility is defined as the inability to conceive after a year-long period of regular unprotected sexual relations; however, couples with known risk factors for infertility are evaluated without having to pass that hurdle. This period is based on the observation that most fertile couples conceive within 1 year of unprotected sexual relations [2]. The initial screening evaluation recommended for the male partner is a reproductive history and two semen analyses [3]. If the results of any of these are abnormal, a more comprehensive evaluation should be performed and referral to a specialist in male fertility is recommended.

The main purpose of the infertility evaluation is to determine whether or not there is a treated cause of infertility. In the big picture, there are two competing management options for male infertility. The first is to identify reversible causes of male infertility and introduce therapies aimed at increasing the fecundity of the male partner through improvement in semen quality. The alternative strategy is to optimize the fecundity of the male partner without altering his semen quality through the use of assisted reproductive technologies (ARTs), such as in vitro fertilization (IVF) with intracytoplasmic injection (ICSI). The latter strategy is the only option in men who have idiopathic infertility or irreversible causes, such as Klinefelter syndrome [4]. Both of these competing management strategies may be used when couples desire multiple children. It is important to remember that infertility is not

This work is supported by grant R01 HD 44258-01 from the National Institutes of Health.

E-mail address: jjarow@jhmi.edu

a disease but rather a presenting symptom of an underlying pathophysiologic process. The underlying process in the male partner is frequently an abnormality of testicular function that does not have a major impact on his general medical health. Yet, some male partners of subfertile couples have serious underlying medical diseases, such as testicular or pituitary tumors [5]. Thus, in addition to determining whether or not the infertility is treatable, it is important to make certain that a serious underlying medical disorder is not present.

Initial evaluation

In an era of cost savings, we try to limit the amount of testing performed on patients and limit the more expensive studies to only those patients in whom the test result is likely to affect management. Considering this, the initial evaluation of the patient identified as being subfertile is limited to confirmatory semen testing and endocrine screening with testosterone and follicle-stimulating hormone (FSH). The confirmatory semen testing is thought to be necessary, because initial studies do not always reflect the true status of the male partner. There may have been collection issues or laboratory quality issues that led to a false result. In the author's experience, approximately 15% of patients referred because of an abnormal result of a semen study turn out to be normal on repetitive testing. Endocrinopathies are rarely present in patients with sperm counts greater than 10 million per milliliter; thus, it is reasonable to reserve endocrine screening for only those patients with severe oligospermia [6].

The evaluation of the male partner of an infertile couple should include a thorough medical and reproductive history. The duration of infertility, details of prior pregnancies initiated, methods of birth control used in the past, and couple's frequency of sexual intercourse as well as the timing of coitus should be recorded. The timing of sexual intercourse does not have to coincide exactly with ovulation, because sperm remain viable within the cervical mucus and crypts for 48 hours or longer. Studies have shown that conception may occur when sexual relations take place up to 5 days before ovulation, but because of the short life span of oocytes, it does not occur if sexual relations are performed the day after ovulation [7].

The sexual history includes assessment of erectile and ejaculatory function as well as questioning the use of vaginal lubricants, because most adversely affect sperm and sperm function. Lubricants that do not impair in vitro sperm motility include peanut oil, safflower oil, vegetable oil, and raw egg white. The developmental history of the patient should also be explored, including testicular descent, timing of puberty, and presence of gynecomastia. The patient's past surgical history may be of particular importance, especially pelvic, retroperitoneal, scrotal, and inguinal procedures that may affect the anatomy or function of the ejaculatory system.

The patient should be questioned for a history of urinary tract infections or sexually transmitted diseases. A history of absent or low-volume ejaculate suggests the possibility of retrograde ejaculation, hypogonadism, ejaculatory duct obstruction, or congenital hypoplasia or the absence of the vas deferens and seminal vesicles [8]. Systemic illnesses may have an adverse effect on male fertility. Ejaculatory dysfunction or erectile abnormalities may develop in patients with diabetes mellitus or multiple sclerosis. Infertility is common in patients with end-stage renal disease. Oligospermia is identified in approximately 60% or more of patients with testicular cancer or lymphoma at the time of diagnosis [9–11]. Chemotherapy or radiation therapy may further impair testicular function. Spermatogenesis may be impaired for up to 3 months after a febrile illness [12]. In patients with abnormal semen analyses and a history of a systemic illness within 3 months of the evaluation, additional semen analysis should be performed over a 3- to 6-month period to assess the patient's baseline fertility status adequately. Anabolic steroid abuse by athletes has been increasing, and anabolic steroids often have a contraceptive effect. Exposure to environmental toxicants, such as pesticides, should be noted, because these may be gonadotoxic. Testicular temperatures are normally 1°F to 2.5°F lower than body temperature. Impaired semen quality and spermatogenesis have resulted from experimental hyperthermia. Similarly, the frequent use of hot tubs has been found to result in a 10% decrease in sperm motility [13]. Therefore, the use of saunas and hot tubs should be discontinued in those patients with suboptimal semen analyses. There is no evidence that the type of underwear worn affects spermatogenesis [14].

The effect of cigarette smoking on spermatogenesis is unclear. A meta-analysis of 21 studies on the effect of cigarette smoking on semen quality revealed that smoking lowered sperm density by 13% to 17%, although 14 of the studies did not document an effect [15]. Smoking may serve as a cofactor for patients with other causes of male infertility, however [16]. Androgen receptor abnormalities should be suspected in patients with a family history of intersex disorders. Many of the genes that affect male reproduction, including the androgen receptor gene, are located on the X chromosome. Therefore, the family history should focus on the phenotype of the maternal uncles. In utero exposure to diethylstilbestrol (DES) causes an increased incidence of epididymal cysts, a slightly increased frequency of cryptorchidism, but little or no effect on semen quality in those men who do not have a history of undescended testis [17]. Finally, the physician should be aware of the results of the wife's fertility evaluation.

The physical examination should be directed toward identifying abnormalities that may be associated with infertility. The patient's habitus and the pattern of virilization should be noted. Abnormalities of secondary sex characteristics may indicate whether there is a congenital endocrine disorder, such as a eunuchoid appearance associated with Klinefelter syndrome. Lack of temporal pattern balding and fine wrinkles on the face may be indicative of an acquired androgen deficiency. Gynecomastia is suggestive of an estrogen/androgen imbalance or an excess of prolactin. Situs inversus raises the possibility of Kartagener syndrome associated with immotile cilia, and thus immotile sperm.

Specific attention should be directed toward the genital examination. The penis should be examined for evidence of hypospadias and severe chordee because both may interfere with proper deposition of semen in the deep vagina near the cervix. The testes should be carefully palpated to determine consistency and to rule out the presence of an intratesticular mass. The dimensions of the testes should be noted. Careful palpation of the epididymis should determine the presence of the head, body, and tail. The possibility of epididymal obstruction is suggested by the presence of induration or cystic dilation of the epididymis. Spermatoceles and epididymal cysts are common findings and do not indicate the presence of obstruction. Examination of the spermatic cords should be performed to identify the presence of the vas deferens on each side and to rule out the presence of a varicocele. A rectal examination should be done to evaluate the prostate and the areas above the prostate for evidence of cystic dilatation of the seminal vesicles.

Semen analysis

After the history and physical examination, appropriate laboratory testing should be conducted. All patients should have two or three semen specimens examined. Specimens collected over a period of several weeks usually give an adequate assessment of baseline spermatogenesis. In those instances in which the initial semen parameters vary markedly, additional specimens may be collected over a 2- to 3-month period, particularly if the patient reports recent exposure to a gonadotoxin or febrile illness. The patient should be given specific instructions for the collection and handling of the semen specimen. Consistent abstinence periods of 2 to 3 days should be used, and the samples should be examined within at least 2 hours of collection. Clean wide-mouth containers should be used for specimen collection, and the specimens should be maintained at room or body temperature by placing the container in a shirt pocket next to the patient's body when transporting it to the laboratory. Masturbation is the preferred method of specimen collection. In those cases in which the patient objects to collecting the specimen in this manner, special condoms (seminal collection devices) without spermatotoxins may be provided, allowing the couple to have intercourse. Coitus interruptus should not be used as an alternative, because it is almost impossible to ensure complete collection when obtaining sperm in this manner. With the exception of absolute azoospermia or asthenospermia, it is not possible to separate patients into sterile and fertile groups based on the semen analysis. As semen parameters decrease in quality, the chance of conception decreases but does not reach zero. When interpreting the semen analysis, it is important to differentiate between average semen parameters and minimal semen parameters needed for normal fertility. Whereas average sperm densities are approximately 70 to 80 million sperm per milliliter in fertile populations [18], conception rates do not decrease significantly until the sperm concentration falls to considerably less than 20 million sperm per milliliter. Each laboratory should define its own set of standard values. In addition, the accuracy and reproducibility of semen analyses are notoriously poor, with coefficients of variation greater than 100% for many laboratories [19]. It is critical that the semen analysis laboratory used performs quality control and proficiency testing to ensure that the coefficient of variation is maintained at less than 15%. The author uses the following criteria for normal for semen analysis interpretation:

- Volume of 1.5 to 5.0 mL
- Sperm density greater than 20 million per milliliter and total sperm count greater than 50 million
- Motility greater than or equal to 50% with forward progression greater than 2.0 on a semiquantitative scale of 0 to 4
- Normal morphology greater than 35% using standard criteria and greater than 14% when strict criteria are employed
- White blood cell count less than 1 million per milliliter
- No evidence of sperm agglutination or red blood cells

Computerized systems have been designed to measure the standard semen analysis parameters and additional parameters not measurable by manual methods. Although these machines allow the production of quantitative data, such as sperm velocity and linearity of movement, that may allow for standardization between laboratories, these benefits have not been realized. Computerized semen analysis methods have not been standardized, and the quantitative data obtained have not been shown to improve prognosis or to affect treatment.

Endocrine testing

The goals of endocrine evaluation of infertile men are to identify a treatable cause of male infertility and to obtain prognostic information regarding the patient's fertility status. The prevalence of reversible endocrinopathies is relatively uncommon, at approximately 3% of men attending infertility clinics. Endocrinopathies, however, are exceedingly rare in men whose sperm concentration is greater than 10 million per milliliter [6]. Therefore, an endocrine evaluation should only be performed in those patients with an abnormal semen examination (sperm concentration less than 10 million per milliliter) or when an endocrinopathy is suspected based on clinical stigmata. These clinical findings include gynecomastia, testicular atrophy, and reduced libido. The hormonal tests that should be obtained on initial endocrine screening are serum testosterone and FSH levels [6]. All these hormones are secreted in a pulsatile fashion [20], but studies have shown that a single determination is usually adequate in clinical practice [21]. Further testing with repeat serum testosterone, luteinizing hormone (LH), and prolactin levels should be obtained only if the values are abnormal on initial testing. Pooled blood samples, which are used to avoid the inaccuracies introduced by pulsatile hormone secretion, are only necessary when the results of a single determination do not coincide with the clinical characteristics of the patient. The patterns of endocrine studies and the resultant diagnosis are depicted in Table 1. Hypogonadism, primary or secondary, is the main pattern being sought in patients with azoospermia. Secondary hypogonadism, low testosterone associated with low gonadotropin levels, is usually correctable, whereas primary hypogonadism, low testosterone associated with high gonadotropin levels, is usually irreversible. One of the major causes of primary hypogonadism is Klinefelter syndrome (47,XXY). Therefore, patients with primary hypogonadism should undergo chromosomal assessment with a karyotype.

Reduction of spermatogenesis, identified as azoospermia or severe oligospermia on semen analysis, usually occurs in the setting of decreased inhibin production by Sertoli cells. This diminishes the negative feedback effect of inhibin on the pituitary gland, resulting in a concomitant increase in FSH production [22]. This test is critical in the differentiation of the causes of azoospermia [23]. Elevated serum FSH is indicative of a significant abnormality of the germinal epithelium and distinguishes testicular abnormalities from hypothalamic-pituitary disease and obstructive azoospermia. Because many patients with spermatogenic abnormalities may have a normal serum FSH level, testicular biopsy is indicated as the final documentation of normal spermatogenesis in those patients with normal or mildly elevated serum FSH levels. Measurement of inhibin has never been shown to be clinically useful [24].

Table 1
Endocrine diagnosis based on the results of serum hormonal testing in male infertility

Diagnosis	Testosterone	Luteinizing hormone	Follicle-stimulating hormone
Secondary hypogonadism (ie, Kallmann syndrome)	↓	↓	↓
Primary hypogonadism (ie, Klinefelter syndrome)	↓	↑	↑
Germ cell failure (ie, Sertoli cell only)	Normal	Normal	↑
Eugonadal (ie, obstruction)↓	Normal	Normal	Normal

Abbreviations: ↓, abnormally low; ↑, elevated.

Hyperprolactinemia has also been reported to cause oligospermia. Serum prolactin levels should be measured in patients with low serum testosterone levels and in patients with symptoms of decreased ejaculate volume, diminished libido, severe headaches, visual field disturbances, or galactorrhea. Prolactin-secreting pituitary tumors are associated with significant elevations of prolactin, typically greater than 50 ng/mL. Mild prolactin elevations are usually functional or associated with medications. Hyperprolactinemia affects spermatogenesis indirectly by inhibiting secretion of LH and FSH by feedback inhibition on the hypothalamus and by destruction of normal pituitary in large tumors. Serum testosterone levels are usually abnormally low in patients with pituitary tumors, but approximately 20% of these patients have borderline normal serum testosterone levels. Thyroid function tests are not routinely obtained but may be indicated when patients have clinical stigmata of thyroid abnormalities. Elevated thyrotropin-releasing hormone (TRH) levels can cause hyperprolactinemia, however. Routine hormone load tests and human chorionic gonadotropin (hCG) and gonadotropin-releasing hormone (GnRH) stimulation tests are rarely needed [25].

Differential diagnosis

After the history, physical examination, and initial laboratory studies, a differential diagnosis should be developed. In addition, more specific testing results in a narrowing of the differential diagnosis and allows the physician to place the patient in a causative category.

Absent or low-volume ejaculate

A dry ejaculate (absent ejaculation) may be caused by retrograde ejaculation or failure of emission. Etiologies include bladder neck surgery, androgen deficiency, retroperitoneal surgery, neurologic abnormalities, and drug therapy. A low-volume ejaculate may be caused by a combination of antegrade and retrograde ejaculation. A low-volume ejaculate in the absence of retrograde ejaculation suggests a lack of seminal vesicle contribution to the semen. These patients should be examined carefully for the presence of the vas deferens, which is often absent when there is agenesis of the seminal vesicles. Partial or complete obstruction of the seminal vesicles also causes a low-volume ejaculate. It is important to remember that incomplete collection of the semen specimen is a common cause of low-volume ejaculates, however. This possibility should be evaluated with the collection of a second specimen or by using a seminal collection condom. A postejaculate urine specimen should be examined to rule out retrograde ejaculation. For patients with absent ejaculation, the finding of more than 5 to 10 sperm per high-powered field in the urine indicates the presence of retrograde ejaculation. In patients with low-volume ejaculates, retrograde ejaculation is suggested by finding more sperm in the urine than in the antegrade semen specimen. In the absence of retrograde ejaculation, ejaculatory duct obstruction or seminal vesicle abnormalities should be evaluated with transrectal ultrasonography (TRUS).

Azoospermia

The main objective during the evaluation of the azoospermic patient is to differentiate those patients with lack of spermatogenesis (nonobstructive azoospermia) from those with active spermatogenesis and ductal obstruction (obstructive azoospermia). All azoospermic semen specimens should be subjected to centrifugation. The finding of sperm rules out complete bilateral ductal obstruction but does not rule out partial obstruction. These patients should then be evaluated for oligospermia. Congenital bilateral absence of the vas deferens (CBAVD) is identified by physical examination. In patients with a palpable vas deferens, the results of endocrine testing should guide further evaluation. Patients with normal hormonal study results (normal or near-normal serum FSH) should undergo diagnostic testicular biopsy. The presence of normal spermatogenesis in the testis is indicative of ductal obstruction. With the availability of IVF combined with ICSI, all patients undergoing testicular biopsy should consider extraction of sperm from the testicular tissue and cryopreservation for use in a future IVF cycle if reconstruction is not possible or not successful. Ductal obstruction should be evaluated by scrotal exploration at a later date, with the vasogram performed at the time of reconstruction rather than at the time of testis biopsy. Correctable abnormalities, such as a varicocele, should be sought in those patients with abnormalities in spermatogenesis on testicular biopsy. Azoospermic patients with small atrophic testes and FSH values greater than two times normal always have nonobstructive azoospermia, and a diagnostic testicular biopsy should not be performed [26]. Nevertheless, occasional sperm can often be found in the testes of patients with nonobstructive azoospermia; therefore, they are still candidates for IVF using sperm derived from the testis (TESE). Azoospermic patients with abnormally low serum testosterone and FSH levels have hypogonadotropic hypogonadism. Patients with CBAVD, a normal FSH level, and normal-sized testes almost always have normal spermatogenesis and do not need a testis biopsy. A renal ultrasound scan should be obtained in these patients, because this condition is associated with unilateral renal agenesis.

Oligospermia

Patients with sperm counts less than 20 million per milliliter generally have defects in other parameters as well. Endocrine screening with serum testosterone and FSH levels should be performed in those patients with sperm concentrations less than 10 million per milliliter [27]. Abnormalities in these studies should prompt a complete hormonal evaluation. Patients with isolated oligospermia and normal results of hormonal studies and physical examinations should be counseled about empiric medical therapies and ARTs, such as intrauterine insemination (IUI) and IVF.

Asthenospermia

Diminished sperm mobility, especially when combined with significant sperm agglutination, raises the possibility of immunologic infertility. These patients should have an antisperm antibody assay, preferably one that measures the presence of antisperm antibodies on the sperm surface (direct assays). Patients with antisperm antibodies, although occasionally treated with immunosuppression, are more commonly directed toward the ARTs, such as IVF. Infection is suspected in the presence of increased numbers of round cells in the semen analysis. A study to differentiate white blood cells from immature germ cells should be obtained in these instances. Patients with significant pyospermia should be evaluated with urethral swabs for *Chlamydia* and *Mycoplasma* as well as a urine analysis to rule out the presence of a urinary tract infection. Although semen cultures for bacteria are often performed, these are commonly contaminated by distal urethral organisms. Varicoceles are commonly found in patients with asthenospermia and are often associated with abnormalities in count and morphology as well. Partial ejaculatory duct obstruction should be considered in those patients with borderline low seminal volumes, low motility, and poor forward progression. Ultrastructural defects should be considered in those cases with motilities less than 5% accompanied by high sperm viability [28].

Defects in morphology

Isolated defects in morphology have become more common with the advent of more strict criteria for sperm morphologic evaluation. Varicoceles and temporary insults to spermatogenesis may be found in some of these patients. Rare ultrastructural defects, such as absent acrosomes, may occasionally be identified.

Multiple seminal defects

Varicoceles are the most common abnormality associated with defects in multiple semen parameters. These patients should be examined for the presence of a clinical varicocele. We do not advocate the use of studies to detect subclinical varicoceles (nonpalpable), such as thermography or color duplex ultrasonography. Other abnormalities in this group of patients include partial ejaculatory duct obstruction and temporary insults to spermatogenesis.

Normal semen parameters

The finding of normal semen parameters raises the possibility of immunologic infertility, incorrect coital habits, or, more commonly, a female factor. The absence of sperm on a postcoital test in the presence of normal semen parameters suggests incorrect coital technique. The presence of normal sperm numbers but reduced motility or a shaking motion on a postcoital test is suggestive of the presence of antisperm antibodies. The most common cause of an abnormal postcoital test result is poor timing to the ovulatory cycle, however, because cervical mucus is normally hostile to sperm, except near the time of ovulation. The finding of a normal postcoital test result raises the possibility of a functional sperm defect. In these cases, sperm function testing, such as the sperm penetration assay or the inducibility of the acrosome reaction, should be considered. Abnormalities on these tests should prompt a re-evaluation in the male patients for correctable abnormalities. Patients with documented sperm function abnormalities and no correctable abnormality should be managed with IVF using ICSI.

Pyospermia

Immature germ cells (spermatocytes) and white blood cells appear quite similar under wet mount microscopy and are known as round cells. These two cell types cannot be differentiated without special stains, which are not generally used during the performance of a routine semen analysis. Unless special stains are performed, the reports should list these cells as round cells. Despite considerable controversy, the presence of greater than 1 million white blood cells per milliliter is considered abnormal and raises the possibility of a genital tract infection or inflammation. Although infertile couples tend to have greater concentrations of white blood cells than fertile populations [29], not all studies of patients with increased numbers of leukocytes in the semen report decreased fertility rates [30]. Most studies suggest detrimental effects of leukocytes on sperm function and semen parameters [31,32].

There are several techniques available to differentiate round cells from leukocytes. Immunohistochemical techniques using monoclonal antibodies directed against white blood cell surface antigens are preferred because they detect all leukocyte types [33]. A relatively simple technique relying on the presence of peroxidase within the white blood cells underestimates the number of leukocytes within semen, because monocytes do not contain this enzyme [34]. The management of pyospermia, in the absence of genital tract infection, has included anti-inflammatory medication, empiric antibiotics, frequent ejaculations, and prostatic massage. These therapies lack proven efficacy, however [35]. Semen processing to remove the white blood cells, combined with IUI or IVF, may be considered.

Radiologic imaging

Radiologic imaging has been used for the evaluation of varicoceles, obstruction of the ductal system, and congenital anomalies of the urogenital tract. Vasal agenesis is one of the more common congenital anomalies associated with male infertility. Vasal agenesis is detectable on physical examination. Radiologic imaging is not required to establish the diagnosis of vasal agenesis, except in the rare circumstance when there is a segmental defect [36,37]. There is a strong association between unilateral vasal agenesis and ipsilateral renal agenesis, however [37]. Therefore, abdominal ultrasonography is indicated in these patients to rule out the presence of renal anomalies.

Varicoceles are the most common reversible cause of male infertility. Although the exact pathophysiology has not yet been determined, the current accepted hypothesis is that varicoceles adversely affect sperm production through elevation of scrotal temperature [38]. Early studies suggested that the size of a varicocele does not have any bearing on the chance of improvement after varicocele repair [39]. Thus, it seemed logical that there may be extremely small varicoceles not detected on physical examination (subclinical varicoceles) that could be identified by a radiologic imaging study. Initial studies used venography for the detection of subclinical varicoceles, and it remains the "gold standard" imaging modality [27]. The expense and invasiveness of venography limited its routine use in the evaluation of infertile men, however. Venography is now only performed on those patients who desire percutaneous management of their varicoceles or have a questionable postoperative recurrence. Scrotal ultrasonography is a relatively inexpensive, noninvasive, readily available imaging modality that was popularized for the detection of varicoceles in the 1980s [40,41]. Exact criteria for the interpretation of this examination remain highly controversial, however, and when compared with angiography and physical examination, the accuracy of scrotal ultrasonography is only slightly better than 50% [42,43]. In addition, most recent studies have demonstrated a direct relation between varicocele size and degree of postvaricocelectomy seminal improvement, questioning the significance of subclinical varicoceles. Therefore, scrotal ultrasonography or any other radiologic imaging modality should only be used to detect clinical varicoceles in patients who are difficult to examine, such as obese patients. In this setting, a venous diameter greater than 3.5 mm, measured with the patient in the supine position and at rest, should be used as the cut point for a positive ultrasonographic examination.

Obstruction of the ductal system of the male genital tract is a relatively uncommon disorder but is usually reversible. Obstruction may occur in the epididymis, vas deferens, or ejaculatory ducts. Historically, vasography was the only imaging study available to evaluate the patency of the ductal system. Today, however, we have many more imaging modalities at our disposal, and the need for vasograms has decreased. Vasography is used to detect obstruction of the vas deferens and the ejaculatory ducts. This procedure should only be performed at the time of reconstructive surgery, because there is a risk of vasal injury and subsequent stenosis or stricture formation of the vas deferens at the vasography site. The indication for a vasogram is normal ejaculate volume (>1.5 mL) azoospermia in a patient with documented spermatogenesis by previous testicular biopsy. Formal vasography entails the injection of dilute non-ionic contrast material through a partial-thickness transverse vasotomy toward the prostate using a 24-gauge angiocatheter. The vasotomy should be closed using standard microsurgical technique unless this site is used for reconstruction. In that case, the vas deferens should be completely transected at this location. Creation of a pneumocystogram and angling the radiographic machine 15° into the pelvis significantly improve the images obtained. There are several alternative approaches to the standard vasogram. One is to use plain saline or colored dyes to assess distal patency. A 2-0 monofilament suture may be passed distally until it no longer passes easily if obstruction is suspected based on the results of the infusion test to determine the location of the blockage. The alternative approach of puncturing the vas deferens under microscopic control using a lymphangiogram needle is also effective and does not damage the vas deferens any more than a vasotomy. Contrast material should never be injected toward the epididymis. Epididymal patency is confirmed by the presence of sperm within the vasal fluid.

TRUS has become the favored imaging modality for the evaluation of the prostate, ejaculatory ducts, seminal vesicles, and vasal ampulla in the infertile male patient. The primary indication for TRUS is low ejaculate volume (<1.5 mL) azoospermia to rule out the presence of ejaculatory duct obstruction [44]. The finding of cystic dilation of the seminal vesicles (>1.5-cm anteroposterior diameter) in an azoospermic patient is strongly suggestive of ejaculatory duct obstruction [26]. Seminal vesicle aspiration using a 20-gauge needle may be performed to confirm the diagnosis of obstruction, document normal spermatogenic activity, and rule out concomitant epididymal obstruction in these patients [28]. In addition, seminal vesiculography, by means of injection of contrast, provides anatomic information regarding the site of obstruction [45]. Because contrast normally refluxes into the vas deferens during seminal vesiculography, this imaging modality can be used as an alternative to vasography to rule out obstruction of the pelvic and inguinal portions of the vas deferens in those patients who have had previous inguinal surgery [46]. MRI has also been used to detect structural abnormalities of the male pelvic organs [47]. MRI is much more expensive, however, and not as readily available as TRUS. Therefore, its use is limited to those patients with gross abnormalities, such as an ectopic ureter, that can be difficult to evaluate by TRUS alone [48]. Some investigators have suggested that TRUS could be used to diagnose partial obstruction of the ejaculatory ducts in oligospermic patients with normal-sized testes and endocrine studies [49]. Partial ejaculatory duct obstruction remains an investigational diagnosis in the absence of specific criteria to establish this diagnosis accurately, however. Therefore, TRUS should not be performed in patients without azoospermia in an effort to diagnose this problem unless it is part of an investigational trial.

Summary

The office evaluation of subfertile men can be accomplished with minimal expense in a short time for most patients. More extensive evaluation using testis biopsy, sperm function testing, and radiologic imaging modalities is necessary only in well-defined subsets of patients. The overriding goal of this evaluation is to identify potentially serious underlying medical conditions and to determine as rapidly as possible whether or not the patient has a reversible cause of male infertility. Yet, with the availability of modern micromanipulation techniques, many patients who were previously labeled as sterile can now have genetically related offspring.

References

[1] Thonneau P, Marchand S, Tallec A, et al. Incidence and main causes of infertility in a resident population (1,850,000) of three French regions (1988–1989). Hum Reprod 1991;(6):811–6.

[2] Tietze C, Guttmacher AF, Rubin S. Time required for conception in 1727 planned pregnancies. Fertil Steril 1950;1:338–46.

[3] Sharlip ID, Jarow JP, Belker AM, et al. Best practice policies for male infertility. Fertil Steril 2002;77:873–82.

[4] Palermo GD, Schlegel PN, Sills ES, et al. Births after intracytoplasmic injection of sperm obtained by testicular extraction from men with nonmosaic Klinefelter's syndrome. N Engl J Med 1998;338:588–90.

[5] Jarow JP. Life-threatening conditions associated with male infertility. Urol Clin North Am 1994;21:409–15.

[6] Sigman M, Jarow JP. Endocrine evaluation of infertile men. Urology 1997;50:659–64.

[7] Wilcox AJ, Weinberg CR, Baird DD. Timing of sexual intercourse in relation to ovulation. Effects on the probability of conception, survival of the pregnancy, and sex of the baby. N Engl J Med 1995;333:1517–21.

[8] Jarow JP. Diagnosis and management of ejaculatory duct obstruction. Tech Urol 1996;2: 79–85.

[9] Carroll PR, Whitmore WF Jr, Herr HW, et al. Endocrine and exocrine profiles of men with testicular tumors before orchiectomy. J Urol 1987;137:420–3.

[10] Nijman JM, Schraffordt KH, Kremer J, et al. Gonadal function after surgery and chemotherapy in men with stage II and III nonseminomatous testicular tumors. J Clin Oncol 1987;5:651–6.

[11] Rustin GJ, Pektasides D, Bagshawe KD, et al. Fertility after chemotherapy for male and female germ cell tumours. Int J Androl 1987;10:389–92.

[12] Buch JP, Havlovec SK. Variation in sperm penetration assay related to viral illness. Fertil Steril 1991;55:844–6.

[13] Procope BJ. Effect of repeated increase of body temperature on human sperm cells. Int J Fertil 1965;10:333–9.

[14] Wang C, McDonald V, Leung A, et al. Effect of increased scrotal temperature on sperm production in normal men. Fertil Steril 1997;68:334–9.

[15] Vine MF, Margolin BH, Morrison HI, et al. Cigarette smoking and sperm density: a meta-analysis. Fertil Steril 1994;61:35–43.

[16] Peng BC, Tomashefsky P, Nagler HM. The cofactor effect: varicocele and infertility. Fertil Steril 1990;54:143–8.

[17] Wilcox AJ, Baird DD, Weinberg CR, et al. Fertility in men exposed prenatally to diethylstilbestrol. N Engl J Med 1995;332:1411–6.

[18] Naghma ER, Sobrero AJ, Fertig JW. The semen of fertile men: statistical analysis of 1300 men. Fertil Steril 1975;26:492–502.

[19] Jequier AM, Ukombe EB. Errors inherent in the performance of a routine semen analysis. Br J Urol 1983;55:434–6.

[20] Kardar A, Pettersson BA. Penile gangrene: a complication of penile prosthesis. Scand J Urol Nephrol 1995;29:355–6.

[21] Knoll LD, Benson RC Jr, Bilhartz DL, et al. A randomized crossover study using yohimbine and isoxsuprine versus pentoxifylline in the management of vasculogenic impotence. J Urol 1996;155:144–6.

[22] DeKretser DM, Burger HG, Hudson B. The relationship between germinal cells and serum FSH levels in males with infertility. J Clin Endocrinol Metab 1974;38:787–93.

[23] Jarow JP, Espeland MA, Lipshultz LI. Evaluation of the azoospermic patient. J Urol 1989;142:62–5.

[24] Lue TF. Veno-occlusive dysfunction of corpora cavernosa: comparison of diagnostic methods. J Urol 1996;155:786–7.

[25] Corke PJ, Watters GR. Treatment of priapism with epidural anaesthesia. Anaesth Intensive Care 1993;21:882–4.

[26] Delcour C, Vermonden J, Darimont M, et al. Treatment of glans hyperemia after penile revascularization by transcatheter embolization. J Urol 1992;147:1106–7.

[27] Villeneuve R, Corcos J, Carmel M. Assisted erection follow-up with couples. J Sex Marital Ther 1991;17:94–100.

[28] Schuler JJ, Gray B, Flanigan DP, et al. Increased penile perfusion and reversal of vasculogenic impotence following femoro-femoral bypass. Br J Surg 1982;69(Suppl):S6–10.

[29] Wolff H, Anderson DJ. Immunohistologic characterization and quantitation of leukocyte subpopulations in human semen. Fertil Steril 1988;49:497–504.

[30] Tomlinson MJ, Barratt CL, Cooke ID. Prospective study of leukocytes and leukocyte subpopulations in semen suggests they are not a cause of male infertility. Fertil Steril 1993;60:1069–75.

[31] Yanushpolsky EH, Politch JA, Hill JA, et al. Is leukocytospermia clinically relevant? Fertil Steril 1996;66:822–5.

[32] Aziz N, Agarwal A, Lewis-Jones I, et al. Novel associations between specific sperm morphological defects and leukocytospermia. Fertil Steril 2004;82:621–7.

[33] Homyk M, Anderson DJ, Wolff H, et al. Differential diagnosis of immature germ cells in semen utilizing monoclonal antibody MHS-10 to the intra-acrosomal antigen SP-10. Fertil Steril 1990;53:323–30.

[34] Endtz AW. A rapid staining method for differentiating granulocytes from "germinal cells" in Papanicolaou-stained semen. Acta Cytol 1974;18:2–7.

[35] Yanushpolsky EH, Politch JA, Hill JA, et al. Antibiotic therapy and leukocytospermia: a prospective, randomized, controlled study. Fertil Steril 1995;63:142–7.

[36] McDougal WS, Jeffery RF. Microscopic penile revascularization. J Urol 1983;129:517–21.

[37] Sidi AA, Cameron JS, Dykstra DD, et al. Vasoactive intracavernous pharmacotherapy for the treatment of erectile impotence in men with spinal cord injury. J Urol 1987;138:539–42.

[38] Datta NS. Corpus cavernosography in conditions other than Peyronie's disease. J Urol 1977;118:588–90.

[39] Bartsch G, Menander-Huber KB, Huber W, et al. Orgotein, a new drug for the treatment of Peyronie's disease. Eur J Rheumatol Inflamm 1981;4:250–9.

[40] Seftel AD, Oates RD, Goldstein I. Use of a polytetrafluoroethylene tube graft as a circumferential neotunica during placement of a penile prosthesis. J Urol 1992;148:1531–3.

[41] Rajfer J, Mehringer M. Cavernosography following clinical failure of penile vein ligation for erectile dysfunction. J Urol 1990;143:514–7.

[42] Dos Reis JM, Glina S, Da Silva MF, et al. Penile prosthesis surgery with the patient under local regional anesthesia. J Urol 1993;150:1179–81.

[43] Sidi AA, Reddy PK, Chen KK. Patient acceptance of and satisfaction with vasoactive intracavernous pharmacotherapy for impotence. J Urol 1988;140:293–4.

[44] Schoenberg HW, Zarins CK, Segraves RT. Analysis of 122 unselected impotent men subjected to multidisciplinary evaluation. J Urol 1982;127:445–7.

[45] Mertens C, Merckx L, Derluyn M, et al. Iatrogenic femoral arteriovenous fistula as a cause of erectile dysfunction. Eur Urol 1994;26:340–1.

[46] Iwai T, Sato S, Muraoka Y, et al. The assessment of pelvic circulation after internal iliac arterial reconstruction: a retrospective study of the treatment for vasculogenic impotence and hip claudication. Jpn J Surg 1989;19:549–55.

[47] Parsons CL, Stein PC, Dobke MK, et al. Diagnosis and therapy of subclinically infected prostheses. Surg Gynecol Obstet 1993;177:504–6.

[48] Williams G, Mulcahy MJ, Hartnell G, et al. Diagnosis and treatment of venous leakage: a curable cause of impotence. Br J Urol 1988;61:151–5.

[49] Kurt U, Ozkardes H, Altug U, et al. The efficacy of anti-serotoninergic agents in the treatment of erectile dysfunction. J Urol 1994;152:407–9.

ELSEVIER
SAUNDERS

Endocrinol Metab Clin N Am
36 (2007) 313–331

ENDOCRINOLOGY
AND METABOLISM
CLINICS
OF NORTH AMERICA

Medical and Surgical Management Male Infertility

Jonathan D. Schiff, MD*,
Michelle L. Ramírez, BA, Natan Bar-Chama, MD

*Department of Urology, Mount Sinai School of Medicine, Mount Sinai Medical Center,
1 Gustave L. Levy P., New York, NY 10029, USA*

Medical treatment for male infertility generally falls under two categories: specific therapy and empiric therapy. In approaching a patient, it is practical to first seek a clear etiology to which a specific strategy can be applied rather than using medication for all infertile patients. When a cause cannot be identified, several hormonal therapies are available. It is difficult to predict who will respond to empiric hormonal treatment of idiopathic infertility, but this choice may prove valuable in conjunction with advanced assisted reproductive techniques.

Specific therapy

Gonadotropins

Hypogonadotropic hypogonadism accounts for less than 1% of all cases of male infertility and is discussed in great detail by Layman elsewhere in this issue. Gonadotropin replacement is the rational treatment and is the only clearly accepted and effective management of associated infertility. Normal male fertility requires adequate levels of intratesticular testosterone and follicle-stimulating hormone (FSH); the latter has been shown to initiate and maintain spermatogenesis [1,2]. FSH administered to men who have hypogonadotropic hypogonadism has demonstrated increases in sperm count, motility, morphology, and testicular volume [3]. Thus, it has been postulated that treatment solely with FSH may be adequate, however prolonged.

This work was supported by the Pfizer/AUA Fellowship in Urology.
* Corresponding author. 1120 Park Avenue, New York, NY 10128.
E-mail address: dr.schiff@gmail.com (J.D. Schiff).

Treatment classically includes human chorionic gonadotropin (hCG), a leuteinizing hormone (LH) analog; human menopausal gonadotropin (hMG), which mimics LH and FSH; or purified FSH. Recombinant human FSH (rhFSH) and hCG have replaced their purified counterparts as the standard treatment for hormonal replacement because they are less expensive and more pure. Moreover, they have exhibited equal efficacy in increasing sperm counts and improving motility, morphology, and pregnancy outcomes [4,5]. Pulsatile GnRH may be used to imitate normal physiology, as in tertiary hypogonadotropic hypogonadism (Kallman syndrome); however, its use is infrequent because administration of the drug involves a portable minipump, an inconvenient, costly practice.

Typically, initial management consists of hCG (intramuscular, subcutaneous, 3000–6000 IU/wk) administered until adequate serum testosterone levels are detected. Although intratesticular testosterone concentration is not normally measured, it has been shown to increase linearly with the dose of hCG [6]. If sperm are undetected after 6 months, concomitant treatment with hMG (75–150 U two or three times weekly) or FSH (50–150 IU three times per week) ensues [7]. Although it takes on average 6 to 9 months before sperm appear in the ejaculate, therapy may be needed for 1 to 2 years, and some patients may not respond at all. Larger baseline testicular volume [8], prior gonadotropin therapy [5], postpubertal status [5], or the absence of bilateral maldescended testes may positively correlate with the patient's response [9] and hasten the time to detect sperm in the ejaculate. Treatment with hCG/hMG has also been reported to be effective in a patient who has anabolic steroid-induced azoospermia [10].

Although spermatogenesis is induced in the majority of patients, sperm counts ordinarily do not reach normal levels and may require assisted reproductive techniques. In a study of 24 men who had isolated hypogonadotropic hypogonadism, 92% became fertile after gonadotropin therapy, resulting in 40 pregnancies, 71% of which occurred with sperm concentrations below 20 million/mL [11]. Small study sizes and insufficient formal comparison studies of treatment modalities make it difficult to predict the likelihood of conceiving. Nevertheless, an increase in pregnancies has been established, and, overall, gonadotropins have proven highly effective in inducing fertility [9,12,13].

Androgens

Exogenous testosterone therapy is detrimental to sperm production and has a contraceptive effect [14]. Meta-analyses of 10 randomized, controlled studies of testosterone and mesterolone demonstrate no effect on sperm production and no increases in pregnancy rates [15]. The theory of a reflex increase in gonadotropins occurring after sudden cessation of androgens, known as the rebound effect, was thought to initiate spermatogenesis. However, this rationale, and an androgenic direct effect on spermatogenesis, is unpersuasive given the lack of efficacy in treating idiopathic infertility. Testosterone rebound therapy is not warranted because the patient's condition may worsen with treatment.

Corticosteroids

The current use of glucocorticoids in male infertility is in the treatment of antisperm antibodies. Various doses of prednisolone have been considered to suppress the inflammatory response, allowing sperm–oocyte interactions to ensue without interference. An increase in pregnancies after prednisolone treatment for more than 3 months has been reported [16]; however, an inconsistent and incomplete meta-analysis of four of the six randomized, controlled studies available revealed no significant enhancement of fertility [17]. Some authors have recommended glucocorticoid treatment before intracytoplasmic sperm injection (ICSI) as the method of choice for patients who have high antisperm antibody titers, although statistical significance is lacking [18,19]. Taking into account adverse events, such as aseptic necrosis of the hip, steroid treatment is not recommended for men with antisperm antibodies.

Antibiotics

The incidence of genital tract infections among men who have infertility varies between 10% and 20% [20]. Often these infections are asymptomatic and difficult to diagnose. When leukocytospermia, defined as greater than one million white blood cells per milliliter, is present in an asymptomatic infertile male on semen analysis, an evaluation for a genital tract infection is recommended [21]. However, 54% of men who have leukocytospermia have no evidence of infection, positive semen cultures may be found in up to 83% of healthy men, and pathogens such as *Ureaplasma urealyticum*, *Proteus mirabilis*, *Mycoplasma hominis*, *Escherichia coli*, and *Enterococcus* are isolated in the same frequency in men who have leukocytospermia and men who do not [22]. The indigenous flora of the male genitourinary tract, contamination during sample collection, and the sexual activity and predilections of the individual need to be considered [22].

Certain organisms are considered pathogenic and warrant treatment. *Chlamydia trachomatis* has been isolated frequently in asymptomatic men who have unexplained infertility and has been found to bind to and penetrate human sperm [23]. *M hominis* and *U urealyticum* have been associated with nongonococcccal urethritis and have been demonstrated to impair human sperm function in vitro [24,25]. *E coli* and *U urealyticum* have been reported to decrease sperm motility [26–28]. Other pathogens include *Neisseria gonorrhoeae*, *Treponema pallidum*, *Mycobacterium tuberculosis*, *Haemophilus ducreyi*, herpes simplex virus I and II, papillomaviruses, and *Trichomonas vaginalis*. Therefore, in men who have overt signs of genitourinary infections (eg, cystitis, urethritis, or prostatitis), semen and urine cultures are performed, and appropriate antibiotic treatment is initiated. In asymptomatic infertile men who have leukocytospermia or in cases of truly unexplained infertility, semen cultures can be considered and appropriate antibiotic treatment instituted depending on the organism isolated.

α-Sympathomimetics and anticholinergics

Ejaculatory dysfunction may take the form of failure of emission or retrograde ejaculation. Reported causes are spinal-cord injury, diabetes mellitus, retroperitoneal surgery, multiple sclerosis, and bladder-neck and prostate surgery. The cause may be psychogenic or idiopathic. Medical therapy for ejaculatory dysfunction is initiated with α-sympathomimetic medications: ephedrine, pseudoephedrine, imipramine, and phenylpropanolamine. When these agents are unsuccessful or contraindicated, ejaculatory dysfunction is often successfully treated with vibratory simulation or electroejaculation. Electroejaculation—the application of transrectal electrical current to stimulate the pelvic nerves—results in approximately 90% of patients producing a semen specimen. These specimens are often suboptimal in quality and are used in conjunction with intrauterine insemination or more advanced assisted reproductive techniques [29,30].

Empiric therapy

Antiestrogens

Clomiphene citrate, a synthetic antiestrogen, is the most commonly used drug in the treatment of idiopathic oligospermia. The rationale for its use is based on the drug's ability to bind estrogen receptors, causing antiestrogen and, to a lesser extent, estrogen effects. This removes the negative feedback inhibition of estrogen at the hypothalamic and pituitary levels, increasing GnRH, LH, and FSH secretion and stimulating testosterone production and spermatogenesis. Due to the peripheral conversion of testosterone, estrogen levels may increase above normal levels. Therefore, monitoring of serum testosterone and estradiol is required to make sure levels do not rise to detrimental levels.

Although clomiphene citrate is widely used, its efficacy has been questioned since the first study yielded poor results in 1966 [31]. Within the past 40 years, numerous controlled and uncontrolled studies have demonstrated conflicting results in sperm counts, morphology, motility, and pregnancy rates. These variations may be in part due to differences in subject parameters, patient selection, sperm counts, and female factors. In a randomized, double-blind, placebo-controlled study of 190 couples by the World Health Organization [32], clomiphene was found to have no significant effect on pregnancy rates or semen characteristics, although multiple studies suggest the converse [33–35]. In a meta-analysis of 10 controlled studies involving 738 men, antiestrogens demonstrated a positive hormonal effect, whereas no improvement in pregnancy rate was observed in trials with known randomization [36]. Tamoxifen citrate, an alternative antiestrogen, has yielded similar results in treating idiopathic oligospermia [36].

Despite mixed fertility outcomes, studies have verified beneficial effects on LH, FSH, and testosterone levels. Therefore, therapy with clomiphene may be more advantageous in men who have mild oligospermia and low serum gonadotropins or increased estrogen. Therapy is less likely to be efficacious in men who have elevated baseline gonadotropins and in men who have remarkably abnormal semen analyses or testicular biopsies.

More recently, with the advancement of assisted reproduction techniques, the goal may not be to improve male fertility directly but to augment spermatogenesis so that in vitro fertilization is possible. Hussein and colleagues [37] studied the effects of clomiphene citrate on sperm production in 42 patients who had nonobstructive azoospermia. After 3 to 9 months of therapy with dose titration to achieve testosterone levels of 600 to 800 ng/dL, 64.3% of patients demonstrated semen analyses containing sperm. Although the remaining patients revealed negative semen analyses, adequate sperm for intracytoplasmic sperm injection was retrieved in 100% of patients via testicular sperm extraction, supporting the use of clomiphene in azoospermatic men undergoing sperm retrieval [37].

Although they are usually self-limited, common side effects of clomiphene include weight gain, blurred vision, hypertension, gastrointestinal disturbances, and insomnia. Clomiphene may improve erectile dysfunction in men who have secondary hypogonadism, but data are limited [38]. Commonly used are daily dose regimens of 25 mg for 25 days with a 5-day rest period; however, doses of 25 mg administered every other day may reduce receptor down-regulation and further improve sperm counts, concentration, and motility [39]. The dose should be titrated to reflect increased testosterone levels within the normal range.

Aromatase inhibitors

Aromatase, a P450 cytochrome enzyme, converts testosterone to estradiol and is discussed in great detail by Carlson and Narula in their article on gynecomastia elsewhere in this issue. Estradiol inhibits gonadotropin secretion and may exert direct effects on intratesticular testosterone production [40]. Consequently, aromatase inhibitors have been used to block the conversion of androgens to estrogen and therefore increase testosterone with the hopes of improving male infertility.

Aromatase inhibitors are steroidal (eg, testolactone) or nonsteroidal (eg, anastrazole), the latter being highly potent and less likely to cause interruption of the adrenal axis beyond aromatase inhibition. Anastrazole was found to be comparable to testolactone in raising testosterone levels and in improving semen parameters but more effective in lowering serum estradiol and increasing testosterone/estradiol ratio. Only in men who had Klinefelter syndrome was anastrozole not significantly effective [41].

Although aromatase inhibitors normalized testosterone/estradiol ratios in oligospermatic men and improved in semen parameters in early, poorly controlled studies [42–44], a double-blind randomized controlled trials of testolactone in 25 idiopathic oligospermatic men showed significant increases only in free testosterone, FSH, and LH, in addition to decreased levels of sex hormone-binding globulin. Free and total estradiol and total testosterone levels showed no significant change, and no improvement was seen in semen parameters [45].

More recently, efforts have been aimed at treating subsets of infertile men, specifically those who have decreased testosterone/estradiol ratios. Semen parameters and testosterone/estradiol ratios improved in a study of 63 hypergonadotropic hypogonadic infertile men, including those who had Klinefelter syndrome or other chromosomal abnormalities, varicoceles, cryptorchidism, and postchemotherapy patients [46]. A certain minimal amount of estrogen may be necessary for normal male reproductive function; the lower testolactone dose in this study (100–200 mg/d, the current standard dose, as opposed to 1–2 g/d in earlier studies) may have contributed to the positive outcome. The results were substantiated in a larger trial [41]. Controlled studies looking at pregnancy rates using aromatase inhibitors are lacking.

There are no absolute contraindications to the use of aromatase inhibitors, but given that elevations in liver enzymes have been described in 7% to 17.7% of patients, caution should be taken in patients who have hepatic disease, and liver function tests should be monitored. Estrogen deficiency may lead to osteopenia or osteoporosis. Other adverse reactions include increases in blood pressure that could be significant in hypertensive patients, rash, paresthesias, malaise, aches, peripheral edema, glossitis, anorexia, nausea/vomiting, and, rarely, alopecia that has resolved spontaneously.

Gonadotropins

Gonadotropins have also been used in the treatment of idiopathic infertility, but randomized controlled trials have observed no significant effect of hCG, hMG, or rhFSH on pregnancy rates or seminal parameters [47,48]. In contrast, many uncontrolled studies with positive outcomes have sparked interest in continued investigations [49,50]. Likewise, the development of rhFSH has prompted reconsideration of FSH treatment [51,52].

FSH may be beneficial in certain subsets of patients, such as those who have normal plasma levels of FSH and inhibin B and a testicular tubular appearance of hypospermatogenesis without maturation disturbances [53,54]. Using cytologic analysis, increased stimulation of spermatogenesis was observed after treatment with FSH 100 IU on alternate days but not at doses of 50 IU, and significant increases in testicular volume and sperm parameters were detected with doses of 150 IU [55].

FSH may be useful in infertile men who have certain defects in sperm structure, such as those who have apoptotic or immature sperm, because treatment seems to improve the quality of sperm micro-organelles [56,57]. A single, randomized, controlled study by Foresta and colleagues [58] has strengthened this hypothesis. Of 112 men who had idiopathic oligospermia and normal FSH concentrations, rhFSH treatment showed no significant improvement in sperm parameters when no distinction was made between decreased and defective spermatogenesis. After subgroup analysis, subjects who had isolated hypospermatogenesis without spermatogenic arrest showed a significant rise in sperm count. A significant increase in spontaneous pregnancies was observed in this subset of patients, eliminating the need for assisted reproductive techniques. Additionally, several controlled studies have found better quality embryos and implantation rates after pretreatment of infertile men undergoing in vitro fertilization (IVF)/intra-cytoplasmic sperm injection (ISCI) [55,59]. These data suggest that the role of FSH in treating idiopathic oligospermia may be most practical in patients who have hypospermatogenesis or those attempting IVF/ISCI, rather than in all idiopathic oligospermic patients without specific selection criteria. However, the current data are controversial.

Alternative therapy

Approximately 30% of men presenting for infertility evaluation use alternative therapies, of which the majority are antioxidants, such as tocopherol (vitamin E), ascorbic acid (vitamin C), acetylcysteine, or glutathione [60]. The role of dietary supplements in erectile dysfunction and prostate health is discussed by Tamler and Mechanick elsewhere in this issue.

Reactive oxygen species (ROS) are involved in innate sperm function, but observations of increased ROS in semen of infertile men coupled with evidence of cellular damage with overproduction of ROS in spermatozoa have brought about the widespread use of antioxidants [61,62]. A number of small studies have suggested a beneficial role of antioxidants, including improved sperm quality and increasing fertilizing capacity. Treatment with tocopherol improved sperm function (sperm–zona pellucida binding capacity) [63] and IVF rates [64]. Increased sperm count, decreased ROS, and an augmented acrosome reaction were reported in men who had oligospermia after treatment with acetylcysteine and retinol (vitamin A) together with tocopherol and essential fatty acids [65]. Folic acid and zinc supplements have been also shown to increase sperm concentration in subfertile men, whereas seminal and hormonal parameters were unaffected [66,67]. More recently, L-carnitine, a vital component of sperm metabolism and maturation, has been shown to improve semen quality, including sperm concentration and motility; however, the majority of positive outcomes have resulted from uncontrolled, unblinded studies [68]. Because overall results are encouraging and side effects are minimal, antioxidants continue to be recommended as adjunctive therapy.

Surgical management of male infertility

The surgical management of male infertility provides many options to the couple with male factor infertility. Problems amenable to surgery include varicoceles, obstruction, or sperm retrieval for IVF with intracytoplasmic sperm extraction.

Testicular dysfunction

Varicoceles

Varicoceles are found in 35% to 40% of men who have primary infertility and in 75% to 80% of men who have secondary infertility but are found in only 15% of the general population [69,70]. The association with infertility has been recognized for more than 50 years [71]. Varicocele causes a duration-dependent decline in semen parameters and testosterone production [72,73].

Venous dilation is thought to impair the counter-current heat exchange mechanism in the scrotum [74]. Pooling of venous blood is likely to cause the increased intratesticular temperature and the progressive, duration-dependent decline in testis function observed in patients who have varicoceles [75,76]. Repair of a varicocele can prevent further testicular damage, improve sperm production, and improve testosterone production [72]. Ligation of a varicocele may help prevent infertility and low testosterone levels after repair [77,78]. Several investigators have sought to determine preoperative characteristics of a varicocele that would predict response to varicocelectomy [79,80]. Patients who had larger varicoceles were found to have greater improvements in semen analysis parameters after the procedure than men who had smaller varicoceles [81]. Semen analysis parameters improved in men who had clinically nonpalpable varicoceles detected by ultrasound, and a cutoff of a venous diameter of 3 mm or reversal of flow have been suggested as operating criteria [82–85].

We use the microsurgical, subinguinal approach to repair varicoceles [86]. We believe that this approach with optical magnification minimizes complications and produces the best results by ligating all of the internal spermatic and cremasteric veins that contribute to the formation of varicoceles. The testicular artery is identified, preventing damage to this structure. Also, cremasteric arteries and lymphatic channels are preserved, which prevents the formation of hydroceles [87]. Use of the operating microscope results in a hydrocele rate of approximately 1% compared with up to a 30% rate of hydrocele formation 6 months postoperatively after conventional inguinal and laparoscopic approaches [88,89]. Recurrences are not uncommon and are seen in up to 15% to 25% of men using nonmicrosurgical approaches but in less than 1% of men using microsurgical approaches [89]. Loupes under 2.5× do not provide enough power to reliably identify the testicular artery or lymphatics. Other methods of varicocele surgery include the conventional inguinal, the retroperitoneal, and the laparoscopic approaches.

Radiologic embolization represents another option to correct varicoceles. In this procedure, the testicular veins are accessed percutaneously, and an alcohol-based sclerosant or coils are used to embolize the veins. Two large investigations demonstrated resolution of varicoceles in 83% of men. Significant improvement after embolization was noted for sperm density, motility, and morphology [90,91].

Surgical ligation of varicoceles reduces intratesticular temperature to the normal range [92] and improves semen parameters and Leydig cell function of the testis.

Several studies have demonstrated improvements in semen parameters, testosterone production, and pregnancy outcomes. Semen parameters improve in 60% to 80% of men after repair [70,85,93]. Bilateral repair in men who have a large unilateral and small contralateral varicocele and repair in younger men may have a greater beneficial effect on sperm parameters and androgen production than repair in older men [94–97].

Obstruction

Although varicoceles cause testicular dysfunction that is associated with infertility, most obstructive causes of male infertility are caused intentionally. Vasectomy is performed on more than 500,000 men per year in the United States to affect "permanent" contraception [98]. Due to a variety of factors, most commonly divorce and remarriage, 3% to 8% of vasectomized men request reversal [99,100]. Injury to the vas is also a common cause of obstruction, most often the result of childhood hernia repair, orchiopexy, or hydrocelectomy [101].

Microsurgical techniques have vastly improved the success rate of surgery to repair vasal or epididymal obstruction. Reversal of vasal obstruction, most likely secondary to vasectomy or an iatrogenic injury, can usually be accomplished by a vasovasostomy. In cases of congenital anomalies or secondary epididymal obstruction, a vas-to-epididymis anastomosis is required. Vasovasostomy is successful in up to 99% of cases, whereas vasoepididymostomy has a success rate of up to 90% [89,102–106].

Vasovasostomy

Microsurgical vasovasostomy, initially described by Owen and Silber in 1975, resulted in significantly improved outcomes compared with older techniques [105,107]. A modified microsurgical, single-layered anastomosis is statistically equivalent to a two-layer technique [102]. Patency and pregnancy rates vary directly with the obstructive interval. Although the overall patency rate was 86% and the pregnancy rate was 51.6%, the results for men with obstruction for less than 3 years were 97% patency with a 76%

pregnancy rate [102]. Others have reported similarly good results with a microsurgical approach to vasectomy reversal [103,108]. The gold standard for vasovasostomy is the microsurgical multilayer sutured technique, which had a success rate of up to 99.5% in a large series [103].

The identification of prognostic features of the vasal fluids helps to guide the surgeon in choosing the type of reconstruction to perform. The best results are achieved when sperm are found in the testicular end of the vas, but high rates of return of sperm to the ejaculate are also achieved with clear watery fluid present or if many sperm heads are found in the fluid [89].

The layers of the anastomosis include a mucosa-to-mucosa layer of six 10-0 nylon sutures, a muscular layer of six 9-0 nylon sutures at the region of the gaps, six additional 9-0 nylon sutures in the serosa between each muscular layer suture, and approximation of the vasal sheath with six 7-0 nylon sutures [103]. This achieves a water-tight anastomosis and prevents the formation of sperm granulomas. The importance of placing these sutures is magnified by the realization that there is no constituent of vasal fluid that promotes the sealing of the anastomotic site internally.

Vasoepididymostomy

Vasovasostomy is not always a feasible option to restore vasal patency. If epididymal obstruction is present, whether primary or secondary to chronic vasal obstruction, a vasoepididymostomy, one of the most technically challenging procedures in all of microsurgery, is required proximal to the obstruction to restore continuity for sperm transport. In the situation of epididymal obstruction, the decision to perform a vasovasotomy or vasoepididymostomy is made intraoperatively and is based on the microscopic examination of the proximal vas fluid and the time of obstruction [109,110].

We recently reported results comparing the four main techniques of vasoepididymostomy [104]. Success and pregnancy rates were not significantly different between groups. All conceptions in the groups where intussusception was used were through intercourse; none required assisted reproductive techniques. Among men who had return of sperm to the ejaculate, the intussusception groups had lower rates of disappearance of sperm from the ejaculate after 12 months ($P < .04$). The newer intussusception techniques offer comparable outcomes in terms of return of sperm to the ejaculate and pregnancy rates compared with the older techniques. The late shutdown rates of sperm in the ejaculate are lower. We also use fewer sutures with these techniques, which eases the performance of this challenging anastomosis.

Sperm retrieval techniques

Many cases of testicular dysfunction are not correctable by medical or surgical means. Reconstruction of the vasal and epididymal systems is also not always possible. In such situations, sperm retrieval for IVF is undertaken. Sperm retrieval with assisted reproduction is an also an appropriate option for men who have poor sperm production, in selected cases of obstruction with female factors, or when only one pregnancy is desired.

A variety of genetic and acquired disorders may cause a man who has obstructive azoospermia to be unreconstructable. For example, in congenital bilateral absence of the vas deferens, patients have mutations in the cystic fibrosis transmembrane conductance regulator gene. This results in defects in the sperm transport system from the mid-epididymis to the seminal vesicles, and most of these men are not candidates for reconstruction [111,112].

Nonobstructive azoospermia describes the situation whereby genetic or environmental factors result in severe depression in spermatogenesis to the point that no sperm are present in the ejaculate. Successful sperm retrieval is possible in the majority these cases [113]. Spermatogenesis in many of these patients is a patchy process, and a technique that exposes and explores the entire testis is critical to optimize success rates for sperm retrieval in these challenging patients.

One subgroup of men who have nonobstructive azoospermia is men who have Klinefelter's syndrome, with an abnormal karyotype of 47 XXY. Before the advent of ICSI, men who had Klinefelter's syndrome were considered sterile. Today, a technique of sperm retrieval with ICSI is the preferred treatment modality in those desiring paternity; with this technique, sperm can be retrieved in over 70% of cases [114,115].

Testicular biopsy

The success of different biopsy methods varies with the cause of infertility. In cases of vasal or epididymal obstruction, various percutaneous techniques are highly successful in terms of retrieving sperm. In cases of primary testicular dysfunction with very low sperm production, open biopsies are the preferred techniques. Of 14 patients who had primary testicular failure as proven by histopathology, only in one case (7.1%) were spermatozoa recovered by multiple aspirations, whereas in nine cases (64.3%) spermatozoa were recovered by open biopsy [116].

Percutaneous aspiration successfully retrieves sperm in cases of unreconstructable obstruction [116] and is substantially less painful than open biopsy techniques and has a faster recovery time. It has a far lower success rate in men who have nonobstructive azoospermia, in whom open biopsy yields much better results [117,118]. Some groups have reported better success rates of sperm retrieval using a percutaneous technique in men who have nonobstructive azoospermia. A recent large series from Jordan found a 53.6% success rate in 84 men [119]. In a series of 291 men, 63 men had successful percutaneous retrievals using a 21-gauge butterfly needle [120]. The remaining 228 men required an open biopsy in this series.

Open biopsy in cases of nonobstructive azoospermia is the preferred means of attempting sperm retrieval. Reports with a multiple biopsy

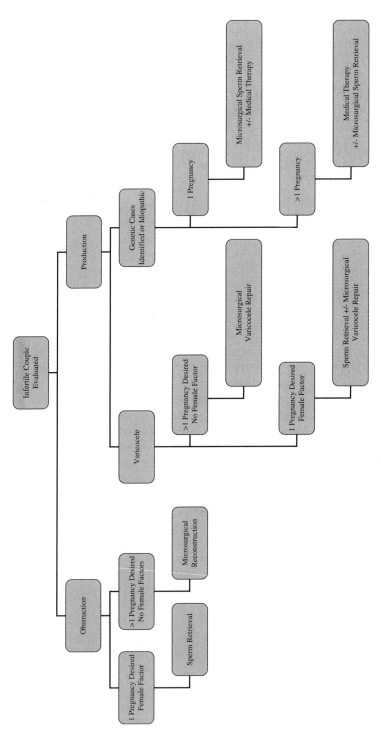

Fig. 1. Algorithm for the treatment of male infertility.

approach reveal successful sperm retrieval in 40% to 50% of cases among men who have nonobstructive azoospermia [118].

Microsurgical sperm retrieval techniques

The technique of microsurgical epididymal sperm aspiration is used to obtain sperm in men who have an intact epididymis. This technique is most commonly used in men who have congenital bilateral absence of the vas deferens or after a long obstructive interval after vasectomy with the desire for only one additional pregnancy. Using this technique, sperm can be aspirated that are suitable for use with ICSI [121,122]. Due to chronic obstruction, the sperm retrieved from these men is often of poor quality and does not fertilize the ovum readily, making ICSI a must.

In men who have nonobstructive azoospermia, the microdissection testicular sperm extraction technique provides the highest yield in terms of sperm retrieval while preserving as much testicular parenchyma as possible [123]. The histology of the testis can often predict the likelihood of successful sperm retrieval; however, even in the worst cases, sperm may be found over 40% of the time [124]. Postchemotherapy, sperm were found in 9 of 20 retrieval attempts in men who had azoospermia [125].

Microsurgical testicular sperm extraction is the most successful technique to retrieve sperm in men who have nonobstructive azoospermia, and it results in the least damage to the testis. Postoperative scarring is substantially lower with this technique compared with open biopsy [126]. The disadvantages of any microsurgical technique are the need for experience and the acquisition of microsurgical skills [127]. These techniques require general anesthesia. In cases of nonobstructive azoospermia, the microsurgical testicular sperm extraction is the procedure of choice for sperm retrieval because it offers the highest success rates with relatively low complications.

Summary

Infertility is a couples' problem, and both partners must be properly evaluated so that the most appropriate therapy can be tailored to the man and the woman. In the vast majority of cases, male infertility is treatable. Whether by medical therapy or surgical means, we can treat the male partner to affect a natural pregnancy or a pregnancy via assisted reproductive techniques. Fig. 1 presents an algorithm that can be used to decide the most appropriate therapy for the male partner of the infertile couple. This is used for guidance, and the specific goals and desires of the individual couple are of paramount importance when deciding on specific therapies.

References

[1] Nieschlag E, Simoni M, Gromoll J, et al. Role of FSH in the regulation of spermatogenesis: clinical aspects. Clin Endocrinol (Oxf) 1999;51(2):139–46.

[2] Moudgal NR, Sairam MR. Is there a true requirement for follicle stimulating hormone in promoting spermatogenesis and fertility in primates? Hum Reprod 1998;13(4):916–9.

[3] Bouloux PM, et al. Induction of spermatogenesis by recombinant follicle-stimulating hormone (puregon) in hypogonadotropic azoospermic men who failed to respond to human chorionic gonadotropin alone. J Androl 2003;24(4):604–11.

[4] Liu PY, et al. Predicting pregnancy and spermatogenesis by survival analysis during gonadotrophin treatment of gonadotrophin-deficient infertile men. Hum Reprod 2002;17(3): 625–33.

[5] Liu PY, et al. Efficacy and safety of recombinant human follicle stimulating hormone (Gonal-F) with urinary human chorionic gonadotrophin for induction of spermatogenesis and fertility in gonadotrophin-deficient men. Hum Reprod 1999;14(6):1540–5.

[6] Coviello AD, et al. Low-dose human chorionic gonadotropin maintains intratesticular testosterone in normal men with testosterone-induced gonadotropin suppression. J Clin Endocrinol Metab 2005;90(5):2595–602.

[7] Isidori A, Latini M, Romanelli F. Treatment of male infertility. Contraception 2005;72(4): 314–8.

[8] Miyagawa Y, et al. Outcome of gonadotropin therapy for male hypogonadotropic hypogonadism at university affiliated male infertility centers: a 30-year retrospective study. J Urol 2005;173(6):2072–5.

[9] Buchter D, et al. Pulsatile GnRH or human chorionic gonadotropin/human menopausal gonadotropin as effective treatment for men with hypogonadotropic hypogonadism: a review of 42 cases. Eur J Endocrinol 1998;139(3):298–303.

[10] Menon DK. Successful treatment of anabolic steroid-induced azoospermia with human chorionic gonadotropin and human menopausal gonadotropin. Fertil Steril 2003;79(Suppl 3):1659–61.

[11] Burris AS, et al. A low sperm concentration does not preclude fertility in men with isolated hypogonadotropic hypogonadism after gonadotropin therapy. Fertil Steril 1988;50(2): 343–7.

[12] Kung AW, et al. Induction of spermatogenesis with gonadotrophins in Chinese men with hypogonadotrophic hypogonadism. Int J Androl 1994;17(5):241–7.

[13] Vicari E, et al. Therapy with human chorionic gonadotrophin alone induces spermatogenesis in men with isolated hypogonadotrophic hypogonadism–long-term follow-up. Int J Androl 1992;15(4):320–9.

[14] World Health Organization. Contraceptive efficacy of testosterone-induced azoospermia and oligozoospermia in normal men. Fertil Steril 1996;65(4):821–9.

[15] Vandekerckhove P, et al. Androgens versus placebo or no treatment for idiopathic oligo/ asthenospermia. Cochrane Database Syst Rev 2000;(2):CD000150.

[16] Omu AE, al-Qattan F, Abdul Hamada B. Effect of low dose continuous corticosteroid therapy in men with antisperm antibodies on spermatozoal quality and conception rate. Eur J Obstet Gynecol Reprod Biol 1996;69(2):129–34.

[17] Kamischke A, Nieschlag E. Analysis of medical treatment of male infertility. Hum Reprod 1999;14(Suppl 1):1–23.

[18] Lombardo F, et al. Antisperm immunity in natural and assisted reproduction. Hum Reprod Update 2001;7(5):450–6.

[19] Shin D, et al. Indications for corticosteroids prior to epididymal sperm retrieval. Int J Fertil Womens Med 1998;43(3):165–70.

[20] Organization WH. WHO laboratory manual for the examination of human semen and semen-cervical mucus interaction. Cambridge (UK): Cambridge University Press; 1992.

[21] Aitken RJ, Baker HW. Seminal leukocytes: passengers, terrorists or good Samaritans? Hum Reprod 1995;10(7):1736–9.

[22] Chan PT, Schlegel PN. Inflammatory conditions of the male excurrent ductal system. Part II. J Androl 2002;23(4):461–9.

[23] Greendale GA, et al. The relationship of Chlamydia trachomatis infection and male infertility. Am J Public Health 1993;83(7):996–1001.

[24] Kohn FM, et al. Influence of urogenital infections on sperm functions. Andrologia 1998; 30(Suppl 1):73–80.

[25] Rose BI, Scott B. Sperm motility, morphology, hyperactivation, and ionophore-induced acrosome reactions after overnight incubation with mycoplasmas. Fertil Steril 1994; 61(2):341–8.

[26] Diemer T, et al. Influence of urogenital infection on sperm function. Curr Opin Urol 2000; 10(1):39–44.

[27] Diemer T, et al. Influence of Escherichia coli on motility parameters of human spermatozoa in vitro. Int J Androl 1996;19(5):271–7.

[28] Nunez-Calonge R, et al. Ureaplasma urealyticum reduces motility and induces membrane alterations in human spermatozoa. Hum Reprod 1998;13(10):2756–61.

[29] Schatte EC, et al. Treatment of infertility due to anejaculation in the male with electroejaculation and intracytoplasmic sperm injection. J Urol 2000;163(6):1717–20.

[30] Sonksen J, Ohl DA. Penile vibratory stimulation and electroejaculation in the treatment of ejaculatory dysfunction. Int J Androl 2002;25(6):324–32.

[31] Mellinger RC, Thompson RJ. The effect of clomiphene citrate in male infertility. Fertil Steril 1966;17(1):94–103.

[32] World Health Organization. A double-blind trial of clomiphene citrate for the treatment of idiopathic male infertility. Int J Androl 1992;15(4):299–307.

[33] Check JH, et al. Empirical therapy of the male with clomiphene in couples with unexplained infertility. Int J Fertil 1989;34(2):120–2.

[34] Paulson DF. Cortisone acetate versus clomiphene citrate in per-germinal idiopathic oligospermia. J Urol 1979;121(4):432–4.

[35] Wang C, et al. Comparison of the effectiveness of placebo, clomiphene citrate, mesterolone, pentoxifylline, and testosterone rebound therapy for the treatment of idiopathic oligospermia. Fertil Steril 1983;40(3):358–65.

[36] Vandekerckhove P, et al. Clomiphene or tamoxifen for idiopathic oligo/asthenospermia. Cochrane Database Syst Rev 2000;(2):CD000151.

[37] Hussein A, et al. Clomiphene administration for cases of nonobstructive azoospermia: a multicenter study. J Androl 2005;26(6):787–91; [discussion: 792–3].

[38] Guay AT, et al. Clomiphene increases free testosterone levels in men with both secondary hypogonadism and erectile dysfunction: who does and does not benefit? Int J Impot Res 2003;15(3):156–65.

[39] Homonnai ZT, et al. Clomiphene citrate treatment in oligozoospermia: comparison between two regimens of low-dose treatment. Fertil Steril 1988;50(5):801–4.

[40] Jones TM, et al. Direct inhibition of Leydig cell function by estradiol. J Clin Endocrinol Metab 1978;47(6):1368–73.

[41] Raman JD, Schlegel PN. Aromatase inhibitors for male infertility. J Urol 2002;167(2 Pt 1): 624–9.

[42] Dony JM, et al. Effect of chronic aromatase inhibition by delta 1-testolactone on pituitary-gonadal function in oligozoospermic men. Andrologia 1986;18(1):69–78.

[43] Itoh N, et al. [Therapeutic efficacy of testolactone (aromatase inhibitor) to oligozoospermia with high estradiol/testosterone ratio]. Nippon Hinyokika Gakkai Zasshi 1991;82(2):204–9 [in Japanese].

[44] Vigersky RA, Glass AR. Effects of delta 1-testolactone on the pituitary-testicular axis in oligospermic men. J Clin Endocrinol Metab 1981;52(5):897–902.

[45] Clark RV, Sherins RJ. Treatment of men with idiopathic oligozoospermic infertility using the aromatase inhibitor, testolactone: results of a double-blinded, randomized, placebo-controlled trial with crossover. J Androl 1989;10(3):240–7.

[46] Pavlovich CP, et al. Evidence of a treatable endocrinopathy in infertile men. J Urol 2001; 165(3):837–41.

[47] Kamischke A, et al. Recombinant human follicle stimulating hormone for treatment of male idiopathic infertility: a randomized, double-blind, placebo-controlled, clinical trial. Hum Reprod 1998;13(3):596–603.

[48] Knuth UA, et al. Treatment of severe oligospermia with human chorionic gonadotropin/human menopausal gonadotropin: a placebo-controlled, double blind trial. J Clin Endocrinol Metab 1987;65(6):1081–7.

[49] Ranieri M, Sturdy J, Marchant S. Follicle-stimulating hormone (pFSH) treatment for male factor infertility with previous failed fertilization in vitro; 1994:19.

[50] Merino G, et al. Sperm characteristics and hormonal profile before and after treatment with follicle-stimulating hormone in infertile patients. Arch Androl 1996;37(3):197–200.

[51] Acosta AA, Khalifa E, Oehninger S. Pure human follicle stimulating hormone has a role in the treatment of severe male infertility by assisted reproduction: Norfolk's total experience. Hum Reprod 1992;7(8):1067–72.

[52] Gromoll J, Simoni M, Nieschlag E. An activating mutation of the follicle-stimulating hormone receptor autonomously sustains spermatogenesis in a hypophysectomized man. J Clin Endocrinol Metab 1996;81(4):1367–70.

[53] Foresta C, et al. Use of recombinant human follicle-stimulating hormone in the treatment of male factor infertility. Fertil Steril 2002;77(2):238–44.

[54] Foresta C, et al. FSH in the treatment of oligozoospermia. Mol Cell Endocrinol 2000; 161(1–2):89–97.

[55] Caroppo E, et al. Recombinant human follicle-stimulating hormone as a pretreatment for idiopathic oligoasthenoteratozoospermic patients undergoing intracytoplasmic sperm injection. Fertil Steril 2003;80(6):1398–403.

[56] Baccetti B, et al. The effect of follicle stimulating hormone therapy on human sperm structure (Notulae seminologicae 11). Hum Reprod 1997;12(9):1955–68.

[57] Ben-Rafael Z, et al. Follicle-stimulating hormone treatment for men with idiopathic oligo-teratoasthenozoospermia before in vitro fertilization: the impact on sperm microstructure and fertilization potential. Fertil Steril 2000;73(1):24–30.

[58] Foresta C, et al. Treatment of male idiopathic infertility with recombinant human follicle-stimulating hormone: a prospective, controlled, randomized clinical study. Fertil Steril 2005;84(3):654–61.

[59] Ashkenazi J, et al. The role of purified follicle stimulating hormone therapy in the male partner before intracytoplasmic sperm injection. Fertil Steril 1999;72(4):670–3.

[60] Zini A, et al. Use of alternative and hormonal therapies in male infertility. Urology 2004; 63(1):141–3.

[61] Alvarez JG, Storey BT. Role of glutathione peroxidase in protecting mammalian spermatozoa from loss of motility caused by spontaneous lipid peroxidation. Gamete Res 1989; 23(1):77–90.

[62] Iwasaki A, Gagnon C. Formation of reactive oxygen species in spermatozoa of infertile patients. Fertil Steril 1992;57(2):409–16.

[63] Kessopoulou E, et al. A double-blind randomized placebo cross-over controlled trial using the antioxidant vitamin E to treat reactive oxygen species associated male infertility. Fertil Steril 1995;64(4):825–31.

[64] Geva E, et al. The effect of antioxidant treatment on human spermatozoa and fertilization rate in an in vitro fertilization program. Fertil Steril 1996;66(3):430–4.

[65] Comhaire FH, et al. The effects of combined conventional treatment, oral antioxidants and essential fatty acids on sperm biology in subfertile men. Prostaglandins Leukot Essent Fatty Acids 2000;63(3):159–65.

[66] Ebisch IM, et al. Does folic acid and zinc sulphate intervention affect endocrine parameters and sperm characteristics in men? Int J Androl 2006;29(2):339–45.

[67] Wong WY, et al. Effects of folic acid and zinc sulfate on male factor subfertility: a double-blind, randomized, placebo-controlled trial. Fertil Steril 2002;77(3):491–8.

[68] Agarwal A, Said TM. Carnitines and male infertility. Reprod Biomed Online 2004;8(4): 376–84.

[69] Gorelick JI, Goldstein M. Loss of fertility in men with varicocele. Fertil Steril 1993;59(3): 613–6.

[70] Kim ED, et al. Varicocele repair improves semen parameters in azoospermic men with spermatogenic failure. J Urol 1999;162(3 Pt 1):737–40.

[71] Russell JK. Varicocele, age, and fertility. Lancet 1957;273(6988):222.

[72] Chehval MJ, Purcell MH. Deterioration of semen parameters over time in men with untreated varicocele: evidence of progressive testicular damage. Fertil Steril 1992;57(1): 174–7.

[73] Su LM, Goldstein M, Schlegel PN. The effect of varicocelectomy on serum testosterone levels in infertile men with varicoceles. J Urol 1995;154(5):1752–5.

[74] Dubin L, Amelar RD. Etiologic factors in 1294 consecutive cases of male infertility. Fertil Steril 1971;22(8):469–74.

[75] Goldstein M, Eid JF. Elevation of intratesticular and scrotal skin surface temperature in men with varicocele. J Urol 1989;142(3):743–5.

[76] Zorgniotti AW, Macleod J. Studies in temperature, human semen quality, and varicocele. Fertil Steril 1973;24(11):854–63.

[77] Younes AK. Improvement of sexual activity, pregnancy rate, and low plasma testosterone after bilateral varicocelectomy in impotence and male infertility patients. Arch Androl 2003;49(3):219–28.

[78] Shah JB. Is there an association between varicoceles and hypogonadism in infertile men. J Urol 2005;173:449.

[79] Eskew LA, et al. Ultrasonographic diagnosis of varicoceles. Fertil Steril 1993;60(4): 693–7.

[80] Takahara M, et al. Relationship between grade of varicocele and the response to varicocelectomy. Int J Urol 1996;3(4):282–5.

[81] Steckel J, Dicker AP, Goldstein M. Relationship between varicocele size and response to varicocelectomy. J Urol 1993;149(4):769–71.

[82] Jarow JP, Ogle SR, Eskew LA. Seminal improvement following repair of ultrasound detected subclinical varicoceles. J Urol 1996;155(4):1287–90.

[83] McClure RD, Hricak H. Scrotal ultrasound in the infertile man: detection of subclinical unilateral and bilateral varicoceles. J Urol 1986;135(4):711–5.

[84] Pierik FH, et al. Improvement of sperm count and motility after ligation of varicoceles detected with colour Doppler ultrasonography. Int J Androl 1998;21(5):256–60.

[85] Schiff JD, Li PS, Goldstein M. Correlation of ultrasound-measured venous size and reversal of flow with Valsalva with improvement in semen-analysis parameters after varicocelectomy. Fertil Steril 2006;86(1):250–2.

[86] Goldstein M, et al. Microsurgical inguinal varicocelectomy with delivery of the testis: an artery and lymphatic sparing technique. J Urol 1992;148(6):1808–11.

[87] Marmar JL, Kim Y. Subinguinal microsurgical varicocelectomy: a technical critique and statistical analysis of semen and pregnancy data. J Urol 1994;152(4):1127–32.

[88] Hassan JM. Hydrocele formation following laparoscopic varicocelectomy. J Urol 2006;175(3 Pt 1):1076–9.

[89] Walsh Goldstein M. Surgical management of male infertility and other scrotal disorders. In: Walsh PC, et al, editors. Campbell's urology. 8 edition. Philadelphia: WB Saunders; 2002. p. 1532–88.

[90] Gazzera C, et al. Radiological treatment of male varicocele: technical, clinical, seminal and dosimetric aspects. Radiol Med (Torino) 2006;111(3):449–58.

[91] Gat Y, et al. Induction of spermatogenesis in azoospermic men after internal spermatic vein embolization for the treatment of varicocele. Hum Reprod 2005;20(4):1013–7.

[92] Wright EJ, Young GP, Goldstein M. Reduction in testicular temperature after varicocelectomy in infertile men. Urology 1997;50(2):257–9.

[93] Madgar I, et al. Controlled trial of high spermatic vein ligation for varicocele in infertile men. Fertil Steril 1995;63(1):120–4.

[94] Hadziselimovic F, et al. Testicular and vascular changes in children and adults with varicocele. J Urol 1989;142(2 Pt 2):583–5 [discussion: 603–5].

[95] Kass EJ, Belman AB. Reversal of testicular growth failure by varicocele ligation. J Urol 1987;137(3):475–6.

[96] Lemack GE, et al. Microsurgical repair of the adolescent varicocele. J Urol 1998;160(1): 179–81.

[97] Scherr D, Goldstein M. Comparison of bilateral versus unilateral varicocelectomy in men with palpable bilateral varicoceles. J Urol 1999;162(1):85–8.

[98] Montie JE, Stewart BH. Vasovasostomy: past, present and future. J Urol 1974;112(1): 111–3.

[99] Cos LR, et al. Vasovasostomy: current state of the art. Urology 1983;22(6):567–75.

[100] Lee HY. A 20-year experience with vasovasostomy. J Urol 1986;136(2):413–5.

[101] Sheynkin YR, et al. Microsurgical repair of iatrogenic injury to the vas deferens. J Urol 1998;159(1):139–41.

[102] Belker AM, et al. Results of 1,469 microsurgical vasectomy reversals by the Vasovasostomy Study Group. J Urol 1991;145(3):505–11.

[103] Goldstein M, Li PS, Matthews GJ. Microsurgical vasovasostomy: the microdot technique of precision suture placement. J Urol 1998;159(1):188–90.

[104] Schiff J, et al. Outcome and late failures compared in 4 techniques of microsurgical vasoepididymostomy in 153 consecutive men. J Urol 2005;174(2):651–5 [quiz: 801].

[105] Silber SJ. Microscopic vasectomy reversal. Fertil Steril 1977;28(11):1191–202.

[106] Silber SJ. Microscopic vasoepididymostomy: specific microanastomosis to the epididymal tubule. Fertil Steril 1978;30(5):565–71.

[107] Owen ER. Microsurgical vasovasostomy: a reliable vasectomy reversal. Aust N Z J Surg 1977;47(3):305–9.

[108] Silber SJ. Pregnancy after vasovasostomy for vasectomy reversal: a study of factors affecting long-term return of fertility in 282 patients followed for 10 years. Hum Reprod 1989; 4(3):318–22.

[109] Chawla A, et al. Should all urologists performing vasectomy reversals be able to perform vasoepididymostomies if required? J Urol 2004;172(3):1048–50.

[110] Thomas AJ. Infertility. New York: Lippincott Williams & Wilkins; 2004. p. 829–30.

[111] Daudin M, et al. Congenital bilateral absence of the vas deferens: clinical characteristics, biological parameters, cystic fibrosis transmembrane conductance regulator gene mutations, and implications for genetic counseling. Fertil Steril 2000;74(6):1164–74.

[112] Stuhrmann M, Dork T. CFTR gene mutations and male infertility. Andrologia 2000;32(2): 71–83.

[113] Chan PT, Schlegel PN. Nonobstructive azoospermia. Curr Opin Urol 2000;10(6):617–24.

[114] Palermo GD, et al. Fertilization and pregnancy outcome with intracytoplasmic sperm injection for azoospermic men. Hum Reprod 1999;14(3):741–8.

[115] Schiff JD, et al. Success of testicular sperm injection and intracytoplasmic sperm injection in men with Klinefelter syndrome. J Clin Endocrinol Metab 2005;90(11):6263–7.

[116] Tournaye H. Surgical sperm recovery for intracytoplasmic sperm injection: which method is to be preferred? Hum Reprod 1999;14(Suppl 1):71–81.

[117] Ezeh UI, Moore HD, Cooke ID. A prospective study of multiple needle biopsies versus a single open biopsy for testicular sperm extraction in men with non-obstructive azoospermia. Hum Reprod 1998;13(11):3075–80.

[118] Friedler S, et al. Testicular sperm retrieval by percutaneous fine needle sperm aspiration compared with testicular sperm extraction by open biopsy in men with non-obstructive azoospermia. Hum Reprod 1997;12(7):1488–93.

[119] Khadra AA, et al. Efficiency of percutaneous testicular sperm aspiration as a mode of sperm collection for intracytoplasmic sperm injection in nonobstructive azoospermia. J Urol 2003;169(2):603–5.

[120] Mercan R, et al. Outcome of testicular sperm retrieval procedures in non-obstructive azoospermia: percutaneous aspiration versus open biopsy. Hum Reprod 2000;15(7):1548–51.

[121] Temple-Smith PD, et al. Human pregnancy by in vitro fertilization (IVF) using sperm aspirated from the epididymis. J In Vitro Fert Embryo Transf 1985;2(3):119–22.

[122] Silber SJ, et al. Conventional in-vitro fertilization versus intracytoplasmic sperm injection for patients requiring microsurgical sperm aspiration. Hum Reprod 1994;9(9):1705–9.

[123] Schlegel PN. Testicular sperm extraction: microdissection improves sperm yield with minimal tissue excision. Hum Reprod 1999;14(1):131–5.

[124] Su LM, et al. Testicular sperm extraction with intracytoplasmic sperm injection for nonobstructive azoospermia: testicular histology can predict success of sperm retrieval. J Urol 1999;161(1):112–6.

[125] Chan PT, et al. Testicular sperm extraction combined with intracytoplasmic sperm injection in the treatment of men with persistent azoospermia postchemotherapy. Cancer 2001; 92(6):1632–7.

[126] Ramasamy R, Yagan N, Schlegel PN. Structural and functional changes to the testis after conventional versus microdissection testicular sperm extraction. Urology 2005;65(6): 1190–4.

[127] Goldstein M, Tanrikut C. Microsurgical management of male infertility. Nat Clin Pract Urol 2006;3(7):381–91.

ELSEVIER
SAUNDERS

Endocrinol Metab Clin N Am
36 (2007) 333–348

ENDOCRINOLOGY
AND METABOLISM
CLINICS
OF NORTH AMERICA

Male Hypogonadism in Systemic Disease

Rita R. Kalyani, MD[a], Sravanya Gavini, BS[a],
Adrian S. Dobs, MD, MHS[a,b,*]

[a]Division of Endocrinology and Metabolism, Johns Hopkins School of Medicine,
1830 E. Monument Street, Baltimore, MD 21287, USA
[b]Department of Medicine, Johns Hopkins School of Medicine, Baltimore, MD, USA

The effect of age on gonadal status has been recognized, but the interaction of systemic illness and androgen deficiency is not as thoroughly understood. Hypogonadism associated with acute and chronic illness is becoming more recognized (Box 1) and can occur as a result of the illness itself or its treatment. Although treating men who have male hypogonadism is standard medical practice, testosterone replacement therapy is still a controversial issue in the context of hypogonadism associated with age or systemic diseases. More studies are needed to delineate the exact mechanisms by which hypogonadism is related to diseases and to determine the long-term effects of testosterone replacement on most systemic illnesses. It is crucial to address these relationships because male hypogonadism may contribute to a reduced quality of life and poorer health outcomes. This article reviews the epidemiology of hypogonadism in common acute and chronic illnesses, the possible mechanisms that cause low testosterone levels (Fig. 1), and the results of replacement studies, if available.

General symptoms of hypogonadism

Hypogonadism is associated with a host of symptoms, including sexual dysfunction, reduced energy, depressed mood, poor concentration and memory, mild anemia, and a diminished sense of well-being [1]. Many of these symptoms are nonspecific and are often present in aging men or in men who have chronic disease. Hypogonadism can also result in decreased lean body mass, loss of bone mineral density, and increased body fat. As an example

---

* Corresponding author. Division of Endocrinology and Metabolism, Johns Hopkins School of Medicine, 1830 E. Monument Street, Baltimore, MD 21287.
    E-mail address: adobs@jhu.edu (A.S. Dobs).

0889-8529/07/$ - see front matter © 2007 Elsevier Inc. All rights reserved.
doi:10.1016/j.ecl.2007.03.014

Box 1. Systemic illnesses associated with hypogonadism

Burn injury
Stroke
Traumatic brain injury
Myocardial infarction
Respiratory illness
Sepsis
Surgical stress
Cancer
Chronic opioid exposure
Chronic renal failure
Chronic liver disease
Rheumatoid arthritis
HIV
Chronic obstructive pulmonary disease
Diabetes
Obesity

---

of the significance of this observation, changes in body composition have been well studied in HIV disease. Reduced lean body mass is found in AIDS wasting and correlates with increased risk of mortality [2]. Thus, male hypogonadism may explain or worsen many signs and symptoms of men who have systemic diseases. It is therefore crucial to diagnose hypogonadism if it is present in patients suffering from systemic diseases and to determine whether or not testosterone replacement is appropriate for alleviating some of these problems.

Laboratory diagnosis of male hypogonadism in the setting of systemic diseases

The Endocrine Society, in their recently published Clinical Practice Guidelines, recommends that when a patient presents with signs and symptoms suggestive of androgen deficiency, measurement of morning serum total testosterone levels should be performed. A patient who has a total testosterone level below 300 ng/dL is likely to be hypogonadal. In patients who have levels between 200 and 400 ng/dL, the test should be repeated along with measurement of free testosterone. Measurement of free testosterone or sex-hormone–binding globulin (SHBG) levels is helpful in determining bioavailable testosterone because many systemic conditions are associated with changes in SHBG levels. Specifically, increases in SHBG can be detected in hepatic cirrhosis, hyperthyroidism, HIV infection, and anticonvulsant use; reductions in SHBG are noted with moderate obesity, low protein states (nephrotic syndrome), hypothyroidism, hyperinsulinism, and glucocorticoid use.

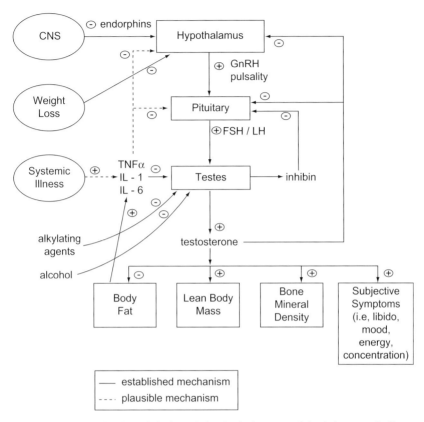

Fig. 1. Mechanism of action of the hypothalamic-pituitary-gonadal axis in systemic disease.

Measurement of leuteinizing hormone (LH) and follicle-stimulating hormone (FSH) is recommended to determine whether androgen deficiency is due to primary testicular failure, in which case the gonadotrophins would be elevated or due to secondary disturbances in the hypothalamus-pituitary-gonadal (HPG) axis, causing low gonadotrophin levels. The two types of hypogonadism can occur together, and this is often the case in many illnesses.

Acute illness

Since the 1970s, hypogonadism has been described in acute illness associated with surgery [3–5], stroke [6], traumatic brain injury [7], myocardial infarction [8], respiratory illness [9], sepsis [10], liver disease [10], and burns [11–13]. In a study of chronically critically ill men requiring mechanical ventilation and intensive nursing care, 96% of patients had bioavailable testosterone levels well below the lower limit of their age range after a median ICU length of stay of 25 days. The bioavailable testosterone values were approximately $11 \pm 11\%$ of the means for normal men in each decade [14]. As many as 90% of men with total body burns of 15% or greater have been found to have hypogonadism [11]. One report found that 24% of patients who had traumatic brain injury had gonadal dysfunction [7].

Primary and secondary hypogonadism have been reported with parallel changes in bioactive and immunoactive LH and FSH in critically ill patients [8,15], and some researchers have suggested that primary hypogonadism may be present to a greater degree in patients who have more severe illness [9]. Exogenous intravenous gonadotropin-releasing hormone (GnRH) pulses can partially or completely overcome hypogonadotropic hypogonadism, supporting a combined hypothalamic-pituitary-gonadal origin [7,16]. Mean free and total testosterone levels were found to fall by approximately half in men who had myocardial infarction, traumatic brain injury, and elective surgery within 24 hours [17]. Normalization of testosterone levels occurred 2 to 8 months after acute brain injury. FSH and LH levels were lower or unchanged. As evidenced by the significant fall of FSH, LH, and estradiol in predominantly postmenopausal women within 24 to 48 hours after the acute event, central hypogonadism occurs with acute illness in both genders [17]. In vivo results suggest that diminished activity of 17,20-desmolase may be a mechanistic explanation for reduced testosterone production within the testis [10]. SHBG levels remain unchanged [10,17].

In patients who have burns, free and total testosterone levels decline rapidly within 24 hours after injury and reach a nadir on average at day 11 or 12, whereas LH levels may remain unchanged or fall below normal by the fourth day [11,12]. Decreased pulsatility of LH release in burn patients has been found, suggesting a plausible mechanism for central hypogonadism in this condition [13]. Another explanation proposed is reduced biologic activity of LH as determined by bioassay techniques [13]. Inhibition of adrenal and testicular C-19–steroid secretion has been suggested by the finding that serum dehydroepiandrosterone sulfate, dehydroepiandrosterone, androstenedione, and testosterone concentrations fall during the first 4 weeks after burn trauma, whereas serum cortisol and 17-hydroxycorticosteroid levels rise in these studies as well [12].

The degree of hypothalamic-pituitary-gonadal axis suppression is related to the severity of illness in critical care patients. Patients who had more severe illness as described by the APACHE score or burns had significantly more profound declines in testosterone levels than those who had relatively mild or moderate illness [9,11]. Severity of head trauma is correlated to hypogonadism, with patients who had the lowest Glasgow Coma Scale score displaying the lowest levels of baseline and peak FSH and testosterone [7]. Chronically ill patients have a more marked reduction in testosterone levels than acutely ill patients [10]. Mean testosterone level among critically ill patients has also been suggested to be a predictor for mortality because surviving patients have significantly higher testosterone levels than nonsurvivors [10].

There is no established role for treatment of critically ill patients with testosterone outside of research protocols, although promising results have been obtained with the use of testosterone and its analogs in burn injuries. In six men who had total body burns of more than 70%, administration of testosterone enanthate 200 mg/wk intramuscularly for as little as 2 weeks resulted in significantly increased protein synthetic efficiency and only half the protein breakdown [18]. The oral testosterone analog oxandrolone has been found to have comparable results to other anabolic agents, such as human growth hormone, in its ability to decrease daily nitrogen loss while improving healing time [19]. These beneficial effects of oxandrolone (20 mg/d) were reproduced in a randomized, double-blinded, placebo-controlled trial in patients who had 40% to 70% total body surface area burns [20]. Positive effects on body weight and lean mass were retained 6 months after discontinuation of oxandrolone [21]. Another study of oxandrolone in burn patients found significantly decreased lengths of stay, although hepatic transaminases warranted monitoring [22]. Table 1 presents an overview of the efficacy of testosterone treatment of men who have hypogonadism and systemic disease.

Chronic illness

Chronic opioid exposure

Long-acting opiate preparations of methadone, morphine sulfate, oxycodone, and fentanyl for the treatment of chronic malignant and nonmalignant pain in men commonly result in opioid-induced androgen deficiency [23]. As many as 5 million men who have chronic nonmalignant pain may have androgen deficiency from opioid use in the United States [24]. In outpatient male patients taking sustained-action oral opioids for nonmalignant pain, as many as 87% of men who have normal erectile function before opioid use reported severe erectile dysfunction or diminished libido after use [25]. Hormone levels were lower in opioid users in a dose-dependent pattern. In a case-control study of 40 cancer survivors who had chronic pain, Rajagopal and colleagues [26] found that chronic opioids users had higher levels of hypogonadism and sexual dysfunction compared with control subjects (90% versus 40%). The prevalence of sexual dysfunction on methadone maintenance was reported to be 14% in one study [27]. High-dose methadone can decrease testosterone levels in male heroin addicts, leading to decreased sexual drive and performance [25,28–30]. Buprenorphine seems not to suppress testosterone levels and may be favored in the treatment of heroin addiction to prevent methadone-induced hypogonadism [31].

Suppression of pulsatile GnRH by the hypothalamus secondarily leads to reduced LH by the pituitary and testosterone by the gonad. Naturally occurring opiates (endorphins) may diminish testosterone levels by inhibiting GnRH. Direct suppressive effects on the pituitary and testes have also been proposed [32,33]. The acute decline in LH levels and testosterone can occur as soon as 1 to 2 hours after administration of a subcutaneous

Table 1
Strength of studies that have shown benefit in treatment of hypogonadism in systemic illness

Disease	Intervention	Strength of benefit	Nature of benefit	Study
Burn injury	IM testosterone injection	****	Protein synthetic efficiency	Ferrando et al, 2001 [18]
	Oxandrolone	*****	Lean body mass, wound healing	Demling and Orgill, 2000 [20]
Cancer	Testosterone patch	****	Fatigue, activity	Howell et al, 2001 [55]
Chronic opioid exposure	Testosterone patch	****	Sexual function, mood	Daniell et al, 2006 [23]
Diabetes/obesity	IM testosterone injection	****	Glycemic control, obesity	Kapoor et al, 2006 [95]
	Oral testosterone undecenoate	****	Glycemic control, obesity, erectile dysfunction	Boyanov et al, 2003 [96]
HIV	IM testosterone injection	*****	Lean body mass, quality of life	Grinspoon et al, 1996 [64]
COPD	IM testosterone injection	***	Lean body mass, bone mineral density	Casaburi et al, 2004 [74]
Chronic liver disease	Testosterone gel	**	Muscle strength, survival	Neff et al, 2004 [82]
Chronic renal failure	Nandrolone decanoate	***	Lean body mass, functionality	Johansen et al, 1999 [88]
Rheumatoid arthritis (no steroids)	Oral testosterone undecanoate	***	RA symptoms, libido	Cutolo et al, 1991 [92]
Rheumatoid arthritis (with steroids)	IM testosterone injection	None	None	Hall et al, 1996 [93]

Relative strength of benefit indicated by number of asterisks (***** = highest). Diabetes and obesity are not formally discussed in this review since they are covered by other authors in this journal.

Abbreviations: COPD, chronic obstructive pulmonary disease; IM, intramuscular; RA, rheumatoid arthritis.

injection of morphine [34]. Opiate antagonists such as naltrexone may partially reverse these effects and may lead to significant elevation in LH levels but no changes in testosterone levels [35]. Tolerance to opiates may develop, and effects on GnRH and gonadoptropin secretion may lessen with time [35].

In a recent 24-week, open–label, pilot study of testosterone patch therapy (5 mg/d for the first 12 weeks, 7.5 mg/d for the second 12 weeks) of 16 men who had androgen deficiency from opioid use [23], free testosterone levels significantly increased. At a dose of 7.5 mg/d, sexual function, mood, and depression scores showed significant improvement, and the patches were well tolerated.

Cancer

Testicular dysfunction can be present in cancer patients pre- or post-treatment. In Hodgkin's disease, approximately one third of patients have oligospermia, and up to 70% of men who have Hodgkin's disease have abnormal semen analysis [36–39]. In testicular cancer, over 50% of men have oligospermia before treatment [37,40].

Explanations for the pathophysiology of testicular dysfunction in Hodgkin's disease are lacking, although proposals have included effects on semen quality or immune-mediated effects [41]. FSH levels are lower than normal, suggesting that pre-treatment hypogonadism may be mediated by the pituitary and the gonad in Hodgkin's disease [36]. In testicular cancer, mechanisms may include local tumor effects, elevation of scrotal temperature, alterations in testicular blood flow, testicular fibrosis, or sperm antibodies [42]. Central hypogonadism may be caused by ectopic adrenocorticotropin hormone–producing tumors or by androgen-producing tumors.

Factors affecting impairment and recovery of spermatogenesis after cytotoxic therapy include the agent used, the dose received, and the age of patient or maturation of the testis at the time of insult [43–46]. The germinal epithelium of the adult testis may be more prone to cytotoxic damage than the prepurbertal testis [47]. Gonadotoxic agents include cyclophosphamide, chlorambucil, mustine, melphalan, busulfan, carmustine, lomustine, cytarabine, vinblastine, procarbazine, and cisplatin [48]. Irradiation dose similarly affects the speed and extent of recovery in radiation-induced testicular damage [49]. Single-dose irradiation with as low as 0.1 Gy can cause oligospermia, and doses above 0.8 Gy result in azoospermia. Recovery to pre-treatment sperm concentrations can take up to 5 years or more for doses of 4 Gy and above. In contrast to cytotoxic injury, irradiation may more severely affect Leydig cell function in the prepubertal testis [50].

Howell and colleagues [51] found that in their cohort of patients treated with mustine, vinblastine, procarbazine, and prednisolone; chlorambucil, vinblastine, procarbazine, prednisolone, etopside, vincristine, and doxorubicin hybrid; or high-dose chemotherapy for a variety of hematologic malignancies, one third of patients had evidence of Leydig cell dysfunction, and 90% of patients had germinal epithelial failure. High cumulative doses of cisplatin (>400 mg/m^2) in patients who have germ cell tumors of the testis are associated with significantly lower mean testosterone levels, lower testoster-one/SHBG ratios, and higher LH levels compared with similar patients not treated with chemotherapy [52]. In bone marrow transplant recipients pre-senting with fatigue, diminished libido, and erectile dysfunction, compensated Leydig cell insufficiency (high LH with normal testosterone levels) was pre-dominant [53].

The use of intramuscular testosterone injections of testosterone cypionate (250 mg 4 times weekly) for 6 months and sildenafil in patients who had erectile dysfunction after bone marrow transplant has been reported with favorable results [54]. Howell and colleagues [55] followed a cohort of 35 men who had LH of 8 IU/L or higher and testosterone levels in the lower range of normal or frankly below normal (testosterone less than 20 nmol/L) after cytotoxic chemotherapy for hematologic malignancy. After 12 months of transdermal testosterone (Andropatch; 2.5-mg patches, 1 to 2 patches/d), significant improvements in physical vigor, low-density lipoprotein choles-terol levels, and activity score were found in the testosterone-treated group versus the placebo group. No significant changes in bone mineral density, mood, or sexual function were observed.

There is a concern that testosterone, as an anabolic agent, may be associated with the proliferation of cancer cells. There are no reports in the literature or evidence that this is true. We do not discuss prostate cancer in this article, in which testosterone may have a permissive effect and would be an absolute contraindication.

HIV

Although the prevalence of hypogonadism ranges from 30% to 50% in men who had HIV wasting before highly active antiretroviral therapy (HAART), it still occurs in about 20% to 25% of HIV-infected men treated with HAART [56,57]. Various mechanisms have been proposed for hypogo-nadism in HIV-infected men, although it is probably a result of a combina-tion of these mechanisms. Primary hypogonadism in HIV-infected men could be caused by testicular atrophy due to opportunistic infections. Nonspecific interstitial inflammation and interstitial fibrosis were observed by De Paepe [58] in 32% of AIDS patients via autopsy examination. In this group of patients, the testes were infected with cytomegalovirus, *Myco-bacterium avium-intracellulare*, and *Toxoplasma*. The autopsies also revealed atrophy due to chemotherapy in patients who had secondary neoplasms. Although therapeutic antifungals such as ketoconazole have been implicated in inhibition of steroidogenesis [59], data about effects of antiretroviral agents are limited and inconclusive [57].

Secondary hypogonadism is more common in HIV-positive patients. Malnutrition and acute and chronic illness in patients who have AIDS can cause significant weight loss and disrupt the HPG axis, causing hypogonad-ism [2]. Cytokines likely affect all levels of the HPG axis [60,61]. Interleukin-1 has been shown to inhibit gonadotrophin release and LH binding to Leydig cells, causing low testosterone levels. Tumor necrosis factor affects the HPG axis and causes a decline in steroidogenesis [60]. Serum hormone binding globulin is reported to be increased as the disease progresses in HIV/AIDS syndrome, resulting in lower bioavailable testosterone [62,63].

Diagnosis and treatment of hypogonadism in HIV-infected men is crucial because androgen deficiency is strongly associated with AIDS wasting syndrome [64–66] and decline in other quality-of-life parameters. A testosterone level below 300 ng/dL is generally used as a cut-off for androgen deficiency, although a measurement of free testosterone and gonadotrophins is recommended [56] to determine which levels of the HPG axis are affected.

Replacement studies with HIV-infected hypogonadal men demonstrate benefit. A randomized, double-blind, placebo-controlled trial of 51 HIV-positive hypogonadal men showed that testosterone replacement increases lean body mass and muscle mass and improves perceived overall well-being and quality of life without reported side-effects to intramuscular testosterone injections [64]. Similar results were reported with a transdermal administration of testosterone by Bhasin and colleagues [67], who reported a favorable moderate increase in red blood cell levels and hemoglobin level in treated patients. Furthermore, Beck depression scores improved significantly in a randomized controlled trial with testosterone replacement after controlling for age, weight, and disease status [68]. Therefore, testosterone replacement in HIV-postive hypogonadal patients can be effective in treating muscle wasting, depression, and other quality-of-life issues.

Chronic obstructive pulmonary disease

The prevalence of hypogonadism in men who have chronic obstructive pulmonary disease (COPD) is about 38% [69]. There are two specific mechanisms that cause hypogonadism: hypoxia and chronic glucocorticoid use. Semple and colleagues [70] reported that patients who have COPD and hypoxia have low testosterone levels. The androgen deficiency becomes more severe with increasing arterial hypoxia and hypercapnia [70,71]. Whether hypoxia causes primary or secondary hypogonadism is unknown. Hypogonadism can also be induced by glucocorticoids that are used for treatment in COPD. Glucocorticoids can directly decrease testosterone biosynthesis in the testis [71] and can affect the HPG axis in numerous ways. They can affect the response of the anterior pituitary to the gonadotrophin-releasing hormone from the hypothalamus and can decrease LH secretion by acting at the negative feedback receptor site, resulting in low testosterone secretion [71,72]. Hypogonadism in patients who have COPD may cause a reduction in quadriceps muscle mass [73] and act together with glucocorticoids to decrease bone density.

Testosterone replacement by intramuscular injection has resulted in an increase in lean body mass and strength in men who have COPD and hypogonadism [74]. Resistance training along with testosterone replacement seems to amplify the effect. Early studies used anabolic agents such as oxandrolone to reverse weight loss associated with COPD [75]. Direct testos-terone replacement is more effective than the use of testosterone analogs because the functionality of patients does not seem to improve despite increases in lean body mass in studies with the testosterone analogs. In a randomized, placebo-controlled trial with men undergoing long-term glucocorticoid treatment, testosterone replacement improved lumbar spine bone mineral density and overall quality of life significantly, whereas nandro-lone decanoate and placebo did not [76]. In addition, testosterone replacement has been shown to improve bone mineral density in men who have asthma who are taking oral glucocorticoids by 5% after 1 year of treatment, com-pared with no change in the placebo group [77,78]. Thus, testosterone replace-ment in hypogonadal men who have COPD or asthma may be recommended to reduce the risk of osteoporosis and to prevent loss of lean body mass.

Chronic liver disease

The prevalence of hypogonadism in chronic liver disease is unknown. In patients who have alcoholic liver disease, primary testicular failure can occur due to defective morphology of Leydig cells caused by ethanol [79] even before clinical signs of hypogonadism are present. The HPG axis is also affected, resulting in a diminished pulsatile secretion of LH [79]. The degree of hypothalamic hypogonadism correlates with the degree of liver damage in cirrhosis [80]. In men who have chronic hepatitis and who have lesser degree of liver damage, the HPG axis is not affected.

The diagnosis can be difficult because the serum level of SHBG is often higher than normal in patients who have chronic liver disease, leading to an overestimate of bioavailable testosterone. Therefore, free testosterone levels should be measured initially to assess the patient's endocrine status because hypogonadism is a significant risk factor for osteoporosis and is predictive of spinal fracture in patients who have chronic liver disease [81].

No studies have investigated bone mineral density with testosterone supplementation in men who have chronic liver disease. A retrospective study showed that testosterone gel improves muscle strength and increases survival in patients undergoing liver transplant who have chronic allograft failure [82]. To reduce the theoretical risk of inducing hepatocellular carcinoma, transdermal testosterone is preferred after discussing the risks and benefits of replacement with the patient. This would reduce exposure of the liver to high levels of testosterone associated with intramuscular injections and lead to more stable serum testosterone levels [81]. Even though testosterone replacement in patients who have chronic liver disease has not been studied thoroughly, it might provide some benefit in reducing the risk of osteoporosis and spinal fracture.

Chronic renal failure

About two thirds of men undergoing hemodialysis for end-stage renal disease have testosterone levels in the hypogonadal range [83,84]. Androgen deficiency and decline in Leydig cell sensitivity to LH is associated with chronic renal failure even with a moderate reduction in glomerular filtration rate [85]. A serum factor present in uremia likely inhibits the LH receptor, thus rendering the Leydig cell less sensitive to LH stimulation [86]. The resultant reduction in testosterone production coupled with increased metabolic clearance of testosterone [87] causes low serum testosterone levels. Secondary hypogonadism also occurs in uremic men when the pulsatile LH secretion is diminished despite reduced negative feedback from low testosterone levels. The pulsatility is present, but the amount of LH released per pulse is reduced [85].

Renal transplantation reverses the combined form of hypogonadism observed in these patients. The use of nandrolone decanoate, a 19-nortestosterone derivative, resulted in a significant increase in lean body mass and physical functionality and in a decrease in fatigue in a randomized controlled trial with patients receiving long-term dialysis [88]. Singh and colleagues [84] reported that using two transdermal testosterone patches instead of one helped achieve mid-normal levels of testosterone in hypogonadal patients undergoing hemodialysis. The effects of testosterone replacement on lean body mass needs further study. Earlier studies demonstrated that although some men might benefit from testosterone replacement, in most men testosterone replacement alone fails to restore libido and erectile function despite restoration of normal serum testosterone levels [85]. A more recent pilot study with 12 patients who were given intramuscular testosterone injections and sildenafil reported a beneficial result [89]. More long-term studies are needed to determine the safety and efficacy of this combination treatment. Although further studies are needed to establish the benefit of testosterone therapy in hypogonadal men who have chronic renal failure, the use of testosterone derivatives might be beneficial in increasing lean body mass and functionality.

Rheumatoid arthritis

Men who have rheumatoid arthritis (RA) have low serum levels of free testosterone and LH [90] due to a hypothalamic/pituitary defect. One possible cause is long-term treatment of RA with nonsteroidal anti-inflammatory drugs, which are known to inhibit gonadotrophin release from the pituitary. Because androgens may be involved in tissue-specific immunosuppressive responses at the level of the synovial tissue in RA, low levels of testosterone may worsen disease activity [91]. Furthermore, androgen deficiency has been implicated in loss of BMD, resulting in osteoporosis in RA.

An open, uncontrolled study with oral testosterone undecenoate administration reported an overall 60% clinical improvement, a reduction of the number of affected joints, lower intake of nonsteroidal anti-inflammatory drugs, and improved libido at the end of 6 months without any relevant side effects [92]. A randomized, double-blind study using testosterone enanthate injections conducted by Hall and colleagues [93] failed to show any significant beneficial effect of testosterone replacement on disease activity and bone density, possibly because the subjects were undergoing steroid treatment for RA, a significant contributor to decreased bone density. Further studies are needed to determine if higher doses of testosterone would be beneficial when patients are undergoing treatment with steroids.

Summary

In relatively healthy men who have hypogonadism, testosterone replacement therapy has been shown to improve sexual function, mood, lean body mass, and bone density. Low serum testosterone in acute and chronic disease is fairly common and is multifactorial due to the combination of weight loss, stress, specific medications, and infections. Few studies have been done evaluating the effects of replacement in such men who have systemic diseases. Little information is available regarding testosterone treatment in the face of acute illness (although benefit in burn patients is likely); therefore, testosterone treatment cannot be routinely recommended. Most data suggest that testosterone can be offered to patients who have chronic disease unless there is a specific contraindication (eg, prostate cancer, breast cancer, or untreated sleep apnea). Testosterone therapy is generally well tolerated [94]. Elevations of hematocrit and prostate-specific antigen levels should be monitored. Although the treatment of hypogonadism in systemic disease is controversial and needs further study, testosterone can be offered to patients who have systemic diseases for symptomatic relief. Although it is unlikely that testosterone will affect the underlying disease, further study is needed to understand the effects of quality of life and maintenance of lean body mass on long-term health outcomes.

References

[1] Bhasin S, Cunningham GR, Hayes FJ, et al. Testosterone therapy in adult men with androgen deficiency syndromes: an endocrine society clinical practice guideline. J Clin Endocrinol Metab 2006;91(6):1995–2010.
[2] Dobs AS, Few WL III, Blackman MR, et al. Serum hormones in men with human immunodeficiency virus-associated wasting. J Clin Endocrinol Metab 1996;81(11):4108–12.
[3] Wang C, Chan V, Yeung RT. Effect of surgical stress on pituitary-testicular function. Clin Endocrinol (Oxf) 1978;9(3):255–66.
[4] Aono T, Kurachi K, Mizutani S, et al. Influence of major surgical stress on plasma levels of testosterone, luteinizing hormone and follicle-stimulating hormone in male patients. J Clin Endocrinol Metab 1972;35(4):535–42.
[5] Nakashima A, Koshiyama K, Uozumi T, et al. Effects of general anesthesia and severity of surgical stress on serum LH and testosterone in males. Acta Endocrinol (Copenh) 1975; 78(2):258–9.
[6] Dimopoulou I, Kouyialis AT, Orfanos S, et al. Endocrine alterations in critically ill patients with stroke during the early recovery period. Neurocrit Care 2005;3(3):224–9.

[7] Dimopoulou I, Tsagarakis S, Theodorakopoulou M, et al. Endocrine abnormalities in critical care patients with moderate-to-severe head trauma: incidence, pattern, and predisposing factors. Intensive Care Med 2004;30(6):1051–7.

[8] Wang C. Effect of acute myocardial infarction on pituitary-testicular function. Clin Endocrinol (Oxf) 1978;9(3):249–53.

[9] Spratt DI, Cox P, Orav J, et al. Reproductive axis suppression in acute illness is related to disease severity. J Clin Endocrinol Metab 1993;76(6):1548–54.

[10] Luppa P. Serum androgens in intensive-care patients: correlations with clinical findings. Clin Endocrinol (Oxf) 1991;34(4):305–10.

[11] Vogel AV, Peake GT, Rada RT. Pituitary-testicular axis dysfunction in burned men. J Clin Endocrinol Metab 1985;60(4):658–65.

[12] Lephart ED, Baxter CR, Parker CR. Effect of burn trauma on adrenal and testicular steroid hormone production. J Clin Endocrinol Metab 1987;64(4):842–8.

[13] Semple CG, Robertson WR, Mitchell R, et al. Mechanisms leading to hypogonadism in men with burn injuries. Br Med J 1987;295(6595):403–7.

[14] Nierman DM, Mechanick JI. Hypotestosteronemia in chronically critically ill men. Crit Care Med 1999;27(11):2418–21.

[15] Spratt DI, Bigos ST, Beitins I, et al. Both hyper- and hypogonadotropic hypogonadism occur transiently in acute illness: bio- and immunoreactive gonadotropins. J Clin Endocrinol Metab 1992;75(6):1562–70.

[16] Van den Berghe G, Weekers F, Baxter RC, et al. Five-day pulsatile gonadotropin-releasing hormone administration unveils combined hypothalamic-pituitary-gonadal defects underlying profound hypoandrogenism in men with prolonged critical care illness. J Clin Endocrinol Metab 2001;86(7):3217–26.

[17] Woolf PD. Transient hypogonadotropic hypogonadism cuased by critical illness. J Clin Endocrinol Metab 1985;60(3):444–50.

[18] Ferrando AA, Sheffield-Moore M, Wolf SE, et al. Testosterone administration in severe burns ameliorates muscle catabolism. Crit Care Med 2001;29(10):1936–42.

[19] Demling RH. Comparison of the anabolic effects and complications of human growth hormone and the testosterone analog, oxandrolone, after severe burn injury. Burns 1999; 25:215–21.

[20] Demling RH, Orgill DP. The anticatabolic and wound healing effects of the testosterone analog oxandrolone after severe burn injury. J Crit Care 2000;15(1):12–7.

[21] Demling RH, Desanti L. Oxandrolone induced lean mass gain during recovery from severe burns is maintained after discontinuation of the anabolic steroid. Burns 2003;29:793–7.

[22] Wolf SE, Edelman LS, Kemalyan N, et al. Effects of oxandrolone on outcome measures in the severely burned: a multicenter prospective randomized double-blind trial. J Burn Care Res 2006;27(2):131–9.

[23] Daniell HW, Lentz R, Mazer NA. Open-label pilot study of testosterone patch therapy in men with opioid-induced androgen deficiency. J Pain 2006;7(3):200–10.

[24] Mazer N, Chapman C, Daniell H, et al. Opioid-induced androgen deficiency in men (OPIAD): an estimate of the potential patient population in the U.S. and Canada [abstract 857]. J Pain 2004;5(Suppl 1):S73.

[25] Daniell HW. Hypogonadism in men consuming sustained-action oral opioids. J Pain 2002; 3(5):377–84.

[26] Rajagopal A, Vassilopoulou-Sellin R, Palmer JL, et al. Symptomatic hypogonadism in male survivors of cancer with chronic exoposure to opioids. Cancer 2004;100(4):851–8.

[27] Brown R, Balousek S, Mundt M, et al. Methadone maintenance and male sexual dysfunction. J Addict Dis 2005;24(2):91–106.

[28] Azizi F, Vagenakis AG, Longcope C, et al. Decreased serum testosterone concentration in male heroin and methadone addicts. Steroids 1973;22(4):467–72.

[29] Cicero TJ, Bell RD, Wiest WG, et al. Function of the male sex organs in heroin and methadone users. N Engl J Med 1975;292(17):882–7.

[30] Mendelson JH, Meyer RE, Ellingboe J, et al. Effects of heroin and methadone on plasma cortisol and testosterone. J Pharmacol Exp Ther 1975;195(2):296–302.

[31] Bliesener N, Albrecht S, Schwagar A, et al. Plasma testosterone and sexual function in men receiving buprenorphine maintenance for opioid dependence. J Clin Endocrinol Metab 2005;90(1):203–6.

[32] Adams ML, Sewing B, Forman JB, et al. Opioid-induced suppression of rat testicular function. J Pharmacol Exp Ther 1993;266(1):323–8.

[33] Blank MS, Fabbri A, Catt KJ, et al. Inhibition of luteinizing hormone release by morphine and endogenous opiates in cultured pituitary cells. Endocrinology 1986;118(5):2097–101.

[34] Cicero TJ. Effects of exogenous and endogenous opiates on the hypothalamic-pituitary-gonadal axis in the male. Fed Proc 1980;39(8):2551–4.

[35] Mendelson JH, Ellingboe J, Kuehnie JC, et al. Heroin and naltrexone effects on pituitary-gonadal hormones in man: interaction of steroid feedback effects, tolerance, and supersensitivity. J Pharmacol Exp Ther 1980;214(3):503–6.

[36] Vigersky RA, Chapman RM, Berenberg J, et al. Testicular dysfunction in untreated Hodgkin's disease. Am J Med 1982;73(4):482–6.

[37] Hendry WF, Stredronska J, Jones CR, et al. Semen analysis in testicular cancer and Hodgkin's disease: pre- and post-treatment findings and implications for cryopreservation. Br J Urol 1983;55(6):769–73.

[38] Viviani S, Ragni G, Santoro A, et al. Testicular dysfunction in Hodgkin's disease before and after treatment. Eur J Cancer 1991;27(11):1389–92.

[39] Shekarriz M, Tolentino MV, Ayzman I, et al. Cryopreservation and semen quality in patients with Hodgkin's disease. Cancer 1995;72(11):2732–6.

[40] Meirow D, Schenker JG. Cancer and male infertility. Hum Reprod 1995;10(8):2017–22.

[41] Barr RD, Clark DA, Booth JD. Dyspermia in men with localized Hodgkin's disease: a potentially reversible immune mediated disorder. Med Hypotheses 1993;40(3):165–8.

[42] Guazzieri S, Lembo A, Ferro G, et al. Sperm antibodies and infertility in patients with testicular cancer. Urology 1985;26(2):139–42.

[43] Da Cunha MF, Meistrich ML, Fuller LM, et al. Recovery of spermatogenesis after treatment for Hodgkin's disease: limiting dose of MOPP chemotherapy. J Clin Oncol 1984; 2(6):571–7.

[44] Meistrich ML, Chawla SP, da Cunha MF, et al. Recovery of sperm production after chemotherapy for osteosarcoma. Cancer 1989;63(11):2115–23.

[45] Pryzant RM, Meistrich ML, Wilson G, et al. Long-term reduction in sperm count after chemotherapy with and without radiation therapy for non-Hodgkin's lymphomas. J Clin Oncol 1993;11(2):239–47.

[46] Watson AR, Rance CP, Bain J. Long term effects of cyclophosphamide on testicular function. Br Med J (Clin Res Ed) 1985;291(6507):1457–60.

[47] Rivkees SA, Crawford JD. The relationship of gonadal activity and chemotherapy-induced gonadal damage. JAMA 1988;259(14):2123–5.

[48] Howell SJ, Shalet SM. Effect of cancer therapy on pituitary-testicular axis. Int J Androl 2002;25:269–76.

[49] Rowley MJ, Leach DR, Warner GA, et al. Effect of graded doses of ionizing radiation on the human testis. Radiat Res 1974;59(3):665–78.

[50] Shalet SM, Tsatsoulis A, Whitehead E, et al. Vulnerability of the human Leydig cell to radiation damage is dependent upon age. J Endocrinol 1989;120(1):161–5.

[51] Howell SJ, Radford JA, Ryder WDJ, et al. Testicular function after cytotoxic chemotherapy: evidence of Leydig cell insufficiency. J Clin Oncol 1999;17(5):1493–8.

[52] Gert A, Muhlbayer D, Hansmann G, et al. The impact of chemotherapy on Leydig cell function in long term survivors of germ cell tumors. Cancer 2001;91(7):1297–303.

[53] Chatterjee R, Kottaridis PD, McGarrigle HH, et al. Patterns of Leydig cell insufficiency in adult males following bone marrow transplantation for hematological malignancies. Bone Marrow Transplant 2001;28(5):497–502.

[54] Chatterjee R, Kottaridis PD, McGarrigle HH, et al. Management of erectile dysfunction by combination therapy with testosterone and sildenafil in recipients of high-dose therapy for hematological malignancies. Bone Marrow Transplant 2002;29(7):607–10.

[55] Howell SJ, Radford JA, Adams JE, et al. Randomized placebo-controlled trial of testosterone replacement in men with mild Leydig cell insufficiency following cytotoxic chemotherapy. Clin Endocrinol (Oxf) 2001;55(3):315–24.

[56] Crum NF, Furtek KJ, Olson PE, et al. A review of hypogonadism and erectile dysfunction among HIV-infected men during the pre- and post-HAART eras: diagnosis, pathogenesis, and management. AIDS Patient Care STDS 2005;19(10):655–71.

[57] Rietschel P, Corcoran C, Stanley T, et al. Prevalence of hypogonadism among men with weight loss related to human immunodeficiency virus infection who were receiving highly active antiretroviral therapy. Clin Infect Dis 2000;31:1240–4.

[58] De Paepe ME, Waxman M. Testicular atrophy in AIDS. Hum Pathol 1989;20(3):210–4.

[59] Pont A, Graybill JR, Craven PC, et al. High-dose ketoconazole therapy and adrenal and testicular function in humans. Arch Intern Med 1984;144:2150–3.

[60] Mylonakis E, Koutkia P, Grinspoon S. Diagnosis and treatment of androgen deficiency in human immunodeficiency virus-infected men and women. Clin Infect Dis 2001;33: 857–64.

[61] Sellmeyer DE, Gruenefeld C. Endocrine and metabolic disturbances in human immunodeficiency virus infection and the acquired immune deficiency syndrome. Endocr Rev 1996;17: 518–32.

[62] Poretsky L, Can S, Zumoff B. Testicular dysfunction in human immunodeficiency virus-infected men. Metabolism 1995;44(7):946–53.

[63] Martin ME, Benassayag C, Amiel C, et al. Alterations in the concentrations and binding properties of sex steroid binding protein and corticosteroid-binding globulin in HIV+ patients. J Endocrinol Invest 1992;15:597–603.

[64] Grinspoon S, Corcoran C, Lee K, et al. Loss of lean body and muscle mass correlates with androgen levels in hypogonadal men with acquired immunodeficiency syndrome and wasting. J Clin Endocrinol and Metab 1996;81(11):4051–8.

[65] Grinspoon S, Corcoran C, Askari H, et al. Effects of androgen administration in men with the AIDS wasting syndrome. Ann Intern Med 1998;129(1):18–26.

[66] Behler C, Shade S, Gregory K, et al. Anemia and HIV in the antiretroviral era: potential significance of testosterone. AIDS Res Hum Retroviruses 2005;21(3):200–6.

[67] Bhasin S, Storer TW, Asbel-Sethi N, et al. Effects of testosterone replacement with a nongenital, transdermal system, androderm, in human immunodeficiency virus-infected men with low testosterone levels. J Clin Endocrinol Metab 1998;83(9):3155–62.

[68] Grinspoon S, Corcoran C, Stanley T, et al. Effects of hypogonadism and testosterone administration on depression indices in HIV-infected men. J Clin Endocrinol Metab 2000; 85(1):60–5.

[69] Laghi F, Antonescu-Turcu A, Collins E, et al. Hypogonadism in men with chronic obstructive pulmonary disease. Am J Respir Care Med 2005;171:728–33.

[70] Semple PD, Beastall GH, Watson WS, et al. Serum testosterone depression associated with hypoxia in respiratory failure. Clin Sci 1980;58:105–6.

[71] Creutzberg EC, Casaburi R. Endocrinological disturbances in chronic obstructive pulmonary disease. Eur Respir J 2003;22(46):76s–80s.

[72] Creutzberg EC, Schols AMWJ. Anabolic steroids. Curr Opin Clin Nutr Metab Care 1999;2: 243–53.

[73] Van Vilet M, Spruit MA, Verleden G, et al. Hypogonadism, quadriceps weakness, and exercise intolerance in chronic obstructive pulmonary disease. Am J Respir Crit Care Med 2005;172:1105–11.

[74] Casaburi R, Bhasin S, Cosentino L, et al. Effects of testosterone and resistance training in men with chronic obstructive pulmonary disease. Am J Respir Crit Care Med 2004;170: 870–8.

[75] Yeh S, DeGuzman B, Kramer T. Reversal of COPD-associated weight-loss using the anabolic agent oxandrolone. Chest 2002;122:421–8.

[76] Crawford BAL, Liu PY, Kean MT, et al. Randomized placebo-controlled trial of androgen effects of on muscle and bone in men requiring long-term systemic glucocorticoid treatment. J Clin Endocrinol Metab 2003;88(7):3167–76.

[77] Biskobing DM. COPD and osteoporosis. Chest 2002;121:609–20.

[78] Reid IR, Wattie DJ, Evans MC, et al. Testosterone therapy in glucocorticoid-treated men. Arch Intern Med 1996;156(11):1133–4.

[79] Bannister P, Handley T, Chapman C, et al. Hypogonadism in chronic liver disease: impaired release of luteinizing hormone. Br Med J 1986;293:1191–4.

[80] Gursoy S, Baskol M, Ozbakir O, et al. Hypothalamo-pituitary gonadal axis in men with chronic hepatitis. Hepatogastroenterology 2004;51:787–90.

[81] Collier JD, Ninkovic M, Compton JE. Guidelines on the management of osteoporosis associated with chronic liver disease. Gut 2002;50:1–9.

[82] Neff GW, O'Brien CB, Shire NJ, et al. Topical testosterone treatment for chronic allograft failure in liver transplant recipients with recurrent hepatitis C virus. Transplant Proc 2004; 36:3071–4.

[83] Johansen KL, Holley JL. Testosterone metabolism and replacement therapy in patients with end-stage renal disease. Semin Dial 2004;17:202–8.

[84] Singh AB, Norris K, Modi N, et al. Pharmacokinetics of a transdermal testosterone system in men with end stage renal disease receiving maintenance hemodialysis and health hypogonadal men. J Clin Endocrinol Metab 2001;86(6):2437–45.

[85] Palmer BF. Sexual dysfunction in uremia. J Am Soc Nephrol 1999;10:1381–8.

[86] Dunkel L, Raivio T, Laine J, et al. Circulating luteinizing hormone receptor inhibitor(s) in boys with chronic renal failure. Kidney Int 1997;5:777–84.

[87] Handelsman DJ, Dong Q. Hypothalamo-pituitary gonadal axis in chronic renal failure. Endocrinol Metab Clin North Am 1993;22(1):145–61.

[88] Johansen KL, Mulligan K, Schambelan M. Anabolic effects of nandrolone decanoate in patients receiving dialysis: a randomized controlled trial. JAMA 1999;281(14):1275–81.

[89] Chatterjee R, Wood S, McGarrigle HH. A novel therapy with testosterone and sildenafil for erectile dysfunction in patients on renal dialysis or after renal transplantation. J Fam Plann Reprod Health Care 2004;30(2):88–90.

[90] Tengstrand B, Carlstrom K, Hafstrom I. Bioavailable testosterone in men with rheumatoid arthritis—high frequency of hypogonadism. Rheumatology 2002;41:285–9.

[91] Cutolo M. Sex hormone adjuvant therapy in rheumatoid arthritis. Rheum Dis Clin North Am 2000;26(4):881–95.

[92] Cutolo M, Balleari E, Giusti M, et al. Androgen replacement therapy in male patients with rheumatoid arthritis. J Rheumatol 1991;34(1):1–5.

[93] Hall GM, Larbre JP, Spector TD, et al. A randomized trial of testosterone therapy in males with rheumatoid arthritis. Br J Rheumatol 1996;35:568–73.

[94] Gruenewald DA, Matsumoto AM. Testosterone supplementation therapy for older men: potential benefits and risks. J Am Geriatr Soc 2003;51:101–15.

[95] Kapoor D, Goodwin E, Channer KS, et al. Testosterone replacement therapy improves insulin resistance, glycemic control, visceral adiposity and hyercholesterolaemia in hypogonadalmen with type 2 diabetes. Eur J Endocrinol 2006;154(6):899–906.

[96] Boyanov MA, Boneva Z, Christov VG. Testosterone supplementation in men with type 2 diabetes, visceral obesity and partial androgen deficiency. Aging Male 2003;6(1):1–7.

ELSEVIER
SAUNDERS

Endocrinol Metab Clin N Am
36 (2007) 349–363

ENDOCRINOLOGY
AND METABOLISM
CLINICS
OF NORTH AMERICA

Androgens, Obesity, and Sleep-Disordered Breathing in Men

Peter Y. Liu, MBBS, FRACP, PhD[a],
Ian D. Caterson, MBBS, FRACP, PhD[b],
Ronald R. Grunstein, MBBS, FRACP, PhD[c],
David J. Handelsman, MBBS, FRACP, PhD[d],*

[a]Department of Andrology, ANZAC Research Institute, Concord Hospital (C64),
University of Sydney, Sydney NSW 2139, Australia
[b]Human Nutrition Unit (G08), Royal Prince Alfred Hospital, University of Sydney,
NSW 2006, Australia
[c]Sleep and Circadian Group, Woolcock Institute, Royal Prince Alfred Hospital (C39),
University of Sydney, NSW 2006, Australia
[d]ANZAC Research Institute, Concord Hospital (C64), University of Sydney,
Sydney NSW 2139, Australia

The widening obesity epidemic and male reproductive function

A worldwide obesity epidemic in genetically predisposed populations, sustained by effortless access to affordable high-caloric food and a sedentary modern lifestyle, threatens health care resources [1–8]. Even seemingly minor energy imbalances can produce massive obesity if sustained over a sufficiently long period [2], particularly if applied over an entire population. One in three Americans is classified as obese, and this number has been steadily rising [9]. Similar trends are apparent across the Pacific ocean, but only one in five Australians are obese [10,11]. These trends are likely to worsen if documented declines in physical activity and larger food intake persist [12,13]. Concern arises because obesity predicts increased mortality [14,15], particularly through its linkage with important comorbidities such as diabetes mellitus, cardiovascular disease, the metabolic syndrome, and obstructive sleep apnea (OSA) [8,16–37].

This work was supported by a postdoctoral fellowship (262025) from the NHMRC (Australia) awarded to PYL.

* Corresponding author.

E-mail address: pliu@mail.usyd.edu.au (D.J. Handelsman).

doi:10.1016/j.ecl.2007.03.002
endo.theclinics.com

A fundamental relationship between energy balance and reproductive function exists from an evolutionary perspective in many mammalian species to ensure that population growth is controlled during times of famine. Epidemiologic evidence also links male reproductive function (and one of its key prerequisites, normal androgen action) with obesity. Reduced fertility has been documented recently in a large cohort of 1329 overweight and obese men [38]. Obese men may have lower sperm concentration [39] and reduced sperm quality [40]. However, such studies relying on semen collection are known to be unrepresentative of the population being studied. Obesity is associated with sexual and erectile dysfunction [41], and weight loss in obese men improves erectile function [42]. These relationships could be further modulated by altered androgen action because the polyglutamate repeat length in exon 1 of the androgen receptor (which is a known functionally relevant polymorphism that influences androgen receptor sensitivity by modulating transactivation efficiency [43–48]) was found to be weakly associated with central obesity in a study of 99 men [49]. Studies in twins suggest that other polygenic factors govern erectile function, but these remain poorly defined [50].

Interventional studies designed to examine the role of androgens in the energy balance of obese men have been largely contradictory and underpowered. One uncontrolled pilot study reported reduced waist/hip circumference and improved insulin sensitivity in eight men treated for 3 months with transdermal testosterone (250 mg in 10 g gel daily) but found no effect in another nine men treated for the same duration with transdermal dihydrotestosterone (250 mg in 10 g gel daily) [51]. The same investigators also reported a double-blind study in which 28 middle-aged men who had abdominal obesity were randomized to receive transdermal placebo, testosterone (125 mg in 5 g gel daily), or dihydrotestosterone (125 mg in 5 g gel daily) gel for 9 months [52]. Compared with treatment with dihydrotestosterone and placebo, testosterone treatment inhibited lipid uptake into adipose tissue, decreased serum triglycerides and lipoprotein lipase activity, reduced visceral fat (as shown by CT scan), and increased insulin sensitivity [52,53]. Another study failed to detect any beneficial effect, but an interim change in study design unblinded treatment assignment and reduced power. Although no consistent testosterone effects were reported, the unplanned change in study design limits interpretation [54].

These preliminary data suggest that testosterone treatment may improve body composition, but studies have been underpowered to detect clinically significant weight changes or changes in adipose tissue depots. Reduced fat mass is supported by ancillary data from 32 older men, seven of whom were obese (body mass index greater than 30), which showed that therapeutic androgen therapy decreased total and abdominal fat [55]. A similar trend was seen in young men who had classical androgen deficiency [56].

Strategies to specifically enhance weight loss in obese men within the framework of the core lifestyle interventions of diet restriction and exercise promotion are needed [57] because obese men have proportionally worse health consequences because abdominal (android) obesity and OSA are more prominent in men and because current antiobesity strategies have generally only been successfully applied to women [30,57,58]. Such methods are likely to succeed because men who participate in weight-loss programs are more likely than women to undergo behavioral modifications [57], and men can lose weight more easily because they require a smaller reduction in energy balance to effect loss of fat [59].

The metabolic syndrome

The metabolic syndrome is a constellation of abdominal obesity, insulin resistance, hypertension, and dyslipidemia, which is variably defined but probably refines and explains many of the health consequences of obesity and highlights the central pathogenic role of visceral (abdominal) obesity and insulin resistance. Whether the syndromic collection of these seemingly diverse factors has consequences beyond those known for each factor alone is debated, leading to the suggestion that a specific diagnosis of the metabolic syndrome is neither useful nor necessary [60]. Furthermore, the World Health Organization, the Third Report of the National Cholesterol Education Program's Adult Treatment Panel, the European Group for study of Insulin Resistance, the American Association of Clinical Endocrinologists, and the International Diabetes Foundation have each advocated slightly different definitions of the metabolic syndrome around similar core features [17,60]. The differences are not trivial because discordant classification occurs in up to 20% of Americans [60]. Nevertheless, approximately one in four American adults has the metabolic syndrome [17], and its definition probably remains a useful contribution to the problem.

Recent epidemiologic data have implicated the role of androgens in the pathogenesis of the metabolic syndrome in men. In non-obese Caucasian men residing in the greater Boston area, sex hormone-binding globulin (SHBG), testosterone, and symptomatic androgen deficiency independently predict development of the metabolic syndrome [61]. These data largely confirm previous data in other populations [62] and extend existing knowledge that SHBG and testosterone predict diabetes mellitus and central adiposity [63–65]. The longitudinal and population-based nature of these cohorts from around the world is an important design strength. Conversely, metabolic syndrome can predict future development of hypogonadism [66]. These data suggest that reproductive function and metabolic syndrome are interlinked, perhaps independently of the aforementioned relationships between reproductive function and obesity.

Abdominal obesity (indicated clinically by waist circumference) is a central component of the metabolic syndrome and may be more important than total fat mass (indicated by body mass index) as a cardiovascular risk marker [67]. Visceral abdominal fat is independently associated with increased blood pressure, waist circumference, triglycerides, fasting plasma glucose, and low high-density lipoprotein cholesterol levels, each of which is an independent risk factor for cardiovascular disease [68]. Visceral abdominal fat is also an independent predictor of all-cause mortality, as shown in a community-based randomly selected nested case-control study [69]. For these reasons, abdominal obesity is the primary target for the treatment of the metabolic syndrome [17]. Androgen therapy reduces visceral abdominal fat in a wider range of men, including those who are older [55], abdominally obese, and middle-aged [51,70] or hypogonadal [56]. This effect is probably potentiated by the greater androgen receptor expression in visceral abdominal rather than subcutaneous fat [71].

Insulin resistance is the other central component of the metabolic syndrome and is associated with shortened lifespan and reduced quality of life [8]. Insulin resistance is associated with obesity, particularly abdominal obesity, and with low serum testosterone concentrations [64,65]. Although testosterone replacement should theoretically decrease insulin resistance by increasing muscle and decreasing (abdominal) fat, interventional studies suggest otherwise (Table 1) [72–77]. Mainly equivocal effects of androgen supplementation on insulin sensitivity have been reported in a wide range of men with or without reproductive disorders (see Table 1). This could be explained by other counteracting effects of testosterone. For example, adiponectin, a fat-secreted hormone, is normally observed with favorable changes in body composition and has beneficial systemic effects, such as improved insulin sensitivity [78]. However, testosterone therapy seems to decrease serum adiponectin concentrations [79,80].

Obstructive sleep apnea

OSA affects approximately 25% of middle-aged men [81]. It is characterized by repeated episodes of nocturnal upper airway occlusion leading to hypoxemia and is commonly associated with sleep fragmentation and loss of normal sleep architecture [82]. Sleepiness, attention deficit, and neurocognitive impairment cumulatively increase accident risk [83,84]. Independent of obesity, men who have OSA have proportionally greater all-cause mortality and stroke [85], cardiovascular mortality [86], hypertension and arrhythmia [87], diabetes mellitus [88], visceral abdominal fat, and insulin resistance [89–93]. These manifestations occur largely due to apnea-associated sleep fragmentation and intermittent hypoxemia, both of which are prevented with the standard therapy, nasal continuous positive airflow pressure (CPAP). This treatment delivers pressurized air to the nose via a nose mask, thereby splinting open the upper airway during sleep and re-establishing normal breathing and sleep patterns.

The male preponderance of OSA provides preliminary evidence that gonadal function is related. This rationale is strengthened by its association with obesity, decreased blood testosterone concentrations, metabolic

Table 1
Effect of androgenic supplementation on insulin sensitivity in men

Study	Subjects	Androgen	No	RCT	Effect
Non-intramuscular					
Liu, 2003 [72]	Normal	Subcutaneous r-hCG	30	+	0
Marin, 1993 [70]	Centrally obese	Transdermal T or DHT	27	+	+ or 0
Marin, 1992 [51]	Centrally obese	Oral T	25	+	+
Intramuscular					
Singh, 2002 [73]	Normal	T	61	+	0
Lovejoy, 1995 [54]	Centrally obese	Oral oxandrolone then intramuscular nandrolone, or intramuscular T	30	–	0 or 0
Hobbs, 1996 [74]	Normal	T or nandrolone	11	–	0 or ±
Saad, 2001 [75]	Pubertal delay	DHT	10	–	0
Arslanian, 1997 [76]	Pubertal delay	T	7	–	0
Tripathy, 1998 [77]	Gonadotropin deficient	T	10	–	0

Abbreviations: DHT, dihydrotestosterone; RCT, randomized, placebo-controlled trial; r-hCG, recombinant human chorionic gonadotropin; T, testosterone; 0, no significant change; ±, equivocal change.

Data from Liu PY, Swerdloff RS, Veldhuis JD. Clinical review 171: the rationale, efficacy and safety of androgen therapy in older men: future research and current practice recommendations. J Clin Endocrinol Metab 2004;89:4789–96.

syndrome, and cardiovascular disease. Men who have OSA have suppressed pituitary-gonadal function; this may be due to recurrent hypoxia, sympathetic overstimulation, or other mechanisms. Low systemic testosterone concentrations in such men (and its reversibility with nasal CPAP therapy) have been long recognized [94] and more recently confirmed in other cohorts [95,96] and by multiple overnight blood sampling of leuteinizing hormone and testosterone concentrations [97]. These studies also implicate the degree of hypoxia and disordered breathing independently of increasing age or obesity in the pathogenesis of pituitary–gonadal dysfunction. The direction of this association and its reversibility have recently been examined for the first time in a randomized sham CPAP, placebo-controlled study of 101 men [96]. Total testosterone and leuteinizing hormone significantly fell in men who had moderate OSA randomized to receive 1 month of subtherapeutic nasal CPAP but did not change in the adequately treated men. Although significant between-group increases in total testosterone and SHBG were seen, the modest changes observed contrast with those found in the earlier, less well controlled report [94] and may be explained by shorter duration of treatment and less severe baseline disease. Nevertheless, the fact that these large studies [94,96] show reversal of OSA-associated hypogonadism with CPAP is consistent with similar trends observed in smaller studies [98,99].

Increased visceral abdominal fat and decreased insulin sensitivity commonly occur together, possibly because visceral abdominal fat strongly determines lipid supply to liver and muscle. Increased intrahepatic and intramyocellular lipid causes insulin resistance [100]. Insulin resistance and diabetes mellitus are associated with OSA in large, population–based, epidemiologic studies [88,89]. Mechanistically, impaired glucose tolerance follows recurrent hypoxia [101]. On one hand, insulin resistance may be related to alterations in autonomic (sympathetic overactivity indicated by increased blood catecholamines) and neuroendocrine function induced by recurrent hypoxemia and sleep fragmentation. On the other hand, excessive release of inflammatory cytokines and adipokines may be responsible [89,102–104]. For these reasons, OSA most likely causes insulin resistance, although few studies have examined whether reversal of sleep-disordered breathing with CPAP can improve insulin sensitivity. Controlled trials (using a no-treatment control group) are not available, and only two studies adequately measured insulin sensitivity by gold standard methods (such as hyperinsulinemic euglycemic clamp or minimal model analysis) [89]. These two uncontrolled studies showed that CPAP improved insulin sensitivity in men with [105] or without diabetes mellitus [106]. In 40 men who had at least moderate OSA (apnea-hypopnea index greater than 20 events/h) without diabetes mellitus, CPAP improved insulin sensitivity (5.75 $\pm$ 4.2 baseline versus 6.79 $\pm$ 4.91 μmol/kg/min; $P = .003$) within 2 days, and this improvement was sustained for 3 months [106]. The rapid improvement in insulin sensitivity was much greater in non-obese men. These data implicate recurrent OSA in the pathogenesis of insulin resistance, which is one of the core components of the metabolic syndrome. Potential mediators involved in this relationship include altered adrenergic function, direct effect of hypoxemia on glucose regulation, and release of proinflammatory cytokines that alter metabolism [89].

Only two longitudinal (uncontrolled) studies have examined the effect of CPAP therapy on visceral abdominal fat in men who have severe OSA [107,108]. In the earlier study of 22 men [107], visceral abdominal fat area decreased by 50 cm^2 after 6 months of CPAP irrespective of any change in total body weight. In a more recent study of 29 men [108], at least 3 months of CPAP decreased visceral abdominal fat by 8% in 19 post-hoc classified regular CPAP users. Randomized, sham-controlled, CPAP-controlled trials are not available but are needed to properly address this question.

The interrelationships among testosterone, obesity, and obstructive sleep apnea

The preceding discussion strongly implicates an interdependence among gonadal function, obesity, and OSA. We propose that low blood testosterone, obesity, and OSA are linked in men by two interrelated cycles (Fig. 1), in which depressed testosterone plays a central role. Decreased testosterone is a metabolic consequence of obesity. Men who are obese have lower serum testosterone concentrations and lower SHBG compared with age-matched, non-obese men, and this may be due to hypothalamic dysfunction [109,110] or increased testosterone metabolic clearance rate [111]. Weight loss restores systemic gonadotropin and testosterone concentrations to the reference range of healthy, young adult men [112]. Increasing obesity predicts lower future serum testosterone [113,114], possibly due to decreased lipolysis of abdominal fat [53]. In a randomized, controlled study of 28 middle-aged, abdominally obese men, 9 months of testosterone therapy inhibited directly measured lipoprotein lipase activity in biopsied abdominal fat. Cross-sectional representative, population-based studies show that increasing abdominal obesity is related to decreasing serum testosterone [115,116]. Conversely, low blood testosterone concentrations predict the future development of obesity, particularly visceral obesity [63,117], and organic androgen deficiency is associated with increased fat mass [118]. Androgen therapy rapidly increases muscle and decreases fat mass in hypogonadal and eugonadal young and older men [119–122].

The apparent bidirectional relationship between low serum testosterone and visceral obesity leads to a vicious cycle whereby low testosterone concentrations contribute to visceral obesity, and visceral obesity further reduces circulating testosterone (see Fig. 1). This suggests that obesity is a state of relative androgen deficiency.

OSA is also associated with morbid obesity and androgen deficiency [94,96,97]. Adequate treatment of OSA by CPAP therapy or with surgery reverses these hormonal deficits, suggesting that OSA causes androgen

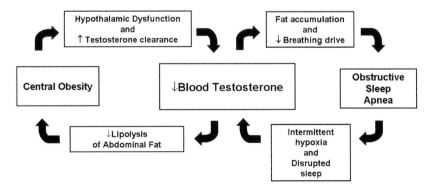

Fig. 1. The inter-relationships among low blood testosterone, obesity, and OSA.

deficiency [94,96,123]. These longitudinal data [94,123] have been verified by an aforementioned randomized, sham-controlled trial of CPAP therapy, which additionally showed a strong negative correlation between OSA severity and blood testosterone [96]. Low systemic testosterone exposure could be the consequence of severe oxygen desaturation [95] or decreased or disrupted sleep [124]. Conversely, decreased testosterone levels alter fat distribution and breathing drive, either of which could further impair sleep breathing [102,125]. Hence, we also propose that there is a vicious cycle of testosterone deficiency and sleep apnea (see Fig. 1).

We and others have shown that high–dose (two to four times the conventional dose), supraphysiologic, short-acting androgen administration acutely increases sleep apnea in a small proportion of hypogonadal and elderly men [122,126]. These systematic reports follow earlier nonrandomized case reports [127–129]. It may be that either either insufficient (by promoting fat gain) or supraphysiologically high testosterone exposure promotes sleep-disordered breathing. More physiologic, lower-dose, and near steady-state testosterone therapy has no negative effects on sleep breathing [119,130], a finding that has been supported by a recent rigorously conducted meta-analysis [131]. Three years of transdermal testosterone patch therapy titrated to maintain a young eugonadal blood testosterone concentration in 96 men over 65 years of age does not adversely affect breathing during sleep [119,132]. Disordered breathing was detected by pulse oximetry (not standard overnight laboratory polysomnography) in this study, indicating that subtle changes in sleep breathing may have been undetected. This observation is pertinent because one third of United States men in this age group will have (largely undiagnosed) OSA [133].

Summary

Impaired gonadal function, obesity, metabolic syndrome, and OSA are interlinked in men by two vicious cycles. Evolving data implicate androgen action in metabolic syndrome and disordered sleep breathing. Future studies confirming the molecular basis for these relationships are needed. Such data have implications for the efficacy and safety of androgen therapy in other populations, such as older men who have relative age-associated androgen deficiency [121].

References

[1] Dal Grande E, Gill T, Taylor AW, et al. Obesity in South Australian adults: prevalence, projections and generational assessment over 13 years. Aust N Z J Public Health 2005; 29(4):343–8.
[2] Haslam DW, James WP. Obesity. Lancet 2005;366(9492):1197–209.
[3] Villareal DT, Apovian CM, Kushner RF, et al. Obesity in older adults: technical review and position statement of the American Society for Nutrition and NAASO, The Obesity Society. Obes Res 2005;13(11):1849–63.

[4] WHO. Obesity: preventing and managing the global epidemic. vol. 1. Geneva (Switzerland): WHO; 2000.

[5] Kuczmarski RJ, Flegal KM, Campbell SM, et al. Increasing prevalence of overweight among US adults. The National Health and Nutrition Examination Surveys, 1960 to 1991. JAMA 1994;272(3):205–11.

[6] Ford ES, Giles WH, Dietz WH. Prevalence of the metabolic syndrome among US adults: findings from the third National Health and Nutrition Examination Survey. JAMA 2002; 287(3):356–9.

[7] Hedley AA, Ogden CL, Johnson CL, et al. Prevalence of overweight and obesity among US children, adolescents, and adults, 1999–2002. JAMA 2004;291(23):2847–50.

[8] Poirier P, Giles TD, Bray GA, et al. Obesity and cardiovascular disease: pathophysiology, evaluation, and effect of weight loss: an update of the 1997 American Heart Association Scientific Statement on Obesity and Heart Disease from the Obesity Committee of the Council on Nutrition, Physical Activity, and Metabolism. Circulation 2006;113(6):898–918.

[9] Ogden CL, Carroll MD, Curtin LR, et al. Prevalence of overweight and obesity in the United States, 1999–2004. JAMA 2006;295(13):1549–55.

[10] Dunstan DW, Zimmet PZ, Welborn TA, et al. Diabesity and associated disorders in Australia 2000· the Final Report of the Australian diabetes, obesity and lifestyle study (AusDiab). Melbourne (Australia): International Diabetes Institute; 2001.

[11] Australian Institute of Health and Welfare (AIHW). Australia's welfare 2005. vol. 1. 7th edition. Canberra (Australia): Australian Institute of Health and Welfare; 2005.

[12] Armstrong T, Bauman A, Davies J. Physical activity patterns of Australian adults: results of the 1999 National Physical Activity Survey. vol. 1. 1st edition. Canberra (Australia): Australian Institute of Health and Welfare; 2000.

[13] Cook P, Rutishauser IHE, Seelig M. Comparable data on food and nutrient intake and physical measurements from the 1983, 1985 and 1995 national nutrition surveys. vol. 1. 1st edition. Canberra (Australia): Commonwealth Department of Health and Aged Care, Canberra; 2001.

[14] Hu FB, Willett WC, Li T, et al. Adiposity as compared with physical activity in predicting mortality among women. N Engl J Med 2004;351(26):2694–703.

[15] Lee I, Manson JE, Hennekens CH, et al. Body weight and mortality: a 27-year follow-up of middle-aged men. JAMA 1993;270(23):2823–8.

[16] Klein S, Burke LE, Bray GA, et al. Clinical implications of obesity with specific focus on cardiovascular disease: a statement for professionals from the American Heart Association Council on Nutrition, Physical Activity, and Metabolism: endorsed by the American College of Cardiology Foundation. Circulation 2004;110(18):2952–67.

[17] Grundy SM, Cleeman JI, Daniels SR, et al. Diagnosis and management of the metabolic syndrome: an American Heart Association/National Heart, Lung, and Blood Institute Scientific Statement. Circulation 2005;112(17):2735–52.

[18] Cassidy AE, Bielak LF, Zhou Y, et al. Progression of subclinical coronary atherosclerosis: does obesity make a difference? Circulation 2005;111(15):1877–82.

[19] Jee SH, Pastor-Barriuso R, Appel LJ, et al. Body mass index and incident ischemic heart disease in South Korean men and women. Am J Epidemiol 2005;162(1):42–8.

[20] Solomon CG, Manson JE. Obesity and mortality: a review of the epidemiologic data. Am J Clin Nutr 1997;66(Suppl 4):1044S–50S.

[21] Grunstein RR, Stenlof K, Hedner J, et al. Impact of obstructive sleep apnea and sleepiness on metabolic and cardiovascular risk factors in the Swedish Obese Subjects (SOS) Study. Int J Obes Relat Metab Disord 1995;19(6):410–8.

[22] NHMRC expert panel on the prevention of obesity and overweight. Acting on Australia's weight: a strategic plan for the prevention of overweight and obesity. vol. 1. Canberra (Australia): Australian Government Publishing Service; 1997.

[23] WHO, IASO, IOTF. The Asia-Pacific perspective: redefining obesity and its treatment. vol. 1. Melbourne (Australia): Health Communications, Australia Pty Ltd; 2000.

[24] WHO. Global strategy on diet, physical activity and health [resolution WHA57.17]. vol. 1. Geneva (Switzerland): WHO; 2004.

[25] Villanova N, Pasqui F, Burzacchini S, et al. A physical activity program to reinforce weight maintenance following a behavior program in overweight/obese subjects. Int J Obes (Lond) 2005;30(4):697–703.

[26] Knowler WC, Barrett-Connor E, Fowler SE, et al. Reduction in the incidence of type 2 diabetes with lifestyle intervention or metformin. N Engl J Med 2002;346(6):393–403.

[27] Pi-Sunyer FX, Aronne LJ, Heshmati HM, et al. Effect of rimonabant, a cannabinoid-1 receptor blocker, on weight and cardiometabolic risk factors in overweight or obese patients: RIO-North America: a randomized controlled trial. JAMA 2006;295(7): 761–75.

[28] Despres JP, Golay A, Sjostrom L. Effects of rimonabant on metabolic risk factors in overweight patients with dyslipidemia. N Engl J Med 2005;353(20):2121–34.

[29] Van Gaal LF, Rissanen AM, Scheen AJ, et al. Effects of the cannabinoid-1 receptor blocker rimonabant on weight reduction and cardiovascular risk factors in overweight patients: 1-year experience from the RIO-Europe study. Lancet 2005;365(9468):1389–97.

[30] Li Z, Maglione M, Tu W, et al. Meta-analysis: pharmacologic treatment of obesity. Ann Intern Med 2005;142(7):532–46.

[31] Maggard MA, Shugarman LR, Suttorp M, et al. Meta-analysis: surgical treatment of obesity. Ann Intern Med 2005;142(7):547–59.

[32] Flier JS. Obesity wars: molecular progress confronts an expanding epidemic. Cell 2004; 116(2):337–50.

[33] Pagotto U, Marsicano G, Cota D, et al. The emerging role of the endocannabinoid system in endocrine regulation and energy balance. Endocr Rev 2006;27(1):73–100.

[34] Barash IA, Cheung CC, Weigle DS, et al. Leptin is a metabolic signal to the reproductive system. Endocrinology 1996;137(7):3144–7.

[35] Novak CM, Kotz CM, Levine JA. Central orexin sensitivity, physical activity, and obesity in diet-induced obese and diet-resistant rats. Am J Physiol Endocrinol Metab 2006;290(2): E396–403.

[36] Sakurai S, Nishijima T, Takahashi S, et al. Low plasma orexin-A levels were improved by continuous positive airway pressure treatment in patients with severe obstructive sleep apnea-hypopnea syndrome. Chest 2005;127(3):731–7.

[37] O'Donnell CP, Tankersley CG, Polotsky VP, et al. Leptin, obesity, and respiratory function. Respir Physiol 2000;119(2–3):163–70.

[38] Sallmen M, Sandler DP, Hoppin JA, et al. Reduced fertility among overweight and obese men. Epidemiology 2006;17(5):520–3.

[39] Jensen TK, Andersson AM, Jorgensen N, et al. Body mass index in relation to semen quality and reproductive hormones among 1,558 Danish men. Fertil Steril 2004;82(4):863–70.

[40] Kort HI, Massey JB, Elsner CW, et al. Impact of body mass index values on sperm quantity and quality. J Androl 2006;27(3):450–2.

[41] Bacon CG, Mittleman MA, Kawachi I, et al. A prospective study of risk factors for erectile dysfunction. J Urol 2006;176(1):217–21.

[42] Esposito K, Giugliano F, Di Palo C, et al. Effect of lifestyle changes on erectile dysfunction in obese men: a randomized controlled trial. JAMA 2004;291(24):2978–84.

[43] Buchanan G, Yang M, Cheong A, et al. Structural and functional consequences of glutamine tract variation in the androgen receptor. Hum Mol Genet 2004;13(16): 1677–92.

[44] Callewaert L, Christiaens V, Haelens A, et al. Implications of a polyglutamine tract in the function of the human androgen receptor. Biochem Biophys Res Commun 2003;306(1): 46–52.

[45] Beilin J, Ball EM, Favaloro JM, et al. Effect of the androgen receptor CAG repeat polymorphism on transcriptional activity: specificity in prostate and non-prostate cell lines. J Mol Endocrinol 2000;25(1):85–96.

[46] Knoke I, Allera A, Wieacker P. Significance of the CAG repeat length in the androgen receptor gene (AR) for the transactivation function of an M780I mutant AR. Hum Genet
1999;104(3):257–61.

[47] Chamberlain NL, Driver ED, Miesfeld RL. The length and location of CAG trinucleotide
repeats in the androgen receptor N-terminal domain affect transactivation function.
Nucleic Acids Res 1994;22(15):3181–6.

[48] Mhatre AN, Trifiro MA, Kaufman M, et al. Reduced transcriptional regulatory compe-
tence of the androgen receptor in X-linked spinal and bulbar muscular atrophy. Nat Genet
1993;5(2):184–8.

[49] Gustafson DR, Wen MJ, Koppanati BM. Androgen receptor gene repeats and indices of
obesity in older adults. Int J Obes Relat Metab Disord 2003;27(1):75–81.

[50] Fischer ME, Vitek ME, Hedeker D, et al. A twin study of erectile dysfunction. Arch Intern
Med 2004;164(2):165–8.

[51] Marin P, Holmang S, Jonsson L, et al. The effects of testosterone treatment on body composition and metabolism in middle-aged obese men. Int J Obes Relat Metab Disord 1992;
16(12):991–7.

[52] Marin P. Testosterone and regional fat distribution. Obes Res 1995;3(Suppl 4):609S–12S.

[53] Marin P, Oden B, Bjorntorp P. Assimilation and mobilization of triglycerides in subcutaneous abdominal and femoral adipose tissue in vivo in men: effects of androgens. J Clin
Endocrinol Metab 1995;80(1):239–43.

[54] Lovejoy JC, Bray GA, Greeson CS, et al. Oral anabolic steroid treatment, but not parenteral androgen treatment, decreases abdominal fat in obese, older men. Int J Obes Relat
Metab Disord 1995;19(9):614–24.

[55] Schroeder ET, Zheng L, Ong MD, et al. Effects of androgen therapy on adipose tissue and
metabolism in older men. J Clin Endocrinol Metab 2004;89(10):4863–72.

[56] Katznelson L, Finkelstein JS, Schoenfeld DA, et al. Increase in bone density and lean body
mass during testosterone administration in men with acquired hypogonadism. J Clin Endocrinol Metab 1996;81(12):4358–65.

[57] Miles A, Rapoport L, Wardle J, et al. Using the mass-media to target obesity: an analysis of
the characteristics and reported behaviour change of participants in the BBC's 'Fighting
Fat, Fighting Fit' campaign. Health Educ Res 2001;16(3):357–72.

[58] Dalle Grave R, Calugi S, Molinari E, et al. Weight loss expectations in obese patients
and treatment attrition: an observational multicenter study. Obes Res 2005;13(11):
1961–9.

[59] Pietrobelli A, Allison DB, Heshka S, et al. Sexual dimorphism in the energy content of
weight change. Int J Obes Relat Metab Disord 2002;26(10):1339–48.

[60] Kahn R, Buse J, Ferrannini E, et al. The metabolic syndrome: time for a critical appraisal:
joint statement from the American Diabetes Association and the European Association for
the Study of Diabetes. Diabetes Care 2005;28(9):2289–304.

[61] Kupelian V, Page ST, Araujo AB, et al. Low sex hormone-binding globulin, total testosterone, and symptomatic androgen deficiency are associated with development of the metabolic syndrome in nonobese men. J Clin Endocrinol Metab 2006;91(3):843–50.

[62] Laaksonen DE, Niskanen L, Punnonen K, et al. Testosterone and sex hormone-binding
globulin predict the metabolic syndrome and diabetes in middle-aged men. Diabetes
Care 2004;27(5):1036–41.

[63] Khaw KT, Barrett-Connor E. Lower endogenous androgens predict central adiposity in
men. Ann Epidemiol 1992;2(5):675–82.

[64] Haffner SM, Shaten J, Stern MP, et al. Low levels of sex hormone-binding globulin and testosterone predict the development of non-insulin-dependent diabetes mellitus in men. Am J
Epidemiol 1996;143:889–97.

[65] Stellato RK, Feldman HA, Hamdy O, et al. Testosterone, sex hormone-binding globulin,
and the development of type 2 diabetes in middle-aged men: prospective results from the
Massachusetts male aging study. Diabetes Care 2000;23(4):490–4.

[66] Laaksonen DE, Niskanen L, Punnonen K, et al. The metabolic syndrome and smoking in relation to hypogonadism in middle-aged men: a prospective cohort study. J Clin Endocrinol Metab 2005;90(2):712–9.

[67] Yusuf S, Hawken S, Ounpuu S, et al. Obesity and the risk of myocardial infarction in 27,000 participants from 52 countries: a case-control study. Lancet 2005;366(9497):1640–9.

[68] Carr DB, Utzschneider KM, Hull RL, et al. Intra-abdominal fat is a major determinant of the National Cholesterol Education Program Adult Treatment Panel III criteria for the metabolic syndrome. Diabetes 2004;53(8):2087–94.

[69] Kuk JL, Katzmarzyk PT, Nichaman MZ, et al. Visceral fat is an independent predictor of all-cause mortality in men. Obes Res 2006;14(2):336–41.

[70] Marin P, Holmang S, Gustafsson C, et al. Androgen treatment of abdominally obese men. Obes Res 1993;1(4):245–51.

[71] Dieudonne MN, Pecquery R, Boumediene A, et al. Androgen receptors in human preadipocytes and adipocytes: regional specificities and regulation by sex steroids. Am J Physiol 1998;274(6 Pt 1):C1645–52.

[72] Liu PY, Wishart SM, Celermajer DS, et al. Do reproductive hormones modify insulin sensitivity and metabolism in older men? A randomized, placebo-controlled clinical trial of recombinant human chorionic gonadotropin. Eur J Endocrinol 2003;148(1):55–66.

[73] Singh AB, Hsia S, Alaupovic P, et al. The effects of varying doses of T on insulin sensitivity, plasma lipids, apolipoproteins, and C-reactive protein in healthy young men. J Clin Endocrinol Metab 2002;87(1):136–43.

[74] Hobbs CJ, Jones RE, Plymate SR. Nandrolone, a 19-nortestosterone, enhances insulin-independent glucose uptake in normal men. J Clin Endocrinol Metab 1996;81(4):1582–5.

[75] Saad RJ, Keenan BS, Danadian K, et al. Dihydrotestosterone treatment in adolescents with delayed puberty: does it explain insulin resistance of puberty? J Clin Endocrinol Metab 2001;86(10):4881–6.

[76] Arslanian S, Suprasongsin C. Testosterone treatment in adolescents with delayed puberty: changes in body composition, protein, fat, and glucose metabolism. J Clin Endocrinol Metab 1997;82(10):3213–20.

[77] Tripathy D, Shah P, Lakshmy R, et al. Effect of testosterone replacement on whole body glucose utilisation and other cardiovascular risk factors in males with idiopathic hypogonadotrophic hypogonadism. Horm Metab Res 1998;30(10):642–5.

[78] Yamauchi T, Kamon J, Waki H, et al. The fat-derived hormone adiponectin reverses insulin resistance associated with both lipoatrophy and obesity. Nat Med 2001;7(8):941–6.

[79] Lanfranco F, Zitzmann M, Simoni M, et al. Serum adiponectin levels in hypogonadal males: influence of testosterone replacement therapy. Clin Endocrinol (Oxf) 2004;60(4):500–7.

[80] Page ST, Herbst KL, Amory JK, et al. Testosterone administration suppresses adiponectin levels in men. J Androl 2005;26(1):85–92.

[81] Young T, Palta M, Dempsey J, et al. The occurrence of sleep-disordered breathing among middle-aged adults. N Engl J Med 1993;328(17):1230–5.

[82] Guilleminault C, Tilkian A, Dement WC. The sleep apnea syndromes. Annu Rev Med 1976;27:465–84.

[83] Teran-Santos J, Jimenez-Gomez A, Cordero-Guevara J. The association between sleep apnea and the risk of traffic accidents. Cooperative Group Burgos-Santander. N Engl J Med 1999;340(11):847–51.

[84] Gordon P, Sanders MH. Sleep.7: positive airway pressure therapy for obstructive sleep apnoea/hypopnoea syndrome. Thorax 2005;60(1):68–75.

[85] Yaggi HK, Concato J, Kernan WN, et al. Obstructive sleep apnea as a risk factor for stroke and death. N Engl J Med 2005;353(19):2034–41.

[86] Marin JM, Carrizo SJ, Vicente E, et al. Long-term cardiovascular outcomes in men with obstructive sleep apnoea-hypopnoea with or without treatment with continuous positive airway pressure: an observational study. Lancet 2005;365(9464):1046–53.

[87] Peppard PE, Young T, Palta M, et al. Prospective study of the association between sleep-disordered breathing and hypertension. N Engl J Med 2000;342(19):1378–84.

[88] Reichmuth KJ, Austin D, Skatrud JB, et al. Association of sleep apnea and type II diabetes: a population-based study. Am J Respir Crit Care Med 2005;172(12):1590–5.

[89] Punjabi NM, Polotsky VY. Disorders of glucose metabolism in sleep apnea. J Appl Physiol 2005;99(5):1998–2007.

[90] Patel SR, White DP, Malhotra A, et al. Continuous positive airway pressure therapy for treating sleepiness in a diverse population with obstructive sleep apnea: results of a meta-analysis. Arch Intern Med 2003;163(5):565–71.

[91] Barbe F, Mayoralas LR, Duran J, et al. Treatment with continuous positive airway pressure is not effective in patients with sleep apnea but no daytime sleepiness: a randomized, controlled trial. Ann Intern Med 2001;134(11):1015–23.

[92] Marshall NS, Neill AM, Campbell AJ, et al. Randomised controlled crossover trial of humidified continuous positive airway pressure in mild obstructive sleep apnoea. Thorax 2005;60(5):427–32.

[93] Grunstein RR. Metabolic aspects of sleep apnea. Sleep 1996;19(Suppl 10):S218–20.

[94] Grunstein RR, Handelsman DJ, Lawrence SJ, et al. Neuroendocrine dysfunction in sleep apnea: reversal by continuous positive airways pressure therapy. J Clin Endocrinol Metab 1989;68(2):352–8.

[95] Gambineri A, Pelusi C, Pasquali R. Testosterone levels in obese male patients with obstructive sleep apnea syndrome: relation to oxygen desaturation, body weight, fat distribution and the metabolic parameters. J Endocrinol Invest 2003;26(6):493–8.

[96] Meston N, Davies RJ, Mullins R, et al. Endocrine effects of nasal continuous positive airway pressure in male patients with obstructive sleep apnoea. J Intern Med 2003; 254(5):447–54.

[97] Luboshitzky R, Aviv A, Hefetz A, et al. Decreased pituitary-gonadal secretion in men with obstructive sleep apnea. J Clin Endocrinol Metab 2002;87(7):3394–8.

[98] Bratel T, Wennlund A, Carlstrom K. Pituitary reactivity, androgens and catecholamines in obstructive sleep apnoea: effects of continuous positive airway pressure treatment (CPAP). Respir Med 1999;93(1):1–7.

[99] Luboshitzky R, Lavie L, Shen-Orr Z, et al. Pituitary-gonadal function in men with obstructive sleep apnea: the effect of continuous positive airways pressure treatment. Neuroendocrinol Lett 2003;24(6):463–7.

[100] Gan SK, Kriketos AD, Poynten AM, et al. Insulin action, regional fat, and myocyte lipid: altered relationships with increased adiposity. Obes Res 2003;11(11):1295–305.

[101] Oltmanns KM, Gehring H, Rudolf S, et al. Hypoxia causes glucose intolerance in humans. Am J Respir Crit Care Med 2004;169(11):1231–7.

[102] Yee B, Liu P, Philips C, et al. Neuroendocrine changes in sleep apnea. Curr Opin Pulm Med 2004;10(6):475–81.

[103] Mills PJ, Kennedy BP, Loredo JS, et al. Effects of nasal continuous positive airway pressure and oxygen supplementation on norepinephrine kinetics and cardiovascular responses in obstructive sleep apnea. J Appl Physiol 2006;100(1):343–8.

[104] Hucking K, Hamilton-Wessler M, Ellmerer M, et al. Burst-like control of lipolysis by the sympathetic nervous system in vivo. J Clin Invest 2003;111(2):257–64.

[105] Brooks B, Cistulli PA, Borkman M, et al. Obstructive sleep apnea in obese noninsulin-dependent diabetic patients: effect of continuous positive airway pressure treatment on insulin responsiveness. J Clin Endocrinol Metab 1994;79(6):1681–5.

[106] Harsch IA, Schahin SP, Radespiel-Troger M, et al. Continuous positive airway pressure treatment rapidly improves insulin sensitivity in patients with obstructive sleep apnea syndrome. Am J Respir Crit Care Med 2004;169(2):156–62.

[107] Chin K, Shimizu K, Nakamura T, et al. Changes in intra-abdominal visceral fat and serum leptin levels in patients with obstructive sleep apnea syndrome following nasal continuous positive airway pressure therapy. Circulation 1999;100(7):706–12.

[108] Trenell MI, Ward JA, Yee BJ, et al. Influence of constant positive airway pressure therapy on lipid storage, muscle metabolism and insulin action in obese patients with severe obstructive sleep apnoea syndrome. Diabetes Obes Metab 2007, in press.

[109] Glass AR, Swerdloff RS, Bray GA, et al. Low serum testosterone and sex hormone binding globulin in massively obese men. J Clin Endocrinol Metab 1977;45:1211–9.

[110] Giagulli VA, Kaufman JM, Vermeulen A. Pathogenesis of the decreased androgen levels in obese men. J Clin Endocrinol Metab 1994;79(4):997–1000.

[111] Petra PH, Stanczyk FZ, Namkung PC, et al. Direct effect of sex-steroid binding protein (SBP) of plasma on the metabolic clearance rate of testosterone in the rhesus macaque. J Steroid Biochem 1985;22(6):739–46.

[112] Strain GW, Zumoff B, Miller LK, et al. Effect of massive weight loss on hypothalamic-pituitary-gonadal function in obese men. J Clin Endocrinol Metab 1988;66(5): 1019–23.

[113] Feldman HA, Longcope C, Derby CA, et al. Age trends in the level of serum testosterone and other hormones in middle-aged men: longitudinal results from the Massachusetts male aging study. J Clin Endocrinol Metab 2002;87(2):589–98.

[114] Gapstur SM, Gann PH, Kopp P, et al. Serum androgen concentrations in young men: a longitudinal analysis of associations with age, obesity, and race. The CARDIA male hormone study. Cancer Epidemiol Biomarkers Prev 2002;11(10 Pt 1):1041–7.

[115] Haffner SM, Karhapaa P, Mykkanen L, et al. Insulin resistance, body fat distribution, and sex hormones in men. Diabetes 1994;43(2):212–9.

[116] Svartberg J, von Muhlen D, Sundsfjord J, et al. Waist circumference and testosterone levels in community dwelling men. The Tromso study. Eur J Epidemiol 2004;19(7): 657–63.

[117] Tibblin G, Adlerberth A, Lindstedt G, et al. The pituitary-gonadal axis and health in elderly men: a study of men born in 1913. Diabetes 1996;45(11):1605–9.

[118] Mooradian AD, Morley JE, Korenman SG. Biological actions of androgens. Endocr Rev 1987;8(1):1–28.

[119] Snyder PJ, Peachey H, Hannoush P, et al. Effect of testosterone treatment on bone mineral density in men over 65 years of age. J Clin Endocrinol Metab 1999;84(6): 1966–72.

[120] Wang C, Swerdloff RS, Iranmanesh A, et al. Transdermal testosterone gel improves sexual function, mood, muscle strength, and body composition parameters in hypogonadal men. J Clin Endocrinol Metab 2000;85(8):2839–53.

[121] Liu PY, Swerdloff RS, Veldhuis JD. Clinical review 171: the rationale, efficacy and safety of androgen therapy in older men: future research and current practice recommendations. J Clin Endocrinol Metab 2004;89(10):4789–96.

[122] Liu PY, Yee BJ, Wishart SM, et al. The short-term effects of high dose testosterone on sleep, breathing and function in older men. J Clin Endocrinol Metab 2003;88(8): 3605–13.

[123] Santamaria JD, Prior JC, Fleetham JA. Reversible reproductive dysfunction in men with obstructive sleep apnea. Clin Endocrinol (Oxf) 1988;28:461–70.

[124] Axelsson J, Ingre M, Akerstedt T, et al. Effects of acutely displaced sleep on testosterone. J Clin Endocrinol Metab 2005;90(8):4530–5.

[125] White DP, Schneider BK, Santen RJ, et al. Influence of testosterone on ventilation and chemosensitivity in male subjects. J Appl Physiol 1985;59(5):1452–7.

[126] Schneider BK, Pickett CK, Zwillich CW, et al. Influence of testosterone on breathing during sleep. J Appl Physiol 1986;61:618–23.

[127] Sandblom RE, Matsumoto AM, Scoene RB, et al. Obstructive sleep apnea induced by testosterone administration. N Engl J Med 1983;308:508–10.

[128] Matsumoto A, Sandblom RE, Schoene RB, et al. Testosterone replacement in hypogonadal men: effects on obstructive sleep apnea, respiratory drives and sleep. Clin Endocrinol (Oxf) 1985;22:713–21.

[129] Millman RP, Kimmel PL, Shore ET, et al. Sleep apnea in hemodialysis patients: the lack of testosterone effect on its pathogenesis. Nephron 1985;40:407–10.

[130] Leibenluft E, Schmidt PJ, Turner EH, et al. Effects of leuprolide-induced hypogonadism and testosterone replacement on sleep, melatonin, and prolactin secretion in men. J Clin Endocrinol Metab 1997;82(10):3203–7.

[131] Calof OM, Singh AB, Lee ML, et al. Adverse events associated with testosterone replacement in middle-aged and older men: a meta-analysis of randomized, placebo-controlled trials. J Gerontol A Biol Sci Med Sci 2005;60(11):1451–7.

[132] Snyder PJ, Peachey H, Hannoush P, et al. Effect of testosterone treatment on body composition and muscle strength in men over 65 years of age. J Clin Endocrinol Metab 1999;84(8): 2647–53.

[133] Young T, Skatrud J, Peppard PE. Risk factors for obstructive sleep apnea in adults. JAMA 2004;291(16):2013–6.

ELSEVIER
SAUNDERS

Endocrinol Metab Clin N Am
36 (2007) 365–377

ENDOCRINOLOGY
AND METABOLISM
CLINICS
OF NORTH AMERICA

Why Men's Hearts Break:
Cardiovascular Effects of Sex Steroids

Brian G. Choi, MD, MBA,
Mary Ann McLaughlin, MD, MPH*

*The Zena and Michael A. Wiener Cardiovascular Institute, The Mount Sinai School
of Medicine, One Gustave L. Levy Place, Box 1030, New York, NY 10029, USA*

Coronary artery disease (CAD) has long been recognized as the leading cause of morbidity and mortality in men [1]. Since 1950, modern medical management of CAD has resulted in a 70% reduction in mortality attributable to CAD (Fig. 1) [2], largely through aggressive management of modifiable factors of cardiovascular risk: hypertension, hyperlipidemia, and smoking cessation [3]. Continued success in the battle against heart disease is mandated because, despite the successes of the past half century, CAD remains the number one killer of Americans [1]. Continuing the downward trend of cardiovascular mortality may require re-examination of the nonmodifiable factors of cardiovascular risk: age and gender [4]. Life expectancy for women exceeds that for men, and one speculated mechanism for this discrepancy has been differences in sex hormone profiles as a contributor to accelerated atherogenesis in men. Heart disease prevalence in women lags behind that in men until postmenopausal age; after that time, women outpace men (Fig. 2) [1], leading to speculation that sex hormone profile differences are contributors to risk. Evidence associates aberrant circulating androgen levels with increased risk for CAD in both genders, but the precise relation remains to be well defined [5].

Impact of hypogonadism on coronary artery disease

The Endocrine Society clinical practice guideline defines hypogonadism in men as a clinical syndrome that results from failure of the testis to produce physiologic levels of testosterone (androgen deficiency) and the normal

Drs. Choi and McLaughlin have an investigator-initiated grant from Solvay Pharmaceuticals.
* Corresponding author.
E-mail address: maryann.mclaughlin@mssm.edu (M.A. McLaughlin).

0889-8529/07/$ - see front matter © 2007 Elsevier Inc. All rights reserved.
doi:10.1016/j.ecl.2007.03.011 *endo.theclinics.com*

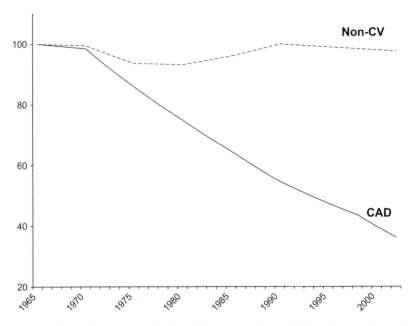

Fig. 1. Age-adjusted death rates in the United States secondary to CAD and noncardiovascular causes (Non-CV) by year, standardized to the 1965 death rate. (*Data from* National Institute of Health. Morbidity and mortality: 2004 chart book on cardiovascular, lung, and blood diseases. Bethesda (MD): US Department of Health and Human Services 2004.)

number of spermatozoa because of disruption of one or more levels of the hypothalamic-pituitary-gonadal (HPG) axis. Although no absolute cutoff value for a testosterone value was determined, the Endocrine Society acknowledged that most medical literature has used a cutoff level for total testosterone of 300 ng/dL and for free testosterone of 5 ng/dL [6]. A cutoff level of 150 ng/dL is commonly used for bioavailable testosterone (which is defined as free testosterone and weakly bound testosterone).

In male adults, levels of total testosterone decrease by approximately 0.8% per year, and because of a progressive rise in sex hormone-binding globulin (SHBG), free testosterone and bioavailable testosterone fall by almost 2% per year, respectively [7]. It is therefore not surprising that the prevalence of hypogonadism is quoted as 20% among the general population of men aged 60 to 69 years [8]. Although it is well established that sex hormone levels decrease in men as they age and hypogonadism is estimated to affect between 19% and 34% of men older than the age of 60 years, those with CAD have lower testosterone levels than age-matched men with normal coronary angiograms [9–11].

There have been eight prospective cohort or nested case-control studies examining the relation between endogenous testosterone and cardiovascular disease incidence in men [12–19], none of which has shown a clear association.

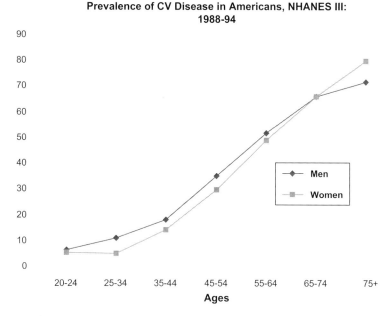

Fig. 2. Epidemiologically, according to the findings of the Third National Health and Nutrition Examination Survey, cardiovascular (CV) disease in women lags behind that in men during the premenopausal years, and then accelerates past that of men in the postmenopausal age, generating the hypothesis that estrogen is cardioprotective or androgens are deleterious. (*Data from* Thom T, Haase N, Rosamond W, et al. Heart disease and stroke statistics-2006 update: a report from the American Heart Association Statistics Committee and Stroke Statistics Subcommittee. Circulation 2006;113:e85–151.)

Previous studies on this issue have had various methodologic shortcomings, including (1) differences in the patient populations that were studied and (2) the hormonal end points that were measured. Patient populations in prospective studies have typically included many individuals with low CAD risk. Therefore, the study designs were underpowered to detect differences in low event rates. Consequently, any potential association between sex hormone levels and cardiovascular mortality was difficult to detect [15]. Moreover, older studies usually focused exclusively on total testosterone. Assessing free and bioavailable testosterone in addition to total testosterone improves accuracy in the diagnosis of hypogonadism [20,21] because their concentration also depends on SHBG, the principal binding protein for circulating testosterone and estradiol. SHBG falls dramatically as a consequence of diabetes, insulin resistance, and obesity [22]. In fact, one study showed that use of free and bioavailable testosterone as opposed to total testosterone decreased false-positive diagnoses of hypogonadism by 36% and false-negative diagnoses by 12% [23].

Estrogen exerts effects on the cardiovascular system in men. Although treatment with high doses of exogenous estradiol has deleterious effects in men, a prospective cohort study from the Framingham Heart Study examining circulating estradiol in men found that those men with the highest estradiol levels had lower risk for cardiovascular events [12]. This association with the cardioprotective effects of estrogen in men may explain a possible association between higher levels of dehydroepiandrosterone (DHEA) and its sulfate conjugate (DHEAS) and a lower incidence of cardiovascular disease. DHEA and DHEAS are weak adrenally produced androgens that may serve as prohormones for downstream estrogenic hormones in men [5,24,25]. Of six prospective cohort studies [12,26–30], one [26] suggested lower DHEAS levels in CAD survivors and two [28,30] showed a trend toward benefit with higher DHEAS. Men found to have defective mutations of estrogen synthesis or estrogen receptors have premature atherosclerosis, which may be consistent with this view that estrogens yield some cardioprotective effect in men [31,32]. Indeed, the most recent prospective cohort study suggests that higher endogenous estrogen is a better predictor of lower cardiovascular disease incidence than testosterone or DHEAS [12].

In spite of an ostensible lack of association between androgens and cardiovascular morbidity and mortality, an effect, although real, may be small and result in preclinical changes. Imaging studies suggest that male hypogonadism may be associated with increased atherosclerosis. In a cohort of Dutch men older than the age of 70 years from the town of Zoetermeer, serial carotid ultrasound revealed that low free testosterone predicted higher intima-media thickness (IMT) of the common carotid artery independent of cardiovascular risk factors [33]. In a different cohort of men aged 40 to 70 years from the Finnish town of Turku, low testosterone again predicted higher IMT independent of age, total cholesterol, body mass index (BMI), blood pressure, and smoking [34]. These findings are corroborated by a similar study of Norwegian men from the town of Tromso, in which low testosterone was associated with more atherosclerosis as assessed by IMT [35]. An explanation for the discrepancy between the cardiovascular events-based epidemiologic studies and the imaging-based ones could be that imaging is a more sensitive measure of the consequences of atherogenesis. Therefore, the disease may not penetrate adequately to increase morbidity and mortality measures, or decreased IMT secondary to high testosterone paradoxically may not result in decreased cardiovascular events by plaque destabilization.

Obesity and sex hormone profile

The connection between obesity and hypogonadism is discussed by Liu and colleagues elsewhere in this issue, but cardiovascular risk cannot be fully appreciated without examining ties to diabetes, hyperlipidemia, and obesity. In untreated hypogonadal men, a disproportional increase in BMI and total fat mass has been observed with advancing age. Administration of testosterone induces an increase in lean body mass and a decrease in fatty tissue [36]. Testosterone therapy is reported to improve insulin resistance and components of the metabolic syndrome in men with low testosterone levels [37].

Obesity is an independent risk factor for CAD as well as a contributor to insulin resistance. At the cellular level, adipocytes contain a high concentration of testosterone receptors [38]. Androgens, acting on adipocytes, stimulate lipolysis, thereby reducing fat storage [39–42]. Plasma testosterone levels show inverse correlations with lipid/lipoprotein profiles, including triglycerides, total cholesterol, and low-density lipoprotein (LDL). Testosterone levels have even stronger inverse correlations with BMI; waist circumference; waist-to-hip ratio (WHR) [43]; amount of visceral fat; and serum levels of leptin, insulin, and free fatty acids (FFAs) [44]. The visceral adipose tissue significantly influences general metabolism through the secretion of adipokines, including tumor necrosis factor (TNF)-α, resistin, interleukin (IL)-6, IL-8, acylation-stimulating protein (ASP), angiotensinogen, and plasminogen activator inhibitor-1 (PAI-1). This combined effect renders the entire body less sensitive to insulin [45], deleteriously affects endothelial function, potentiates the development of atherosclerosis [46], and, by way of inflammatory pathways, contributes to making diabetes mellitus (DM) an important risk factor for CAD.

In men, the main source of estrogen production is adipose tissue, in which a portion of testosterone is converted to estrogen by means of the enzyme cytochrome P450 aromatase [47]. The extent of this conversion seems to be governed mostly by sheer fat mass [48]. Higher serum estrogen levels, in turn, negatively feed back on the pituitary output of gonadotropins. This condition, common in men with central adiposity [49,50], is referred to as hyperestrogenic hypogonadotropic hypogonadism [23].

The hypogonadism-dependent increase in insulin resistance through weight gain and increased visceral fat has been confirmed by clinical studies [51]. In addition, low testosterone levels predict the development of the metabolic syndrome even in lean subjects [52,53]. In this hypoandrogenic population, replenishment with testosterone leads to a reduction in body weight, leptin levels, and insulin levels. Moreover, a meta-analysis of sex hormone levels and risk of DM suggests that high testosterone levels in men are associated with a 42% lower risk of DM [54]. Treatment of eugonadal obese men with testosterone decreased their visceral fat mass and, in turn, improved their insulin sensitivity and corrected dyslipidemia [55].

The metabolic effects of low testosterone levels are best illustrated in profoundly hypogonadal men. Although one small study with an experimentally induced brief episode of hypogonadism showed favorable increases in high-density lipoprotein (HDL) that dissipated with testosterone replacement [56,57], in more robust studies, men receiving therapeutic androgen ablation therapy for prostate cancer were found to have disadvantageous lipid profiles. Importantly, hypogonadism is associated with an increased incidence of hyperglycemia and type 2 diabetes mellitus (T2DM) [58–60].

Patients with Klinefelter syndrome, another group of profoundly hypogonadal patients, die from complications of DM at a rate that is almost six times that of the general population [61,62]. These findings indicate that low testosterone in men is an important contributor to the metabolic syndrome, obesity, T2DM, and dyslipidemia, all of which are risk factors for CAD.

Myocardium

Androgens at supraphysiologic doses taken by male bodybuilders have been associated with the development of left ventricular hypertrophy [63], heart failure [64] and dilated cardiomyopathy [65]. A randomized, double-blind, placebo-controlled trial of physiologic doses of transdermal testosterone in 76 men with heart failure found that men who received androgen supplementation had increased exercise capacity, however, as measured by a symptom-limited walk test and improved New York Heart Association functional class [66]. The mechanism for this improvement was unclear, because left ventricular ejection fraction was unchanged between the groups, although some experimental models suggest that exogenous testosterone decreases muscle fatigue in response to exercise by mechanisms yet to be elucidated [67,68]. Therefore, a peripheral effect of exogenous testosterone on the skeletal musculature may be the source of this benefit. Conversely, experimental animal models suggest that testosterone may be detrimental in terms of myocardial remodeling after myocardial infarction (MI). In a mouse MI model, elevated testosterone was associated with increased myocardial inflammation after ischemic injury, thereby adversely affecting myocardial healing and early remodeling [69]. Even a single dose of testosterone after ischemia-reperfusion in the isolated rat heart increased apoptosis and decreased myocardial function recovery [70]. Furthermore, blocking endogenous testosterone by castration or by flutamide injection improved myocardial recovery after ischemia-reperfusion in a similar model [71].

Testosterone and thrombosis

Prospective studies have identified various hemostatic biomarkers as increasing cardiovascular risk [72]. MI risk increases with rising plasma levels of the thrombogenic factors fibrinogen and factor VII as well as with increased plasma levels of the fibrinolysis inhibitor PAI-1 and tissue plasminogen activator (t-PA). Testosterone has been found to shift the hemostatic balance toward decreased coagulation. In a study of 32 healthy men who received supraphysiologic doses of testosterone (doubling circulating testosterone levels) as part of a contraception trial, a sustained 15% to 20% decrease in fibrinogen over 52 weeks of treatment was noted [73,74]. The antithrombotic effects were underscored by significant decreases of the procoagulatory PAI-1, protein S, and protein C as well as by increases in antithrombin III and β-thromboglobulin. This observation has not been uniformly observed, and in a study by Smith and colleagues [75], physiologic testosterone supplementation in 46 men with CAD resulted in no significant effect on fibrinogen or t-PA.

Although the aforementioned studies indicate beneficial or neutral effects of testosterone supplementation on hemostasis, the potentially detrimental effects on platelets are better understood. In a randomized, double-blind, placebo-controlled study of exogenous testosterone given to 16 healthy male volunteers, testosterone administration resulted in increased expression of platelet thromboxane-A2 receptor and significantly increased platelet aggregation response. Therefore, antiplatelet therapy, ideally with aspirin, given its anti–thromboxane-A2 effects, but also possibly with a thienopyridine, is mandatory in the patient with CAD taking exogenous testosterone.

Cardiovascular effects of exogenous testosterone

Because men with coronary heart disease (CHD) have lower serum levels of bioavailable testosterone than men of a similar age with normal coronary angiograms [10], administration of exogenous testosterone to those with CAD has been considered for treatment of CAD. Animal studies from the authors' group and others have shown that low testosterone is associated with a greater atherosclerotic burden and replacement with testosterone improves aortic atherosclerosis. This observation is only partly explained by a lipid effect [76–79]. Although the burden of atherosclerosis may be reduced with elevated testosterone, it may paradoxically result in increased cardiovascular events from increased plaque instability. In vitro data show that in macrophages derived from men, androgen treatment upregulates proatherogenic genes associated with lipoprotein processing, cell-surface adhesion, extracellular signaling, and coagulation and fibrinolysis [80]. Also, exogenous DHEA increases human macrophage foam cell formation in vitro [81], which may lead to increased vulnerability to plaque rupture if this effect exists in vivo.

Testosterone has also been shown in numerous studies to be a vasodilator. In a recent placebo-controlled trial, testosterone replacement in hypogonadal men was shown to improve time to ischemic threshold, as assessed by treadmill exercise testing at 4 and 12 weeks [82]. Prior studies had also shown a beneficial effect on exercise-induced ischemia in men with CAD but not in exclusively hypogonadal men [83–85].

Endothelial function

Decreased vascular responsiveness is an early marker of atherosclerosis, which may be the result of impaired flow-mediated nitric oxide release from endothelium muscle relaxation in response to nitric oxide. Impaired vasodilation contributes to angina and promotes coronary plaque rupture and thromboses [86,87]. In vitro and in vivo studies have found testosterone to be a coronary vasodilator [88–90].

Flow-mediated dilation, measured in the brachial artery, has been used to investigate endothelial-dependent arterial dilation. Arterial compliance, or elasticity, can be measured by pulse wave velocity (PWV). Decreased central arterial compliance worsens coronary artery perfusion and increases cardiac workload [91]. Human studies have shown that intravenous administration of testosterone to men with CAD improved endothelial function, as measured by brachial flow-mediated dilation [92].

Inflammation and coagulation

In cell culture studies, testosterone has been found to reduce the expression of proinflammatory cytokines, such as TNFα, IL-1, and IL-6, in human vascular endothelium and monocytes [93,94]. TNFα is a proinflammatory cytokine increased in inflammatory and infective states. Atherosclerosis is a disease of chronic inflammation. Serum TNFα is known to be increased during acute coronary syndromes and, to a lesser degree, in chronic angina [95]. One study in hypogonadal men determined that treatment with testosterone did reduce TNFα [96].

Recent studies have explored the impact of testosterone supplementation on cardiovascular physiology. Webb and colleagues [97] studied the effect of testosterone on exercise tolerance and showed that a single intravenous bolus of testosterone increased the time for ischemic changes to be detected by exercise tolerance test (ETT). This same group detected angiographically that injected testosterone caused increased coronary vasodilation [89]. Although these observations required pharmacologic doses of testosterone to demonstrate an effect, increases of up to 17% in coronary artery blood flow were seen even with the administration of only physiologic levels of testosterone. Rosano and colleagues [85] have also confirmed these findings by demonstrating an increase in exercise tolerance after one-time intravenous infusion of testosterone. Total exercise time on ETT rose by 16%, and time until electrocardiographic (ECG) signs of ischemia increased by 23% in men with established CAD. In a randomized, placebo-controlled, double-blind study investigating the effects of testosterone cypionate (200 mg administered intramuscularly weekly) on ETT in men (n = 25 in each group), the ischemic changes after a standard two-step exercise test (16 measurements in all) decreased by 32% and 51% from baseline after 4 and 8 weeks in the treated group compared with no change in the placebo group [84]. Similarly, in an unblinded crossover study, Wu and Weng [98] demonstrated symptomatic relief in 69% and improved resting ECG signs in 75% of 62 men with CAD who received 4 weeks of oral testosterone undecenoate. English and colleagues [83] explored the benefits of transdermally administered physiologic doses of testosterone and noted that treated patients in a 12- week, placebo-controlled, double-blind trial (n = 50) demonstrated delayed occurrence of ST segment depression on ETT. This effect was more pronounced with increased duration of the study, leading to an increase of 16% by the study's conclusion. Several reports have highlighted the clinical meaningfulness of direct and indirect effects of testosterone on the endothelium by means of inflammatory markers. Malkin and colleagues [66] noted a reduction in TNFα with testosterone supplementation in hypogonadal men with CAD. Finally, Guler and colleagues [99] showed that 3 weeks of testosterone supplementation before stent implantation led to a marked decrease in numerous inflammatory markers.

In summary, the effects of sex steroids on the cardiovascular system are complex. In addition to their direct actions, influences on lipids and on inflammatory and thrombolytic systems must be considered. Ongoing studies by the authors' group and others should further elucidate the cardiovascular effects of testosterone supplementation in men at risk for coronary events.

References

[1] Thom T, Haase N, Rosamond W, et al. Heart disease and stroke statistics—2006 update: a report from the American Heart Association Statistics Committee and Stroke Statistics Subcommittee. Circulation 2006;113:e85–151.

[2] Morbidity and mortality: 2004 chart book on cardiovascular, lung, and blood diseases. In: Bethesda (MD): National Heart, Lung, and Blood Institute; 2004.

[3] Choi BG, Vilahur G, Viles-Gonzalez JF, et al. The role of high-density lipoprotein cholesterol in atherothrombosis. Mt Sinai J Med 2006;73:690–701.

[4] Executive Summary of the Third Report of the National Cholesterol Education Program (NCEP) Expert Panel on Detection, Evaluation, and Treatment of High Blood Cholesterol in Adults (Adult Treatment Panel III). JAMA 2001;285:2486–97.

[5] Wu FC, von Eckardstein A. Androgens and coronary artery disease. Endocr Rev 2003;24: 183–217.

[6] Bhasin S, Cunningham GR, Hayes FJ, et al. Testosterone therapy in adult men with androgen deficiency syndromes: an Endocrine Society clinical practice guideline. J Clin Endocrinol Metab 2006;91(6):1049–57.

[7] Feldman HA, Longcope C, Derby CA, et al. Age trends in the level of serum testosterone and other hormones in middle-aged men: longitudinal results from the Massachusetts male aging study. J Clin Endocrinol Metab 2002;87:589–98.

[8] Cunningham GR. Testosterone replacement therapy for late-onset hypogonadism. Nat Clin Pract Urol 2006;3:260–7.

[9] Dobrzycki S, Serwatka W, Nadlewski S, et al. An assessment of correlations between endogenous sex hormone levels and the extensiveness of coronary heart disease and the ejection fraction of the left ventricle in males. J Med Invest 2003;50:162–9.

[10] English KM, Mandour O, Steeds RP, et al. Men with coronary artery disease have lower levels of androgens than men with normal coronary angiograms. Eur Heart J 2000;21:890–4.

[11] Sieminska L, Wojciechowska C, Swietochowska E, et al. Serum free testosterone in men with coronary artery atherosclerosis. Med Sci Monit 2003;9:CR162–6.

[12] Arnlov J, Pencina MJ, Amin S, et al. Endogenous sex hormones and cardiovascular disease incidence in men. Ann Intern Med 2006;145:176–84.

[13] Barrett-Connor E, Khaw KT. Endogenous sex hormones and cardiovascular disease in men. A prospective population-based study. Circulation 1988;78:539–45.

[14] Cauley JA, Gutai JP, Kuller LH, et al. Usefulness of sex steroid hormone levels in predicting coronary artery disease in men. Am J Cardiol 1987;60:771–7.

[15] Contoreggi CS, Blackman MR, Andres R, et al. Plasma levels of estradiol, testosterone, and DHEAS do not predict risk of coronary artery disease in men. J Androl 1990;11:460–70.

[16] Harman SM, Metter EJ, Tobin JD, et al. Longitudinal effects of aging on serum total and free testosterone levels in healthy men. Baltimore Longitudinal Study of Aging. J Clin Endocrinol Metab 2001;86:724–31.

[17] Hautanen A, Manttari M, Manninen V, et al. Adrenal androgens and testosterone as coronary risk factors in the Helsinki Heart Study. Atherosclerosis 1994;105:191–200.

[18] Phillips GB, Yano K, Stemmermann GN. Serum sex hormone levels and myocardial infarction in the Honolulu Heart Program. Pitfalls in prospective studies on sex hormones. J Clin Epidemiol 1988;41:1151–6.

[19] Yarnell JW, Beswick AD, Sweetnam PM, et al. Endogenous sex hormones and ischemic heart disease in men. The Caerphilly prospective study. Arterioscler Thromb 1993;13:517–20.

[20] de Ronde W, van der Schouw YT, Muller M, et al. Associations of sex-hormone-binding globulin (SHBG) with non-SHBG-bound levels of testosterone and estradiol in independently living men. J Clin Endocrinol Metab 2005;90:157–62.

[21] Rosner W. Plasma steroid-binding proteins. Endocrinol Metab Clin North Am 1991; 20:697.

[22] Lewis JG, Shand BI, Elder PA, et al. Plasma sex hormone-binding globulin rather than corticosteroid-binding globulin is a marker of insulin resistance in obese adult males. Diabetes Obes Metab 2004;6:259–70.

[23] Dhindsa S, Prabhakar S, Sethi M, et al. Frequent occurrence of hypogonadotropic hypogonadism in type 2 diabetes. J Clin Endocrinol Metab 2004;89:5462–8.

[24] Ebeling P, Koivisto VA. Physiological importance of dehydroepiandrosterone. Lancet 1994; 343:1479–81.

[25] Hayashi T, Esaki T, Muto E, et al. Dehydroepiandrosterone retards atherosclerosis formation through its conversion to estrogen: the possible role of nitric oxide. Arterioscler Thromb Vasc Biol 2000;20:782–92.

[26] Barrett-Connor E, Goodman-Gruen D. The epidemiology of DHEAS and cardiovascular disease. Ann N Y Acad Sci 1995;774:259–70.

[27] Berr C, Lafont S, Debuire B, et al. Relationships of dehydroepiandrosterone sulfate in the elderly with functional, psychological, and mental status, and short-term mortality: a French community-based study. Proc Natl Acad Sci U S A 1996;93:13410–5.

[28] Kiechl S, Willeit J, Bonora E, et al. No association between dehydroepiandrosterone sulfate and development of atherosclerosis in a prospective population study (Bruneck Study). Arterioscler Thromb Vasc Biol 2000;20:1094–100.

[29] Tilvis RS, Kahonen M, Harkonen M. Dehydroepiandrosterone sulfate, diseases and mortality in a general aged population. Aging (Milano) 1999;11:30–4.

[30] Trivedi DP, Khaw KT. Dehydroepiandrosterone sulfate and mortality in elderly men and women. J Clin Endocrinol Metab 2001;86:4171–7.

[31] Maffei L, Murata Y, Rochira V, et al. Dysmetabolic syndrome in a man with a novel mutation of the aromatase gene: effects of testosterone, alendronate, and estradiol treatment. J Clin Endocrinol Metab 2004;89:61–70.

[32] Sudhir K, Chou TM, Messina LM, et al. Endothelial dysfunction in a man with disruptive mutation in oestrogen-receptor gene. Lancet 1997;349:1146–7.

[33] Muller M, van den Beld AW, Bots ML, et al. Endogenous sex hormones and progression of carotid atherosclerosis in elderly men. Circulation 2004;109:2074–9.

[34] Makinen J, Jarvisalo MJ, Pollanen P, et al. Increased carotid atherosclerosis in andropausal middle-aged men. J Am Coll Cardiol 2005;45:1603–8.

[35] Svartberg J, von Muhlen D, Mathiesen E, et al. Low testosterone levels are associated with carotid atherosclerosis in men. J Intern Med 2006;259:576–82.

[36] Rolf C, von Eckardstein S, Koken U, et al. Testosterone substitution of hypogonadal men prevents the age-dependent increases in body mass index, body fat and leptin seen in healthy ageing men: results of a cross-sectional study. Eur J Endocrinol 2002;146:505–11.

[37] Simon D, Charles MA, Lahlou N, et al. Androgen therapy improves insulin sensitivity and decreases leptin level in healthy adult men with low plasma total testosterone: a 3-month randomized placebo-controlled trial. Diabetes Care 2001;24:2149–51.

[38] Pedersen SB. Studies on receptors and actions of steroid hormones in adipose tissue. Dan Med Bull 2005;52:258.

[39] Marin P, Arver S. Androgens and abdominal obesity. Baillieres Clin Endocrinol Metab 1998;12:441–51.

[40] Marin P, Lonn L, Andersson B, et al. Assimilation of triglycerides in subcutaneous and intraabdominal adipose tissues in vivo in men: effects of testosterone. J Clin Endocrinol Metab 1996;81:1018–22.

[41] Marin P, Oden B, Bjorntorp P. Assimilation and mobilization of triglycerides in subcutaneous abdominal and femoral adipose tissue in vivo in men: effects of androgens. J Clin Endocrinol Metab 1995;80:239–43.

[42] Rebuffe-Scrive M, Marin P, Bjorntorp P. Effect of testosterone on abdominal adipose tissue in men. Int J Obes 1991;15:791–5.

[43] Svartberg J, von Muhlen D, Sundsfjord J, et al. Waist circumference and testosterone levels in community dwelling men. The Tromso Study. Eur J Epidemiol 2004;19:657–63.

[44] Dunajska K, Milewicz A, Szymczak J, et al. Evaluation of sex hormone levels and some metabolic factors in men with coronary atherosclerosis. Aging Male 2004;7:197–204.

[45] Rondinone CM. Adipocyte-derived hormones, cytokines, and mediators. Endocrine 2006; 29:81–90.

[46] Murdolo G, Smith U. The dysregulated adipose tissue: a connecting link between insulin resistance, type 2 diabetes mellitus and atherosclerosis. Nutr Metab Cardiovasc Dis 2006; 16(Suppl 1):S35–8.

[47] Deslypere JP, Verdonck L, Vermeulen A. Fat tissue: a steroid reservoir and site of steroid metabolism. J Clin Endocrinol Metab 1985;61:564–70.

[48] Gennari L, Masi L, Merlotti D, et al. A polymorphic CYP19 TTTA repeat influences aromatase activity and estrogen levels in elderly men: effects on bone metabolism. J Clin Endocrinol Metab 2004;89:2803–10.

[49] de Boer H, Verschoor L, Ruinemans-Koerts J, et al. Letrozole normalizes serum testosterone in severely obese men with hypogonadotropic hypogonadism. Diabetes Obes Metab 2005;7: 211–5.

[50] Hayes FJ, Seminara SB, Decruz S, et al. Aromatase inhibition in the human male reveals a hypothalamic site of estrogen feedback. J Clin Endocrinol Metab 2000;85:3027–35.

[51] Svartberg J, Jenssen T, Sundsfjord J, et al. The associations of endogenous testosterone and sex hormone-binding globulin with glycosylated hemoglobin levels, in community dwelling men. The Tromso Study. Diabetes Metab 2004;30:29–34.

[52] Kupelian V, Page ST, Araujo AB, et al. Low sex hormone-binding globulin, total testosterone, and symptomatic androgen deficiency are associated with development of the metabolic syndrome in nonobese men. J Clin Endocrinol Metab 2006;91:843–50.

[53] Muller M, Grobbee DE, den Tonkelaar I, et al. Endogenous sex hormones and metabolic syndrome in aging men. J Clin Endocrinol Metab 2005;90:2618–23.

[54] Ding EL, Song Y, Malik VS, et al. Sex differences of endogenous sex hormones and risk of type 2 diabetes: a systematic review and meta-analysis. JAMA 2006;295:1288–99.

[55] Marin P, Holmang S, Jonsson L, et al. The effects of testosterone treatment on body composition and metabolism in middle-aged obese men. Int J Obes Relat Metab Disord 1992; 16:991–7.

[56] Bagatell CJ, Knopp RH, Rivier JE, et al. Physiological levels of estradiol stimulate plasma high density lipoprotein 2 cholesterol levels in normal men. J Clin Endocrinol Metab 1994; 78:855–61.

[57] Bagatell CJ, Knopp RH, Vale WW, et al. Physiologic testosterone levels in normal men suppress high-density lipoprotein cholesterol levels. Ann Intern Med 1992;116: 967–73.

[58] Basaria S, Muller DC, Carducci MA, et al. Hyperglycemia and insulin resistance in men with prostate carcinoma who receive androgen-deprivation therapy. Cancer 2006;106:581–8.

[59] Bataille V, Perret B, Evans A, et al. Sex hormone-binding globulin is a major determinant of the lipid profile: the PRIME study. Atherosclerosis 2005;179:369–73.

[60] Braga-Basaria M, Muller DC, Carducci MA, et al. Lipoprotein profile in men with prostate cancer undergoing androgen deprivation therapy. Int J Impot Res 2006;18(5):494–8.

[61] Bojesen A, Juul S, Birkebaek NH, et al. Morbidity in Klinefelter syndrome: a Danish register study based on hospital discharge diagnoses. J Clin Endocrinol Metab 2006;91: 1254–60.

[62] Swerdlow AJ, Higgins CD, Schoemaker MJ, et al. Mortality in patients with Klinefelter syndrome in Britain: a cohort study. J Clin Endocrinol Metab 2005;90:6516–22.

[63] Karila TA, Karjalainen JE, Mantysaari MJ, et al. Anabolic androgenic steroids produce dose-dependent increase in left ventricular mass in power athletes, and this effect is potentiated by concomitant use of growth hormone. Int J Sports Med 2003;24:337–43.

[64] Nieminen MS, Ramo MP, Viitasalo M, et al. Serious cardiovascular side effects of large doses of anabolic steroids in weight lifters. Eur Heart J 1996;17:1576–83.

[65] Ferrera PC, Putnam DL, Verdile VP. Anabolic steroid use as the possible precipitant of dilated cardiomyopathy. Cardiology 1997;88:218–20.

[66] Malkin CJ, Pugh PJ, West JN, et al. Testosterone therapy in men with moderate severity heart failure: a double-blind randomized placebo controlled trial. Eur Heart J 2006;27: 57–64.

[67] Tamaki T, Uchiyama S, Uchiyama Y, et al. Anabolic steroids increase exercise tolerance. Am J Physiol Endocrinol Metab 2001;280:E973–81.

[68] Van Zyl CG, Noakes TD, Lambert MI. Anabolic-androgenic steroid increases running endurance in rats. Med Sci Sports Exerc 1995;27:1385–9.

[69] Cavasin MA, Tao ZY, Yu AL, et al. Testosterone enhances early cardiac remodeling after myocardial infarction, causing rupture and degrading cardiac function. Am J Physiol Heart Circ Physiol 2006;290:H2043–50.

[70] Crisostomo PR, Wang M, Wairiuko GM, et al. Brief exposure to exogenous testosterone increases death signaling and adversely affects myocardial function after ischemia. Am J Physiol Regul Integr Comp Physiol 2006;290:R1168–74.

[71] Wang M, Tsai BM, Kher A, et al. Role of endogenous testosterone in myocardial proinflammatory and proapoptotic signaling after acute ischemia-reperfusion. Am J Physiol Heart Circ Physiol 2005;288:H221–6.

[72] Choi BG, Vilahur G, Ibanez B, et al. Measures of thrombosis and fibrinolysis. Clin Lab Med 2006;26(3):655–78.

[73] Anderson RA, Ludlam CA, Wu FC. Haemostatic effects of supraphysiological levels of testosterone in normal men. Thromb Haemost 1995;74:693–7.

[74] Andersson B, Marin P, Lissner L, et al. Testosterone concentrations in women and men with NIDDM. Diabetes Care 1994;17:405–11.

[75] Smith AM, English KM, Malkin CJ, et al. Testosterone does not adversely affect fibrinogen or tissue plasminogen activator (tPA) and plasminogen activator inhibitor-1 (PAI-1) levels in 46 men with chronic stable angina. Eur J Endocrinol 2005;152:285–91.

[76] Alexandersen P, Haarbo J, Byrjalsen I, et al. Natural androgens inhibit male atherosclerosis: a study in castrated, cholesterol-fed rabbits. Circ Res 1999;84:813–9.

[77] Arad Y, Badimon JJ, Badimon L, et al. Dehydroepiandrosterone feeding prevents aortic fatty streak formation and cholesterol accumulation in cholesterol-fed rabbit. Arteriosclerosis 1989;9:159–66.

[78] Hak AE, Witteman JC, de Jong FH, et al. Low levels of endogenous androgens increase the risk of atherosclerosis in elderly men: the Rotterdam study. J Clin Endocrinol Metab 2002; 87:3632–9.

[79] van den Beld AW, Bots ML, Janssen JA, et al. Endogenous hormones and carotid atherosclerosis in elderly men. Am J Epidemiol 2003;157:25–31.

[80] Ng MK, Quinn CM, McCrohon JA, et al. Androgens up-regulate atherosclerosis-related genes in macrophages from males but not females: molecular insights into gender differences in atherosclerosis. J Am Coll Cardiol 2003;42:1306–13.
[81] Ng MK, Nakhla S, Baoutina A, et al. Dehydroepiandrosterone, an adrenal androgen, increases human foam cell formation: a potentially pro-atherogenic effect. J Am Coll Cardiol 2003;42:1967–74.
[82] Malkin CJ, Pugh PJ, Morris PD, et al. Testosterone replacement in hypogonadal men with angina improves ischaemic threshold and quality of life. Heart 2004;90:871–6.
[83] English KM, Steeds RP, Jones TH, et al. Low-dose transdermal testosterone therapy improves angina threshold in men with chronic stable angina: a randomized, double-blind, placebo-controlled study. Circulation 2000;102:1906–11.
[84] Jaffe MD. Effect of testosterone cypionate on postexercise ST segment depression. Br Heart J 1977;39:1217–22.
[85] Rosano GM, Leonardo F, Pagnotta P, et al. Acute anti-ischemic effect of testosterone in men with coronary artery disease. Circulation 1999;99:1666–70.
[86] De Caterina R. Endothelial dysfunctions: common denominators in vascular disease. Curr Opin Lipidol 2000;11:9–23.
[87] Viles-Gonzalez JF, Choi BG, Fuster V, et al. Peroxisome proliferator-activated receptor ligands in atherosclerosis. Expert Opin Investig Drugs 2004;13:1393–403.
[88] Jones RD, Pugh PJ, Jones TH, et al. The vasodilatory action of testosterone: a potassium-channel opening or a calcium antagonistic action? Br J Pharmacol 2003;138:733–44.
[89] Webb CM, McNeill JG, Hayward CS, et al. Effects of testosterone on coronary vasomotor regulation in men with coronary heart disease. Circulation 1999;100:1690–6.
[90] Yue P, Chatterjee K, Beale C, et al. Testosterone relaxes rabbit coronary arteries and aorta. Circulation 1995;91:1154–60.
[91] Woolam GL, Schnur PL, Vallbona C, et al. The pulse wave velocity as an early indicator of atherosclerosis in diabetic subjects. Circulation 1962;25:533–9.
[92] Ong PJ, Patrizi G, Chong WC, et al. Testosterone enhances flow-mediated brachial artery reactivity in men with coronary artery disease. Am J Cardiol 2000;85:269–72.
[93] D'Agostino P, Milano S, Barbera C, et al. Sex hormones modulate inflammatory mediators produced by macrophages. Ann N Y Acad Sci 1999;876:426–39.
[94] Hatakeyama H, Nishizawa M, Nakagawa A, et al. Testosterone inhibits tumor necrosis factor-alpha-induced vascular cell adhesion molecule-1 expression in human aortic endothelial cells. FEBS Lett 2002;530:129–32.
[95] Ridker PM, Rifai N, Pfeffer M, et al. Elevation of tumor necrosis factor-alpha and increased risk of recurrent coronary events after myocardial infarction. Circulation 2000;101:2149–53.
[96] Malkin CJ, Pugh PJ, Jones RD, et al. The effect of testosterone replacement on endogenous inflammatory cytokines and lipid profiles in hypogonadal men. J Clin Endocrinol Metab 2004;89:3313–8.
[97] Webb CM, Adamson DL, de Zeigler D, et al. Effect of acute testosterone on myocardial ischemia in men with coronary artery disease. Am J Cardiol 1999;83:437–9.
[98] Wu SZ, Weng XZ. Therapeutic effects of an androgenic preparation on myocardial ischemia and cardiac function in 62 elderly male coronary heart disease patients. Chin Med J (Engl) 1993;106:415–8.
[99] Guler N, Batyraliev T, Dulger H, et al. The effects of short term (3 weeks) testosterone treatment on serum inflammatory markers in men undergoing coronary artery stenting. Int J Cardiol 2005;109(3):339–43.

ELSEVIER
SAUNDERS

Endocrinol Metab Clin N Am
36 (2007) 379–398

ENDOCRINOLOGY
AND METABOLISM
CLINICS
OF NORTH AMERICA

Androgenetic Alopecia

Nina Otberg, MD[a], Andreas M. Finner, MD[b],
Jerry Shapiro, MD, FRCPC[a],*

[a]Department of Dermatology and Skin Science, University of British Columbia,
835 West 10th Avenue, Vancouver, BC V5Z 4E8, Canada
[b]Department of Dermatology, University Clinic, Leipziger Street 44,
39120 Magdeburg, Germany

Androgenetic alopecia (AGA), or male pattern hair loss, is the most common form of alopecia in men and can be seen as a genetically determined event. The development and occurrence of AGA depends on an interaction of endocrine factors and genetic predisposition [1].

Hair plays an important role in human social and sexual communication. Men who have visible hair loss are perceived as older and less physically and socially attractive. Men who have hair loss are reported to be annoyed by the discovery of their condition and have poor self-image, a feeling of being older, and a loss of self-confidence [2–10]. Although AGA can be seen as a physiologic process, millions of dollars are spent every year on hair restoration products [7].

Egyptian papyruses from 4000 years ago report the social and psychologic importance of hair and contain recipes for different formulations for the treatment of hair loss. Aristotle (384–322 BC) recognized that baldness does not occur in eunuchs or before sexual maturity and tied libido to the degree of hair loss [7,11]. In the nineteenth century, Viennese dermatologists assumed a relationship between seborrhea, pityriasis capitis, and AGA [7,8]. Others proposed that AGA was secondary to seborrheic dermatitis due to *Pityrosporum ovale*, scalp coverage, occlusion, or cerebral congestion [9]. Finally, a lack of hair care or the presence of a toxin in the air were invoked [10].

The modern understanding of AGA started with the studies by Hamilton [11] in 1942, who established that male pattern hair loss is a physiologic process induced in genetically predisposed hair follicles under the influence of androgens. Normal levels of androgen in men are sufficient to lead to the manifestation of AGA, which is genetically determined for the individual [9].

* Corresponding author.
E-mail address: jerry.shapiro@vch.ca (J. Shapiro).

0889-8529/07/$ - see front matter © 2007 Elsevier Inc. All rights reserved.
doi:10.1016/j.ecl.2007.03.004

Clinical features and classification

The gradual replacement of strong, thick, pigmented terminal hair by fine vellus-like hair on the scalp of adult men who have AGA occurs in certain patterns. In 1951, Hamilton [12] produced the first grading scale for Caucasian men and women, ranging from type I to VIII. Type I represents the prepubertal scalp with terminal hair growth on the forehead and all over the scalp, and types VII and VIII show a confluence of the balding areas and leave hair only around the back and the sides of the head. Norwood [13] modified the classification to include variations on the middle grades: IIIa, IVa and Va show a more prominent gradual receding of the middle portion of the frontal hair line, and type III vertex is characterized by a loss of hair mainly in the tonsure area and a frontotemporal recession but never exceeds that of type III. Rook and colleagues [14] used a scale of five grades of alopecia and described different variants of balding in different ethnic groups and both genders. Class A represents the Caucasian variant with the eventual persistence of a central lock; class B describes the Asian variant of AGA, characterized by a denuding of the frontal hair line and diffuse thinning in the frontoparietal area; class C describes a mediterranean or latin variant, which corresponds to the Hamilton scale; and class D represents the female pattern with diffuse thinning and for the most part persistence of the frontal hair line.

Fig. 1 shows the Norwood-Hamilton classification. The Norwood-Hamilton-scale is used for the assessment of efficacy of drugs for hair restoration in clinical trials.

Prevalence

Estimates of the prevalence of AGA vary widely. Several authors have reported an incidence greater than 96% in Caucasian men [12,14–16]. Sixty-two percent of Caucasian men 20 to 40 years of age have bitemporal recession, and 54% of Caucasian men over 30 years of age are affected with AGA [17]. The prevalence of male pattern baldness increases with age [18]: 53% of men 40 to 49 years of age show moderate to extensive hair loss (Norwood/Hamilton type III or greater), in contrast to 16% of men 18 to 29 years of age. Hair loss classified as type III or greater is found in 42% of men 18 to 49 years of age [19]. The risk of developing AGA increases with a positive family history in the father, the mother, or the maternal grandfather [20].

Ethnic differences

Hamilton [12] found that most Chinese men retained the frontal hairline after puberty and that baldness was less common, was less extensive, and started later in life compared with Caucasians. Japanese men develop male pattern hair loss approximately 10 years later in life and have a 1.4 times

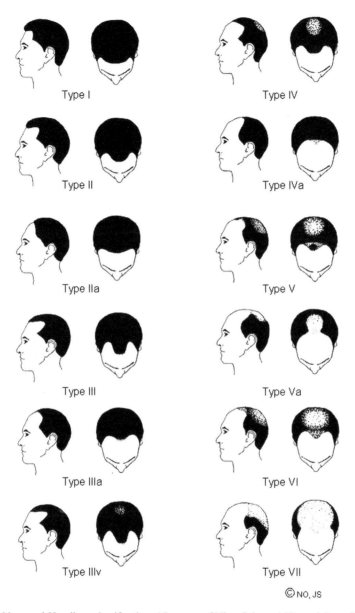

Fig. 1. Norwood-Hamilton classification. (*Courtesy of* Nina Otberg, MD, and Jerry Shapiro, MD, Vancouver, British Columbia, Canada.)

lower incidence in each decade compared with Caucasians [21]. Other researchers found a prevalence of 87% in the East Indian population, 61% in the Chinese population [22], 14.1% in Korean men [23], and 38.5% of male pattern hair loss type III or higher in Thailand [24]. AGA is four times less frequent in men of African origin than in Caucasians [25].

Diagnostics

The diagnosis of AGA in men is usually not difficult. The hair loss in AGA is nonscarring and shows a preservation of the follicular ostia. It is characterized by its special pattern; by a variation in hair shaft diameter; and by the occurrence of miniaturized, vellus-like hairs that sometimes can be seen only with a magnifier or a dermatoscope.

Basic qualitative tests, such as the hair pull test, contrast paper, and dermoscopy, can easily be used as a tool during a hair consultation. A hair pull test, which is usually used as a quick assessment of the activity of the hair loss, is usually negative [26]. The pull test can be positive in an active stage of AGA with a high telogen count in the involved area. To perform a hair pull test, the investigator grasps around 50 to 60 hairs between the thumb, the index, and the middle fingers close to the skin surface. The hairs are gently but firmly pulled from proximal to distal ends. If three or more hairs can be pulled out, the test is considered positive. The presence of variation in hair shaft diameter and miniaturized hair can be seen with a contrast paper placed in a parted area of the scalp. The hair can closely be examined against this backdrop [26]. Dermoscopic examination of the scalp skin helps to identify the presence of follicular ostia and the occurance of miniaturized hair. To monitor AGA in men, standardized overview photos are helpful as a qualitative assessment of the progression of the hair loss and as therapy control.

For routine diagnostics, a scalp biopsy is usually not necessary. A scalp biopsy allows a definitive diagnosis because it provides information on histologic features, the number of terminal and vellus hairs per area, and the number of anagen and telogen hairs. The scalp biopsy is an invasive method and leaves a small scar on the scalp of the patient.

For accurate therapy monitoring, it is reasonable to use quantitative tests such as trichogram and trichoscan. The trichogram, or classical hair-root examination, is a semi-invasive, standardized, light-microscopic technique. It involves the plucking of approximately 50 hairs. The hairs are placed on a glass slide, and the morphologic features of each individual root are examined with light microscopy. This technique allows the calculation of an exact ratio of growing (anagen) and resting (telogen) hair and hair at the regression phase (catagen). Toxically damaged hair (dystrophic hair) can be identified. The latter develops as a consequence of a disruption of the hair growth phase after infections, after organic diseases, or from different drugs. Usually the hairs are pulled out next to each other. As a result, the plucked scalp area is barely visible, and the plucking is less painful. The disadvantage of this technique is that a hair count is not possible. A hair count of terminal hair is possible only if the hairs are epilated in a predefined circle area. This technique is more painful and leaves the patient with a bald area for a couple of weeks. A vellus hair count is not possible with the trichogram technique.

The trichoscan is a modification of the classical trichogram and a photo-trichogram. It is a noninvasive, photographic method whereby the density of terminal and vellus hair and the ratio of growing to nongrowing hair on the scalp of the patient can be evaluated [27]. For the trichoscan, the hair in a circle area of 1.8 cm in diameter is clipped to a defined length and dyed black. Digital images are taken, and a software-program calculates the density of terminal and vellus hair. The technique is applicable only for patients who have light skin types (I–III). Laboratory work-up is usually not necessary unless there is concomitant diffuse hair loss [27]. Every patient who has AGA should be asked about the intake of anabolic steroids. An excellent overview on alopecia related to other etiologies and its differential diagnosis is given by Springer and colleagues [28].

Histology

Cross sections of 4-mm punch biopsies are considered to be one the most useful techniques for studying the pathologic features of AGA [29]. The main histologic characteristic of AGA is the miniaturization of terminal hair follicles and their transformation to vellus-like follicles. The number of hair follicles per area remains the same. Hair with various bulb depths and shaft diameters can be found in skin sections. The anagen phase becomes shorter, and a higher telogen count can be found in the balding scalp because the telogen phase of the hair cycle is prolonged in the miniaturization process of the hair follicles. With further progression of hair loss, the fraction of terminal hair decreases. The earliest histologic change is a nonspecific focal perivascular basophilic degeneration in the lower third of the connective tissue sheath of otherwise normal anagen follicles. This is followed by a perifollicular lymphocytic infiltrate at the level of the sebaceous duct. Multinucleated giant cells may occur with this condition [30]. The basophilic sclerotic remains of the connective tissue sheath of the formerly deep-seated terminal hair follicle are found below miniaturized follicles [9]. They are also referred to as fibrotic streamers and are always present in miniaturized follicles. Sebaceous glands persist even when the hair is greatly miniaturized or can even be enlarged [31].

Pathogenesis

Changes in hair cycle in androgenetic alopecia

The progression of patterned balding in men is the result of a gradual transformation of pigmented, thick scalp hair (terminal hair) into fine, colorless, almost invisible vellus-like hair follicles [32]. A normal hair cycle of the scalp hair involves a long growing period (anagen) of 2 to 6 years on average, a short transitory period of approximately 2 to 3 weeks (catagen), and a resting period (telogen) of around 12 weeks [33]. A normal anagen/telogen ratio for the scalp hair is 9:1, although seasonal variations can be found [34].

In AGA, the duration of the anagen phase decreases with each passage though the hair cycle. Because the duration of the anagen phase is the main determination of hair length, the maximum length of the new anagen hair is shorter than of its predecessor [35]. The proportion of telogen hair increases, leading to thinner, finer hair with every cycle [36]. The time between shedding of the hair and anagen regrowth becomes longer, leading to a reduction of present hair on the scalp [33].

The role of androgens

Hamilton [11] observed that baldness did not develop in 10 eunuchoids, in 10 men castrated at puberty, and in 34 men castrated during adolescence. After administration of testosterone, baldness developed in predisposed individuals. When testosterone was discontinued, the baldness did not progress, although it did not reverse. Castration performed before puberty prevented the development of a beard, whereas castration performed between 16 and 20 years of age partly prevented the full development of the beard, and castration performed after 20 years of age had no effect on beard development. Neither a correlation between baldness and testosterone levels nor a correlation between libido and testosterone levels has been established [9,18].

The skin is an endocrine target tissue for androgen hormone action, similar to the ovaries, testes, and adrenal glands [37]. The circulating androgens dihydroepiandrosterone sulfate (DHEA-S) and androstenedione are produced predominantly in the adrenal glands, and testosterone and 5α-dihydrotestosterone (DHT) are synthesized mainly in the gonads [38]. DHEA-S and androstenedione have a relatively weak androgen potential. They can be metabolized to more potent androgens, such as testosterone and DHT. The androgen metabolic pathways are shown in Fig. 2.

The six enzymes involved in the androgen metabolism in the skin are steroid sulfatase, 3β-hydroxysteroid dehydrogenase/$\Delta^{5\text{-}4}$-isomerase, 17β-hydroxysteroid dehydrogenase, 5α-reductase, 3α-hydroxysteroid dehydrogenase, and aromatase [39]. Steroid sulfatase metabolizes DHEA-S to dehydroepiandrostenone, which is converted to androstenedione by Isoenzyme 1 of 3β-hydroxysteroid dehydrogenase/$\Delta^{5\text{-}4}$-isomerase [40]. Androstenedione can be activated by 17β-hydroxysteroid dehydrogenase, which is found in the outer root sheath cells, to testosterone. Anagen hair mainly expresses high levels of isotype 2, which leads to an inactivation of the potent sex steroids, whereas moderate levels of isotype 1 support the formation of active androgens [41]. 5α-reductase irreversibly converts testosterone to DHT, which is the most potent naturally occurring androgen in the skin and plays the key role in AGA [42]. In balding scalp, a predominance of

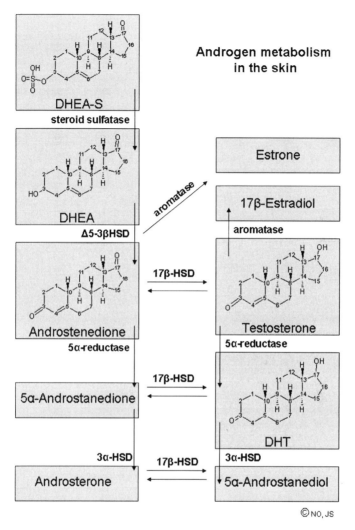

Fig. 2. Metabolism of androgens in human skin. (*Courtesy of* Nina Otberg, MD and Jerry Shapiro, MD, Vancouver, British Columbia, Canada.)

5α-reductase isotype 1 over isotype 2 can be found, whereas in the prostate, the two enzymes have been found to be present in equal proportions [43]. 3α-Hydroxysteroid dehydrogenase inactivates androgens [38]. Finally, aromatase can convert testosterone and androstenedione to estradiol and estrone [39]. Aromatase concentration is five times higher in female scalp skin compared with male scalp skin and may bring about the differences in male and female patterns of balding.

All enzymes can be localized in the sebaceous glands and different parts of the hair follicle of scalp skin. Therefore, the pilosebaceous unit has the potential to mediate androgen action without relying on elevated systemic levels or on the production of testosterone or DHT [44].

Androgen activation and deactivation are mainly intercellular events mediated by binding to a single nuclear receptor. The androgen receptor, as a polymeric complex that includes the heat-shock proteins (hsp) hsp90, hsp70, and hsp56, is initially located in the cytoplasm [38].

Complex enzyme mechanisms, such as phosphorylation and sulfhydryl reduction of the androgen receptor, are necessary for the activation of the ligand-receptor complex [45]. The androgen–androgen receptor complex is transported into the nucleus and ligates to promoter DNA sequences of androgen-regulated genes [38]. The resulting signaling cascade can lead to inhibition or stimulation of messenger proteins or receptors. These messengers alter cellular processes, mediating hair growth or miniaturization [46]. In vitro, testosterone and DHT induce apoptosis in dermal papilla cells in a dose-dependent and time-related manner [47,48]. Androgen-dependent hair follicles release insulin-like growth factor (IGF)-1 after stimulation with testosterone, and IGF-1 induces 5α-reductase [49].

Genetics

The development of AGA shows a strong genetic involvement. The risk of MPHL increases significantly with a positive family history [20]. The occurrence of ethnic difference supports the importance of genes in male pattern hair loss. The nature of inheritance remains unclear. Autosomal-dominant inheritance and a link to polycystic ovary syndrome through the variation of the CYP17 gene on chromosome 10q24.3 have been suggested [50,51]. Other researchers feel that a polygenic inheritance of the trait is far more likely [52].

The observation that patients who have pseudohermaphroditism due to 5α-reductase-2 deficiency do not develop male pattern hair loss suggests an involvement of the genes SRD5A1 on chromosome 5 and SRD5A2 on chromosome 2. No association of the 5α-reductase isoenzymes with male pattern baldness has been established [53,54].

The expression of IGF-1 in the dermal papilla is thought to play an important role in the development of patterned balding. Older men who have vertex balding show higher plasma levels of IGF-1 and lower circulating levels of IGF binding protein 3. A decreased expression of IGF-1 was found in the balding scalp tissue [55,56]. The hairless gene on chromosome 8 is not involved in the development of male pattern baldness [57].

Garton and colleagues [58] reported a possible association of a polymorphism in the gene for ornithine decarboxylase, a regulatory enzyme in the polyamine biosynthesis known to play an important role in the regulation of the hair cycle. In humans, there are two functionally distinct alleles of ornithine decarboxylase. The authors found a common occurrence of the major and weaker allele in balding men and suggested that this polymorphism might be associated with AGA.

Other researchers have developed the hypothesis that a deficiency of steroid sulfatase, which leads to X-linked recessive ichthyosis, precludes the development of AGA [59]. Steroid sulfatase plays an important role in androgen metabolism. Trüeb and Meyer [60] found that AGA occurs as often in patients who have X-linked recessive ichthyosis as in the normal population.

There are two pathways for the steroid biosynthesis. The Delta5 pathway depends on steroid sulfate activity, whereas the Delta4 pathway does not and therefore can produce androgenetic alopecia in men who have X-linked recessive ichthyosis [61].

An X-linked adrenoleukodystrophy mutation has been discussed as a gene locus within the polygenic spectrum of genes responsible for AGA [62]. This X-chromosomal involvement in the development of AGA stresses the importance of the maternal line in the inheritance.

A polymorphism in the androgen receptor gene (q12 in the X chromosome) may be responsible for the development and extent of AGA. A higher expression of the androgen receptor gene was found in balding scalp [63]. A functional mutation in or near the androgen receptor may explain these higher levels of gene expression in balding scalp [64]. A significant correlation exists between the A allele and protection against AGA [65], and genetic variability in the androgen receptor gene is the cardinal prerequisite for the development of early-onset AGA [66].

Risk factors and associations with other diseases

Early-onset vertex balding seems to be a marker for early-onset coronary heart disease, especially in young men who have hypertension or dyslipidemia [67–69]. Men 19 to 50 years of age who have early AGA (occurring before 35 years of age) have an increased incidence of hyperinsulinemia and disorders associated with insulin resistance, such as obesity, hypertension, and dyslipidemia [70].

The incidence of prostate cancer is greater in men who have male pattern baldness [71], particularly of the vertex [49]. The pathophysiology of these findings is unknown. Further studies are necessary to investigate the role of shared androgen pathways in coronary heart disease, insulin-resistance, and prostate cancer.

Treatment

AGA is a progressive condition with a decrease in hair density of approximately 6% of hair fiber per year [36]. Increased shedding can occur periodically, and the extent of hair loss depends on the genetic predisposition. Two pharmaceutical treatments have been approved for the therapy of AGA in men: oral finasteride and topical minoxidil.

Finasteride

Finasteride is a synthetic azo-steroid that has been used for the treatment of AGA in men since 1997. It is a potent and highly sensitive selective 5α-reductase type-2 inhibitor [72]. It binds irreversibly to the 5α-reductase isoenzyme 2 and inhibits the conversion of testosterone to DHT. Finasteride has a pharmacologic half-life of around 8 hours. Finasteride (1 mg/d) reduces the concentration of DHT in scalp and serum by over 60% [72]. The dose-response curve is nonlinear; higher doses do not lead to significantly increased suppression of DHT or greater clinical benefits [73]. Hair count increased significantly in patients who have vertex alopecia or frontal AGA in several randomized controlled trials [74,75]. From these studies, it can be concluded that finasteride can stabilize hair loss in 80% of patients who have vertex hair loss and in 70% of patients who have frontal hair loss. The chance of mild to moderate regrowth is 61% on the vertex and 37% on the frontal scalp [76]. After 24 months of continuous use, 66% of the patients experienced a certain amount (approximately 10%–25% of the hair the patient lost previously) of hair regrowth in the vertex area [77]. Most of the patients had no further hair loss. Continued use beyond 2 years does not seem to promote continued hair regrowth. Instead, the hair density stabilizes with the retention of the newly acquired hair [78]. If successful, the treatment should be continued indefinitely because the balding process continues once treatment ceases [35]. Side effects are rare and include decreased libido in 1.8% of the recipients versus 1.3% in the placebo group, erectile dysfunction in 1.3% of the recipients versus 0.7% in the placebo group, and decreased ejaculate volume in 0.8% of patients versus 0.4% in the placebo group [79,80]. Finasteride (1 mg/d) does not affect spermatogenesis or semen production in men 19 to 41 years of age [81]. Prostate volume and prostate-specific antigen (PSA) are barely affected in younger men [81], but finasteride can decrease PSA levels by 50% in older men [82]. Therefore, a baseline PSA should be obtained in men over 40 years of age, and screening cutoff values for these patients need to be adjusted [76]. No long-term side effects are known. A large randomized controlled trial over 7 years with 5 mg of finasteride showed that finasteride prevents or delays the appearance of prostate cancer in general but may slightly increase the chance of high-risk prostate cancer.

Minoxidil

Minoxidil is a biologic response modifier that has been shown to halt AGA in many patients and regrow hair to a certain extent. For men, it is used as a 2% and a 5% topical treatment in a lotion form, and, more recently, it has been used in a foam preparation. It is recommended for patients who prefer a topical treatment or who want to use it in combination with finasteride [76,83]. Minoxidil is a piperidinopyrimidine derivative originally used as an oral antihypertensive. Hypertrichosis was observed as a side effect, which led to development of a topical preparation.

The 2% and 5% solutions are available as over-the-counter medication for men. In 2006, 5% minoxidil foam was approved by the US Food and Drug Administration. The mechanism of action is not fully understood [84]. It has been shown to have a mitogenic, nonhormonal effect on epidermal cells leading to prolonged survival time [85] and has been shown to induce increased proliferation of hair follicles in vitro [86].

Action on dermal papilla blood supply by vasodilation or via vascular endothelial growth factor–induced vascularization has been suggested [87,88]. However, improved hair survival was demonstrated in the absence of blood supply [89]. Other proposed venues of action are lysine hydroxylase [90] and prostaglandin synthase [91]. A change of intracellular calcium homeostasis has been invoked because minoxidil is converted to minoxidil-sulfate [92], a potassium channel agonist. Increased potassium channel permeability leads to impaired entry of calcium into cells, thus decreasing epidermal growth factors and enhancing hair growth [93].

The efficacy of minoxidil has been shown in several clinical studies. Outcome parameters included hair counts, global photography, and hair weight. The increase in hair counts probably reflects a reversal of miniaturized hairs to thicker, visible, terminal hairs. These hairs need to grow to a certain length to lead to a visible difference. Although studies have been performed on the vertex, the drug also works on the frontal scalp, especially if hairs have not completely miniaturized to vellus-like status. In men using the 2% solution, moderate to dense regrowth can be expected in 30% to 35% of patients as assessed by hair counts and weight [94]. In a study comparing the 5% solution with the 2% solution and placebo in men, the group using the 5% solution had 45% greater hair growth and earlier onset [95]. After treatment is discontinued, hair counts soon return to baseline, or, more exactly, patients reach a stage as if they had never used the medication [96].

Side effects include contact dermatitis in 6.5% of patients and facial hypertrichosis in 3% to 5% of women [97]. Most patients do not have a true contact allergy to minoxidil, but some patients experience an irritation from propylene glycol and may benefit from using 2% lotion or other delivery methods, such as the foam. Only minimal amounts of minoxidil are systemically absorbed, and serum levels are too low to have hemodynamic effects in normotensive or hypertensive patients. Nevertheless, less than 1 in 1000 patients may experience tachycardia and decreased blood pressure. Patients who have hypotension or heart problems should therefore be cautious and should use the medication with approval from their cardiologist. Cardiac effects suggested in earlier studies could not definitively be linked to minoxidil and may be related to the aforementioned increased incidence of coronary heart disease in men who have AGA [67].

Patients should be warned about some increased shedding in the first months of treatment. This positive sign seems to indicate anagen induction with earlier "molting" of telogen hairs from the follicles.

Topical minoxidil solution is used twice daily (1 mL or 25 drops twice a day) on a dry scalp. The hair is parted five times, and five drops per part are applied directly to the fronto-parietal and vertex scalp, preferably by using a dropper. The lotion can be spread with the fingers; massage is not necessary. The patient can then apply styling products. The lotion should stay on the scalp for at least 4 hours before the next shower. Studies have shown 75% absorption during that period [98].

The patient should be informed that this is a life-long treatment. It takes 4 to 6 months before the medication takes effect, and the maximum effect can be expected after 1 year. In a 5-year follow-up study, hair counts plateaued slightly below the 1-year levels but well above baseline [99]. Patients who have terminal or moderately miniaturized hair are better treatment candidates.

Open trials indicate superior efficacy of combining finasteride and minoxidil treatment [100,101]. For patients wanting to switch from minoxidil to finasteride, a 4-month overlap is recommended to avoid hair loss before the effect of the oral treatment starts.

Hair restoration surgery

Hair restoration is the most successful and permanent treatment for AGA in suitable candidates. It includes hair transplantation (HT) and, in skillful hands, scalp reduction surgery. Suitable candidates for HT are those with reasonable expectations, a donor supply that is adequate to cosmetically improve the recipient area coverage, and those without contraindications for surgery. Other forms of hair loss (telogen effluvium, alopecia areata, or active cicatricial alopecia) and concomitant scalp conditions such as actinic keratosis should be excluded. Younger patients, especially those under 25 years of age, and those with early AGA are usually not good candidates. An exact diagnosis should be made, including the stage and progression of AGA. Obtaining a family history and using old photos may be helpful to estimate the activity of the condition. A realistic result and the difficulty of predicting the exact outcome should be discussed with the patient. Designing the hairline, assessing the donor and recipient areas, and discussing graft number and placing with the patient are major parts of the consultation. The most dramatic change in cosmetic appearance is achieved in patients who have stages Hamilton-Norwood VI and VII and in patients who have anterior accentuation of balding (subtypes IIIa and IVa).

With recent advancements in technique and combination with medical treatment, more patients may benefit from the surgical option. Larger numbers of smaller grafts are moved per session, and results have thus become natural [102,103]. It is possible and advisable to distribute small grafts in between pre-existing hairs and thus account for future hair loss. Rational use of the donor area with strip harvesting or follicular unit extraction makes several sessions possible if patients experience progressive hair loss. On the other hand, the procedure has become more complex and requires more manpower and experience, which makes it more expensive.

Up-to-date, quantitative evidence in hair restoration surgery based on randomized controlled trials is insufficient. This may be due to many reasons, such as high variation in techniques, problems in measuring hair growth, and difficult patient recruitment [104].

Surgical treatment should be combined with medical treatment in patients who have pre-existing hair in androgen-dependent areas and progressive AGA. A study comparing patients who underwent surgery with and without finasteride treatment showed better results in the combination group [105]. Minoxidil may also improve and accelerate results of the surgery [106,107].

HT is based on the principle of donor dominance as shown by androgen-independent follicles retaining their properties when they are transplanted into androgen-dependent areas. The donor supply is limited by the area of the strip (the size of the "safe zone," scalp elasticity) and the density of donor hair.

HT is an outpatient procedure and may take up to 10 hours, depending on various factors, especially the number of grafts. Tumescence anesthesia is used for the donor and recipient areas, sometimes combined with nerve blocks.

The most commonly used technique is strip harvesting. It allows for a relatively fast removal of large numbers of hairs, leaving a fine line as a scar. The strip is harvested by double-bladed knives or freehand with a scalpel, alternatively with blunt spreading instruments after a superficial incision. The scar is covered by adjacent hairs, which should be at least 1 inch in length. Thus, the patient can no longer have a short ("buzz") hair cut after the procedure.

The strip is dissected into follicular units ("families" of hairs growing together in one connective tissue sheath) under magnification. This leads to much lower transection rates and smaller grafts with less interfollicular tissue. This allows for smaller recipient sites (ie, slits or holes) and higher densities with a better chance of growth. Dissection quality and speed rely on the skills of the staff and greatly determine the result and duration of the procedure. Careful graft handling is another highly important component; the grafts must always stay wet. Cooling and special storage solutions are frequently used.

Follicular unit extraction is a recently developed technique that involves separately harvesting individual follicular units using small punches [103]. Advantages include less extensive surgery, no long scar, and less staff needed for microscopic dissection. Patients who have a low donor density or scalp elasticity may be candidates. Disadvantages are lower graft numbers, the need for several sessions, multiple fine pin-point scars, and more time and physical effort for the surgeon.

The recipient sites are made with solid-core needles or spear-like blades of various sizes and with different tips. The size, direction, and angulation of the incision should be adjusted to graft size and location. Most surgeons start with an acute frontal angle that increases when going backward on the scalp. Varying the direction of the hair (eg, coronal versus sagittal or oblique) and changing the orientation of the blade (parallel versus perpendicular) have been proposed by many researchers [108].

Creating the hairline and making the hairline incisions are the most critical and demanding parts of the procedure. The hairline should be designed according to the patient's face and following several esthetic rules. It should never be too low and is placed horizontally to the ground or slightly upward toward the fronto-temporal apex. Usually, small and fine hairs are placed in a staggered order. Most surgeons prefer a more irregular hairline with a denser packed zone immediately to the posterior.

The grafts can be spread out evenly over the recipient area or can be packed denser on the frontal part, depending on donor supply, possible subsequent sessions, and patient demands. It may be advised to leave out the vertex area and concentrate on the fronto-parietal scalp; a transition zone with smaller grafts should also be created toward the vertex. Graft placement is usually performed with jeweler's forceps. Bleeding and popping of grafts may complicate this step. The patient should be warned about risks of the surgery, the time line before regrowth (6 months or more), and the initial loss of transplanted hair and a portion of pre-existing hair in the recipient area (shock loss). Some patients may require additional sessions, but this is limited by their donor supply. In advanced stages with inadequate donor supply, a hairpiece may be the cosmetically better option. Stem-cell research holds some promise in the treatment of alopecia and may play a role in the future [109,110].

Fig. 3 shows a 36-year-old patient before and after hair transplantation. A total of 1540 grafts were transplanted to the frontal, parietal, and vertex area.

Summary

AGA, or male pattern hair loss, affects approximately 50% of the male population. AGA is an androgen-related condition in genetically predisposed individuals. DHT has been identified as the upregulated mediator, but its exact mode of action on the dermal papilla is not fully understood. Polymorphisms in the androgen receptor gene and other genes may play a role.

There is no treatment to completely reverse AGA in advanced stages, but with medical treatment (eg, finasteride, minoxidil, or a combination of

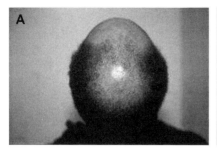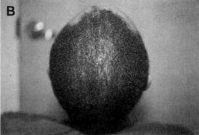

Fig. 3. Patient before (*A*) and after (*B*) transplantation of 1540 grafts.

both), the progression can be arrested and partly reversed in the majority of patients who have mild to moderate AGA. Combination with hair restoration surgery leads to the best results in suitable candidates. Physicians who specialize in male health issues should be familiar with this common condition and all the available approved treatment options.

References

[1] Hanneken S, Ritzmann S, Nothen MM, et al. Androgenetic alopecia: current aspects of a common phenotype. Hautarzt 2003;54(8):703–12.

[2] Terry RL, Davis JS. Components of facial attractiveness. Percept Mot Skills 1976;42:918.

[3] Cash TF. The psychology of hair loss and its implications for patient care. Clin Dermatol 2001;19(2):161–6.

[4] Maffei C, Fossati A, Rinaldi F, et al. Personality disorders and psychopathologic symptoms in patients with androgenetic alopecia. Arch Dermatol 1994;130(7):868–72.

[5] Wells PA, Willmoth T, Russell RJ. Does fortune favour the bald? Psychological correlates of hair loss in males. Br J Psychol 1995;86(Pt 3):337–44.

[6] David B, Himmelberger D, Rhodes T, et al. The effects of hair loss in European men: a survey in four countries. Eur J Dermatol 2000;10(2):122–7.

[7] Trüeb RM. Von der hippokratischen glatze zum gen-shampoo: fortschritte der trichologie im jahrtausendwechsel. Aktuelle Dermatologie 1998;24(4):101–7 [in German].

[8] Hebra F, Kaposi M. On diseases of the skin including the exanthemata. London: The New Sydenham Society; 1874 [Tay W, transl.].

[9] Simpson NB, Barth JH. Hair patterns: hirsuties and androgenetic alopecia: the diseases of the hair and scalp. Oxford (England): Blackwell Science; 1997. p. 95–101.

[10] Galewsky E. Trichokinesis. In: Jadassohn, editor. Erkrankungen der haare and des haarbodens, handbuch der haut-and geschlechtskrankheiten. 1st edition. Berlin: Springer-Verlag; 1932. p. 204–6.

[11] Hamilton JB. Male hormone stimulation is prerequisite and an incitant in common baldness. Am J Anat 1942;71(3):451–80.

[12] Hamilton JB. Patterned loss of hair in man: types and incidence. Ann N Y Acad Sci 1951;53(3):708–28.

[13] Norwood OT. Male pattern baldness: classification and incidence. South Med J 1975;68(11):1359–65.

[14] Rook A, Wilkinson DS, Ebling FJG. Textbook of dermatology. 2nd edition. Oxford (England): Blackwell Scientific; 1972.

[15] Dawber RPR, de Berker D, Wojnarowska F. Disorders of hair. In: Textbook of dermatology. 6th edition. London: Blackwell Science; 1998. p. 869–913.

[16] Gan DCC, Sinclair RD. Prevalence of male and female pattern hair loss in Maryborough. J Investig Dermatol Symp Proc 2005;10:184–9.

[17] Smith MA, Wells RS. Male-type alopecia, alopecia areata, and normal hair in women. Arch Dermatol 1964;89:155–8.

[18] Severi G, Sinclair R, Hopper JL, et al. Epidemiology and health services research androgenetic alopecia in men aged 40-69 years: prevalence and risk factors. Br J Dermatol 2003; 149(6):1207–13.

[19] Rhodes T, Girman CJ, Savin RC, et al. Prevalence of male pattern hair loss in 18-49 year old men. Dermatol Surg 1998;24(12):1330–2.

[20] Chumlea WC, Rhodes T, Girman CJ, et al. Family history and risk of hair loss. Dermatology 2004;209(1):33–9.

[21] Takashima I, Iju M, Sudo M. Alopecia androgenetica: its incidence in Japanese and associated conditions. Hair research: status and future aspects. New York: Springer-Verlag; 1981. p. 287–93.

[22] Tang PH, Chia HP, Cheong LL, et al. A community study of male androgenetic alopecia in Bishan, Singapore. Singapore Med J 2000;41(5):202–5.

[23] Paik JK, Yoon JB, Sim WY, et al. The prevalence and types of androgenetic alopecia in Korean men and women. Br J Dermatol 2001;145(1):95–9.

[24] Pathomvanich D, Pongratananukul S, Thienthaworn P, et al. A random study of Asian male androgenetic alopecia in Bangkok, Thailand. Dermatol Surg 2002;28(9):804–7.

[25] Setty LR. Hair patterns of scalp of white and Negro males. Am J Phys Anthropol 1970; 33(1):49–55.

[26] Shapiro J. Hair loss: principles of diagnosis and management of alopecia. 1st edition. London: Martin Dunitz; 2001.

[27] Hoffmann R. TrichoScan: combining epiluminescence microscopy with digital image analysis for the measurement of hair growth in vivo. Eur J Dermatol 2001;11(4):362–8.

[28] Springer K, Brown M, Stulberg DL. Common hair loss disorders. Am Fam Physician 2003; 68(1):93–102.

[29] Whiting DA. Diagnostic and predictive value of horizontal sections of scalp biopsy specimens in male pattern androgenetic alopecia. J Am Acad Dermatol 1993;28(5):755–63.

[30] Domnitz JM, Silvers DN. Giant cells in male pattern alopecia: a histologic marker and pathogenetic clue. J Cutan Pathol 1979;6:108–12.

[31] Kligman AM. The comparative histopathology of male-pattern baldness and senescent baldness. Clin Dermatol 1988;6(4):108–18.

[32] Camacho FM, Randall VA, Price VH. Hair and its disorders: biology, pathology and management. London: Martin Dunitz; 2000.

[33] Courtois M, Loussouarn G, Hourseau C, et al. Hair cycle and alopecia. Skin Pharmacol 1994;7(1–2):84–9.

[34] Randall VA, Ebling FJ. Seasonal changes in human hair growth. Br J Dermatol 1991; 124(2):146–51.

[35] Ellis JA, Sinclair R, Harrap SB. Androgenetic alopecia: pathogenesis and potential for therapy. Expert Rev Mol Med 2004;4(22):1–11.

[36] Rushton DH, Ramsay ID, Norris MJ, et al. Natural progression of male pattern baldness in young men. Clin Exp Dermatol 1991;16(3):188–92.

[37] Camacho F, Montagna W. Trichology: diseases of the pilosebaceus follicle. 1st edition. Madrid: Aula Medica; 1997.

[38] Zouboulis CC, Degitz K. Androgen action on human skin- from basic research to clinical significance. Exp Dermatol 2004;13(s4):5–10.

[39] Sawaya ME, Price VH. Different levels of 5 alpha-reductase Type I and II, aromatase, and androgen receptor in hair follicles of women and men with androgenetic alopecia. J Invest Dermatol 1997;109:296–300.

[40] Fritsch M, Orfanos CE, Zouboulis CC. Sebocytes are the key regulators of androgen homeostasis in human skin. J Invest Dermatol 2001;116(5):793–800.
[41] Courchay G, Boyera N, Bernard BA, et al. Messenger RNA expression of steroidogenesis enzyme subtypes in the human pilosebaceous unit. Skin Pharmacol 1996;9(3):169–76.
[42] Grino PB. Testosterone at high concentrations interacts with the human androgen receptor similarly to dihydrotestosterone. Endocrinology 1990;126(2):1165–72.
[43] Harris G, Azzolina B, Baginsky W, et al. Identification and selective inhibition of an isozyme of steroid 5 alpha-reductase in human scalp. Proc Natl Acad Sci U S A 1992; 89(22):10787–91.
[44] Sawaya ME, Hordinsky MK. Advances in alopecia areata and androgenetic alopecia. Adv Dermatol 1992;7:211–26.
[45] Cheung-Flynn J, Prapapanich V, Cox MB, et al. Physiological role for the cochaperone FKBP52 in androgen receptor signaling. Mol Endocrinol 2005;19(6):1654–66.
[46] Frieden IJ, Price VH. Androgenetic alopecia. In: Thiers BH, Dobson RL, editors. Pathogenesis of skin disease. 1st edition. New York: Churchill Livingstone; 1986. p. 41–55.
[47] Winiarska A, Mandt N, Kamp H, et al. Effect of 5alpha-dihydrotestosterone and testosterone on apoptosis in human dermal papilla cells. Skin Pharmacol Physiol 2006;19(6):311–21.
[48] Itami S, Sonoda T, Kurata S, et al. Mechanism of action of androgen in hair follicles. J Dermatol Sci 1994;7:S98–103.
[49] Giles GG, Severi G, Sinclair R, et al. Androgenetic alopecia and prostate cancer: findings from an Australian case-control study 1. Cancer Epidemiol Biomarkers Prev 2002;11(6): 549–53.
[50] Bergfeld WF. Androgenetic alopecia: an autosomal dominant disorder. Am J Med 1995; 98(1A):95S–8S.
[51] Carey AH, Waterworth D, Patel K, et al. Polycystic ovaries and premature male pattern baldness are associated with one allele of the steroid metabolism gene CYP17. Hum Mol Genet 1994;3(10):1873–6.
[52] Kuster W, Happle R. The inheritance of common baldness: two B or not two B? J Am Acad Dermatol 1984;11(5):921–6.
[53] Imperato-McGinley J. 5alpha-reductase-2 deficiency and complete androgen insensitivity: lessons from nature. Adv Exp Med Biol 2002;511:121–31.
[54] Ellis JA, Stebbing M, Harrap SB. Genetic analysis of male pattern baldness and the 5alpha-reductase genes. J Invest Dermatol 1998;110(6):849–53.
[55] Tang L, Bernardo O, Bolduc C, et al. The expression of insulin-like growth factor 1 in follicular dermal papillae correlates with therapeutic efficacy of finasteride in androgenetic alopecia. J Am Acad Dermatol 2003;49(2):229–33.
[56] Platz EA, Pollak MN, Willett WC, et al. Vertex balding, plasma insulin-like growth factor 1, and insulin-like growth factor binding protein 3. J Am Acad Dermatol 2000;42(6): 1003–7.
[57] Hillmer AM, Kruse R, Macciardi F, et al. The hairless gene in androgenetic alopecia: results of a systematic mutation screening and a family-based association approach. Br J Dermatol 2002;146(4):601–8.
[58] Garton RA, McMichael AJ, Sugarman J, et al. Association of a polymorphism in the ornithine decarboxylase gene with male androgenetic alopecia. J Am Acad Dermatol 2005; 52(3):535–6.
[59] Happle R, Hoffmann R. Absence of male-pattern baldness in men with X-linked recessive ichthyosis? A hypothesis to be challenged. Dermatology 1999;198(3):231–2.
[60] Trüeb RM, Meyer JC. Male-pattern baldness in men with X-linked recessive ichthyosis. Dermatology 2000;200(3):247–9.
[61] Axt-Gadermann M, Schlichting M, uuml ster W. Male-pattern baldness is common in men with X-linked recessive ichthyosis. Dermatology 2003;207(3):308–9.
[62] König A, Happle R, Tchitcherina E, et al. An X-linked gene involved in androgenetic alopecia: a lesson to be learned from adrenoleukodystrophy. Dermatology 2000;200(3):213–8.

[63] Hibberts NA, Howell AE, Randall VA. Balding hair follicle dermal papilla cells contain higher levels of androgen receptors than those from non-balding scalp. J Endocrinol 1998;156(1):59–65.

[64] Ellis JA, Stebbing M, Harrap SB. Polymorphism of the androgen receptor gene is associated with male pattern baldness. J Invest Dermatol 2001;116(3):452–5.

[65] Hayes VM, Severi G, Eggleton SA, et al. The E211 G> A androgen receptor polymorphism is associated with a decreased risk of metastatic prostate cancer and androgenetic alopecia. Cancer Epidemiol Biomarkers Prev 2005;14(4):993–6.

[66] Hillmer AM, Hanneken S, Ritzmann S, et al. Genetic variation in the human androgen receptor gene is the major determinant of common early-onset androgenetic alopecia. Am J Hum Genet 2005;77(1):140–8.

[67] Herrera CR, D'Agostino RB, Gerstman BB, et al. Baldness and coronary heart disease rates in men from the Framingham Study. Am J Epidemiol 1995;142(8):828–33.

[68] Lotufo PA, Chae CU, Ajani UA, et al. Male pattern baldness and coronary heart disease. The Physicians' Health Study: American Medical Association. All Rights Reserved. Applicable FARS/DFARS Restrictions Apply to Government Use; 2000.

[69] Matilainen VA, Makinen PK, Keinanen-Kiukaanniemi SM. Early onset of androgenetic alopecia associated with early severe coronary heart disease: a population-based, case-control study. J Cardiovasc Risk 2001;8(3):147–51.

[70] Matilainen V, Koskela P, Keinänen-Kiukaanniemi S. Early androgenetic alopecia as a marker of insulin resistance. Lancet 2000;356(9236):1165–6.

[71] Hawk E, Breslow RA, Graubard BI. Male pattern baldness and clinical prostate cancer in the epidemiologic follow-up of the First National Health and Nutrition Examination Survey. Cancer Epidemiol Biomarkers Prev 2000;9(5):523–7.

[72] Drake L, Hordinsky M, Fiedler V, et al. The effects of finasteride on scalp skin and serum androgen levels in men with androgenetic alopecia. J Am Acad Dermatol 1999;41(4):550–4.

[73] Roberts JL, Fiedler V, Imperato-McGinley J, et al. Clinical dose ranging studies with finasteride, a type 2 5alpha-reductase inhibitor, in men with male pattern hair loss. J Am Acad Dermatol 1999;41(4):555–63.

[74] Leyden J, Dunlap F, Miller B, et al. Finasteride in the treatment of men with frontal male pattern hair loss. J Am Acad Dermatol 1999;40(6):930–7.

[75] McClellan KJ, Markham A. Finasteride: a review of its use in male pattern hair loss. Drugs 1999;57(1):111–26.

[76] Bolduc C, Shapiro J. Management of androgenetic alopecia. Am J Clin Dermatol 2000; 1(3):151–8.

[77] Trial RC. Efficacy and tolerability of finasteride 1 mg in men aged 41 to 60 years with male pattern hair loss. Eur J Dermatol 2003;13(2):150–60.

[78] Whiting DA. Advances in the treatment of male androgenetic alopecia: a brief review of finasteride studies. Eur J Dermatol 2001;11(4):332–4.

[79] Price VH. Treatment of hair loss. N Engl J Med 1999;341(13):964–73.

[80] Kaufman KD, Olsen EA, Whiting D, et al. Finasteride in the treatment of men with androgenetic alopecia. Finasteride Male Pattern Hair Loss Study Group. J Am Acad Dermatol 1998;39(4):578–89.

[81] Overstreet JW, Fuh VL, Gould J, et al. Chronic treatment with finasteride daily does not affect spermatogenesis or semen production in young men. J Urol 1999;162(4): 1295–300.

[82] Pannek J, Marks LS, Pearson JD, et al. Influence of finasteride on free and total serum prostate specific antigen levels in men with benign prostatic hyperplasia. J Urol 1998;159(2): 449–53.

[83] Olsen EA, Messenger AG, Shapiro J, et al. Evaluation and treatment of male and female pattern hair loss. J Am Acad Dermatol 2005;52(2):301–11.

[84] Messenger AG, Rundegren J. Minoxidil: mechanisms of action on hair growth. Br J Dermatol 2004;150(2):186–94.

[85] Cohen RL, Alves M, Weiss VC, et al. Direct effects of minoxidil on epidermal cells in culture. J Invest Dermatol 1984;82:90–3.

[86] Buhl AE, Waldon DJ, Kawabe TT, et al. Minoxidil stimulates mouse vibrissae follicles in organ culture. J Invest Dermatol 1989;92:315–20.

[87] Wester RC, Maibach HI, Guy RH, et al. Minoxidil stimulates cutaneous blood flow in human balding scalps: pharmacodynamics measured by laser doppler velocimetry and photopulse plethysmography. J Invest Dermatol 1984;82:515–7.

[88] Lachgar S, Charveron M, Gall Y, et al. Minoxidil upregulates the expression of vascular endothelial growth factor in human hair dermal papilla cells. Br J Dermatol 1998;138: 407–11.

[89] Price VH, Menefee E, Strauss PC. Changes in hair weight and hair count in men with androgenetic alopecia, after application of 5% and 2% topical minoxidil, placebo, or no treatment. J Am Acad Dermatol 1999;41(5):717–21.

[90] Hautala T, Heikkinen J, Kivirikko KI, et al. Minoxidil specifically decreases the expression of lysine hydroxylase in cultured human skin fibroblasts. Biochem J 1992;283:51–4.

[91] Michelet JF, Commo S, Billoni N, et al. Activation of cytoprotective prostaglandin synthase-1 by minoxidil as a possible explanation for its hair growth-stimulating effect. J Invest Dermatol 1997;108:205–9.

[92] Buhl AE, Waldon DJ, Baker CA, et al. Minoxidil sulfate is the active metabolite that stimulates hair follicles. J Invest Dermatol 1990;95:553–7.

[93] Buhl AE, Waldon DJ, Conrad SJ, et al. Potassium channel conductance: a mechanism affecting hair growth both in vitro and in vivo. J Invest Dermatol 1992;98:315–9.

[94] Olsen EA, DeLong ER, Weiner MS. Long-term follow-up of men with male pattern baldness treated with topical minoxidil. J Am Acad Dermatol 1987;16(3):688–95.

[95] Olsen EA, Dunlap FE, Funicella T, et al. A randomized clinical trial of 5% topical minoxidil versus 2% topical minoxidil and placebo in the treatment of androgenetic alopecia in men. J Am Acad Dermatol 2002;47(3):377–85.

[96] Olsen EA, Weiner MS. Topical minoxidil in male pattern baldness: effects of discontinuation of treatment. J Am Acad Dermatol 1987;17(1):97–101.

[97] Shapiro J, Price VH. Hair regrowth; therapeutic agents. Dermatol Clin 1998;16(2): 341–56.

[98] Ferry JJ, Shepard JH, Szpunar GJ. Relationship between contact time of applied dose and percutaneous absorption of minoxidil from a topical solution. J Pharm Sci 1990;79(6): 483–6.

[99] Olsen EA, Weiner MS, Amara IA, et al. Five-year follow-up of men with androgenetic alopecia treated with topical minoxidil. J Am Acad Dermatol 1990;22(4):643–6.

[100] Khandpur S, Suman M, Reddy BS. Comparative efficacy of various treatment regimens for androgenetic alopecia in men. J Dermatol 2002;29(8):489–98.

[101] Alert F. An open, randomized, comparative study of oral finasteride and 5% topical minoxidil in male androgenetic alopecia. Dermatology 2004;209:117–25.

[102] Unger WP. Hair transplantation: current concepts and techniques. J Investig Dermatol Symp Proc 2005;10(3):225–9.

[103] Bernstein RM, Rassman WR. Follicular unit transplantation: 2005. Dermatol Clin 2005; 23(3):393–414.

[104] Swinehart JM. Patient recruitment and enrollment into clinical trials: a discussion of specific methods and disease state. Journal of Clinical Research and Pharmacoepidemiology 1991;5(1):35–47.

[105] Leavitt M, Pm L, Rao NA, et al. Effects of finasteride (1 mg) on hair transplant. Dermatol Surg 2005;31(10):1268–76.

[106] Avram MR, Cole JP, Chase C, et al. The potential role of minoxidil in the hair transplantation setting. Dermatol Surg 2002;28(10):894–900.

[107] Bouhanna P. Topical minoxidil used before and after hair transplantation. J Dermatol Surg Oncol 1989;15(1):50–3.

[108] Martinick JH. The latest developments in surgical hair restoration. Facial Plast Surg Clin North Am 2004;12(2):249–52.

[109] Cotsarelis G. Epithelial stem cells: a folliculocentric view. J Invest Dermatol 2006;126(7): 1459–68.

[110] Moore KA, Lemischka IR. Stem cells and their niches. Science 2006;311(5769):1880–5.

ELSEVIER
SAUNDERS

Endocrinol Metab Clin N Am
36 (2007) 399–419

ENDOCRINOLOGY
AND METABOLISM
CLINICS
OF NORTH AMERICA

Osteoporosis in Men

Luigi Gennari, MD[a], John P. Bilezikian, MD[b,c],*

[a]Department of Internal Medicine, Endocrine-Metabolic Sciences and Biochemistry,
University of Siena, Siena 53100, Italy
[b]Department of Medicine, Division of Endocrinology, College of Physicians and Surgeons,
Columbia University, 630 West 168th Street, New York, NY 10032, USA
[c]Department of Pharmacology, College of Physicians and Surgeons, Columbia University,
630 West 168th Street, New York, NY 10032, USA

Osteoporosis is a worldwide major public health problem. It is defined as a skeletal disorder of compromised bone strength predisposing to an increased risk of fracture [1]. Most studies on metabolic bone diseases over the past decade have focused on the pathogenesis, diagnosis, and treatment of osteoporosis in women. Nevertheless, recent epidemiological and observational studies have shown that osteoporosis in men is an increasingly important clinical issue. In part because the world population is aging, it is estimated that the total number of hip fractures in men in 2025 will be similar to current estimates in women [2,3]. To highlight this point, the 2004 Invest in Your Bones Campaign of the International Osteoporosis Foundation was fully dedicated to the problem of osteoporosis in men.

Epidemiology

The number of men afflicted with osteoporosis is unknown. Unfortunately, the yardstick by which we determine the presence of osteoporosis, namely bone mineral density (BMD), is not as well standardized in men as it is in women. In fact, there are few prospective studies defining the relationship between BMD and fracture risk in men. Data from the Framingham Study cohort [4] suggest that this relationship is different from the relationship in women. Because men experience fractures at a relatively higher absolute BMD, many men who have osteoporosis would not be considered to be at risk if one used absolute bone density as the standard. In

* Corresponding author. College of Physicians and Surgeons, 630 W. 168th Street, New York, NY 10032.
E-mail address: JPB2@columbia.edu (J.P. Bilezikian).

0889-8529/07/$ - see front matter © 2007 Elsevier Inc. All rights reserved.
doi:10.1016/j.ecl.2007.03.008

contrast, in 2004, Schuitt and colleagues [5] reported from the Rotterdam Study that men older than 55 years showed a relationship between absolute BMD and risk of hip and other nonvertebral fractures that was similar to women. A meta-analysis of available cohort studies including the results from the Netherlands cohort came to similar conclusions [6]. If one uses relative risk, however, it is clear that for every standard deviation reduction in BMD, men will have the same fold-increase in risk as women. The big difference is that the number of fractures will be fewer since fracture incidence is less. Even though uncertainties remain about whether to use absolute or relative risk in diagnosing male osteoporosis, the International Society for Clinical Densitometry recommends that we use the male database and the T-score of less than −2.5 to diagnose osteoporosis in men. By applying these standards, according to the World Health Organization (WHO), it is estimated that 1 to 2 million men in the United States have osteoporosis (T-score < −2.5) and another 8 to 13 million have osteopenia (T-score between −1.0 and −2.5). The respective age-adjusted prevalence figures are impressive: 6% for osteoporosis and 47% for osteopenia. On the other hand, if one applies the female reference standard to men (BMD > −2.5 SD below peak bone mass for women), the numbers become much smaller, namely 0.3 to 1 million men with osteoporosis (age-adjusted prevalence, 4%) and 4 to 9 million with osteopenia (age-adjusted prevalence, 33%). These latter figures are not consistent with epidemiological data. Although controversy exists over what database to use, it is clear that men, like women, are at substantial risk for developing osteoporosis throughout the world. In a recent prospective study of more than 5000 men from the MrOS cohort, hip BMD was a strong predictor of hip fracture [7]. The relationship between hip BMD and hip fracture risk seemed to be even stronger than that observed in a large prospective study of women (relative risk [RR] 3.2-fold versus 2.1-fold increased risk per SD decrease in BMD in males versus females, respectively). It is therefore clear, that the BMD measurement can be used to define risk in men, as it is used to define risk in women.

Aging in men, like aging in women, is associated with dramatic increases in fracture risk. The exponential increase in risk occurs approximately 1 decade later than in women. It has been estimated that the lifetime risk of a man suffering an osteoporotic fracture is actually greater than his likelihood of developing prostate cancer [8]. About one in every four to five hip fractures in people older than 50 occurs in men [3]. Overall, one in five men over the age of 50 will have an osteoporosis-related fracture in their remaining lifetime [9–11]. These figures are likely to vary according to the country studied. For example, a recent study in Australia suggests that one in three men over 60 will suffer a fracture due to osteoporosis [12].

Importantly, the morbidity and the mortality from hip fractures are higher in men than in women. In fact, it has been reported that after the hip fracture, fatality rates among those over 75 years is 20.7% in men versus 7.5% in women. Since the age-specific incidence of hip fractures is increasing

[13] and the projected number of hip fractures worldwide by 2025 in men has been calculated to be 1.16 million [14] versus 0.5 million reported in 1990 [3], these projections point to much greater deaths in the future due to the hip fracture and its complications.

Men are also at risk for vertebral fractures. Some reports indicate that the incidence of vertebral fractures in men is as high as half that seen in women, an estimate that is much higher than the 10-fold difference that has been perceived in the past [15]. In a large multinational survey aimed to determine the prevalence of vertebral osteoporosis across different populations in Europe (EVOS), the overall prevalence of vertebral deformity was similar in both sexes, 15.1% in males and 17.2% in females [16]. One explanation is that unsuspected vertebral fractures as determined radiologically are common in men, particularly in their fifties and sixties. In contrast to the hip and vertebral fractures, forearm fractures are uncommon in men and do not increase with age [17,18].

Causes and pathophysiology of osteoporosis in men

To explain the differences in incidence rates between sexes, there are factors that tend to protect men, at least in the years when osteoporosis is becoming common in women. One important point is that, unlike women, men do not have a midlife loss in sex steroid hormone production. When women experience the menopause, estrogen levels fall abruptly and the remodeling rate of bone increases. This process is associated with accelerated bone loss and a subsequent increase in fracture risk. In contrast to women, men do not have a "menopause" unless they have a disorder (hypogonadism) or a therapeutic castration for a disease like prostate cancer. In the middle-aged man, therefore, bone loss proceeds slowly. Moreover, in men, bone loss is characterized during this period as trabecular thinning [19–21]. Loss of bone by trabecular thinning does not cause as much loss of strength in the vertebral body than an equivalent loss of bone by trabecular perforation. Trabecular perforation is more characteristic of high bone turnover states, such as the menopause-related bone loss in women. Another factor that provides relative protection in men is the fact that men achieve 8% to 10% more peak bone mass than women. This greater accrual of peak bone mass is determined by convention dual energy x-ray absorptiometry (DXA), a technology that measures areal density (g/cm^2). Larger areal density confers a mechanical advantage because forces are distributed more widely over the surface of bone. It is important to note, however, that true bone density, a volumetric index (vBMD, g/cm^3), is similar among the sexes at peak bone age. Greater areal density in men is likely to be attributable to the effect of androgens in increasing bone size by periosteal apposition, a mechanism that becomes operative at puberty and continues throughout life. A recent study by peripheral quantitative computed tomography (pQCT) in an age- and sex-stratified population of 373 women and

323 men, showed 35% to 42% larger bone area in young adult men than women [22]. Bone area was found to be higher at central sites in both sexes but more so at peripheral sites in men. This is consistent with the view that the degree of periosteal apposition is likely to be site-specific. Average decreases in trabecular vBMD were greater in women than in men at central sites (55% versus 46%), but were similar at peripheral sites (24% versus 26%). Consistent with menopausal-induced increases in bone turnover as well as with the actions of androgens that maintain cortical density, cortical vBMD decreased more in women than men. Thus, gender-specific differences in the net gain and loss from endosteal and periosteal surfaces are likely to be site-specific. They account, at least in part, for the difference observed between men and women. It is important to introduce a cautionary note with regard to the data available, virtually all of which is cross-sectional. Detailed, prospective studies are needed to clearly define gender differences in densitometric, geometric, and other aspects of bone strength with advancing age.

The causes of bone loss in men are thought to be related to genetics, environmental, hormonal, and disease-specific factors (Box 1). As in females, osteoporosis in males can be attributable to specific, underlying etiologies requiring careful clinical evaluation. Approximately, 50% of men with osteoporosis are diagnosed with an underlying "secondary" cause. This leaves a large percentage of men whose osteoporosis is not explained, so-called "primary" or "idiopathic" osteoporosis. Most of the men in this category are less than 65 to 70 years of age. Of course, there are men over 70 with osteoporosis in which the cause is not known. The older the patient, however, the more we are likely to relate the osteoporosis to age and not to a specific or unknown cause. Clearly, the younger the patient, the more likely it is that other explanations are needed to account for the condition.

Most men with idiopathic osteoporosis present a rather typical clinical and histomorphometric phenotype that differs from age-related osteoporosis. They often show normal or slightly increased bone resorption but decreased bone formation [23,24]. In keeping with this knowledge, a recent in vitro study of bone cells derived from men with idiopathic osteoporosis demonstrated osteoblast dysfunction with decreased osteocalcin production and increased production of factors stimulating osteoclast activation [25]. However, the category that we call idiopathic osteoporosis is clearly a heterogeneous one with many different clinical phenotypes described [26]. For example, osteoporotic men with hypercalciuria with or without accelerated bone resorption have been noted [27–29]. The mechanisms of bone loss in these men with hypercalciuria are still not clear, but they are likely to differ from the idiopathic osteoporosis variant associated with osteoblast dysfunction.

The three major causes of secondary osteoporosis in men are alcohol abuse, glucocorticoid excess (either endogenous Cushing's syndrome or, more commonly, chronic glucocorticoid therapy), and hypogonadism [29–31].

Box 1. Major causes of osteoporosis in men

Primary osteoporosis
- Idiopathic osteoporosis
- Age-related osteoporosis

Secondary osteoporosis
- Alcoholism
- Hormonal disorders
  Hypogonadism
  Cushing's syndrome
  Hyperthyroidism
  Hyperparathyroidism (1° and 2°)
- Gastrointestinal disorders
  Malabsorption syndromes
  Inflammatory bowel disease, gluten entheropathy
  Primary biliary cirrhosis
  Post gastrectomy
- Hypercalciuria
- Chronic obstructive pulmonary disease
- Transplantation osteoporosis
- Neuromuscular disorders
- Systemic illnesses
  Rheumatoid arthritis
  Multiple myeloma
  Other malignancies
  Mastocytosis
- Medication/drug-related
  Glucocorticoids
  Anticonvulsants
  Thyroid hormone
  Chemotherapeutics

In many series, these etiologies account for 40% to 50% of all men with osteoporosis. Other causes are also important to rule out, such as primary hyperparathyroidism, excessive thyroid hormone exposure (either hyperthyroidism or overtreatment with thyroid hormone), gastrointestinal disorders, chronic obstructive pulmonary disease, neuromuscular disorders such as Parkinson disease, multiple myeloma or other malignancies, and use of other drugs (anticonvulsants, high-dose chemotherapeutics, selective serotonin reuptake inhibitors) [29,32,33]. As in women, the presence of risk factors such as tobacco use, physical inactivity, leanness, low calcium intake, and reduced grip strength during midlife may contribute to accelerate bone remodeling, thereby modifying the age-related pattern of bone loss or superimposing on the underlying secondary cause and thus increasing fracture risk [32,34]. Moreover, in the largest population-based study of BMD in older US men performed to date, the strongest factor determining BMD was race/ethnicity. African American men showed 12% higher hip and 6% higher spine BMD than Caucasian men, a finding consistent with previous findings in both men and women [35]. The higher bone mass among African American men was not explained by weight or other historical or lifestyle factors and was sufficiently large to account for their lower risk of fracture. Asian men had lower BMD than Caucasian men in age-adjusted analysis, but this difference was entirely explained by body weight.

Genetic factors are likely to play a major role in male as well as in female osteoporosis [36,37]. Comparisons of mono- and dizygotic twins demonstrated that up to 80% of the variance in BMD might be under genetic control [38]. Epidemiological data from a variety of sources have defined a parental history of fractures (either maternal or paternal) as a major risk factor for osteoporosis in both sexes [39–41]; however, the specific genes involved have not yet been well delineated. The genetic effect may also be gender- and site-specific, with different genes regulating bone density at different skeletal sites in males and females. Most of the work implicating certain genes in osteoporosis have focused on women and include polymorphisms in the vitamin D receptor, the estrogen receptor, and the collagen type I a1 gene [38]. More recent genetic studies have provided intriguing evidence for the possibility that polymorphisms in genes for IGF-I, LRP5, and CYP19 aromatase may predict BMD variability and fracture risk in males more than females [42–45].

Among many attractive hypotheses to account for the mechanism(s) of bone loss in male osteoporosis, a decrease in sex steroid hormone production and/or sensitivity is supposed to play a major role. Hypogonadism is considered to be an important cause of bone loss in women and men. Even though men do not undergo an equivalent of the menopause, both estrogen and androgen levels, and particularly their bioavailable fractions, decline slowly but progressively after 50 to 60 years of age [46–49], apparently as a result of complex alterations in reproductive physiology, secondary causes of gonadal dysfunction and lifestyle factors, or increases in the levels of sex hormone binding globulin [50–52]. Nevertheless, a broad variation in the levels of sex steroid concentrations has also been described in older men, and only a modest amount of the variability in levels was explained by age, suggesting the importance of additional components [53]. To date, the level of testosterone and estradiol that represents sufficiency in the male is unknown and may vary among individuals and between target tissues.

Androgens, the dominant male sex steroid class, have long been assumed to be critical for the growth and the maintenance of the male skeleton;

however, both observational and interventional studies recently have confirmed that estrogens are even more important in the growth and the maintenance of bone mass in men. Since the discovery of osteoporosis and longitudinal bone growth in a young man with an inactivating mutation in the ERα gene, several clinical and experimental lines clearly indicate a dominant role of estrogen over androgen for the initiation of the pubertal growth spurt and growth plate fusion at the end of puberty, as well as for longitudinal bone growth, attainment of peak bone mass, and normal bone remodeling in young males. Certainly, androgens are also important for bone growth in males, especially for periosteal bone expansion and the acquisition of increased bone size, points that distinguish men from women, as described earlier. Androgens are also likely to be important for muscle mass, and consequently, for increasing bone mass.

An important role for estrogens in maintaining male skeletal mass was also suggested by cross-sectional observations in middle-aged and elderly men. It was shown that BMD is more directly related to declining estrogen levels than declining androgen levels [54–60]. Both total and bioavailable serum estradiol concentrations appeared significantly and directly related to bone mass. Serum estradiol levels were more robust predictors of BMD than serum testosterone levels, even in a sample of androgen-deficient men from the Framingham Study [59]. These cross-sectional data were confirmed in longitudinal studies. Over a 2-year period, Slemenda and colleagues [54] described lower estradiol levels in men losing BMD at more than 1% per year as compared with men with higher estradiol levels and lower rates of bone loss. Elderly men with bioavailable estradiol levels below the median value of 40 pmol/L showed higher rates of bone loss at the mid-radius and ulna than men with bioavailable estradiol levels above the median [48]. A similar longitudinal 4-year study of 200 elderly Italian men [49] confirmed and extended these observations by showing a negative correlation between estrogen levels and bone turnover markers or rates of bone loss at the lumbar spine and the distal femur. In the same study, the ratio between estradiol and testosterone, presumed to be an indirect index of aromatase activity, increased significantly with age and was higher in normal than in osteoporotic subjects [49]. These observations illustrate an important role for estrogen in the maintenance of bone mass in aging men.

Considerable indirect evidence also suggests that a threshold value for estrogen in the male skeleton is needed to control bone remodeling and to maintain bone mass [48,49,61]. In a cross-sectional analysis from the MINOS Study, men in the lowest quartile for bioavailable estradiol level showed significantly lower BMD at multiple sites as compared with men in the upper three estradiol quartiles [55]. Moreover, in two longitudinal studies in elderly males, rates of bone loss at different skeletal sites were unrelated to serum estradiol levels if they were above the median value, but clearly associated with estradiol levels if they were below the median value [48,49]. The threshold concentration of bioavailable estradiol appears to be remarkably similar across all studies, ranging from 40 to 55 pmol/L. This apparent threshold value is higher than typical estradiol concentrations for postmenopausal women who are not receiving exogenous estrogens. On the other hand, premenopausal women and young men are typically above this apparent threshold level. Because about 40% to 50% of middle-aged men have estradiol levels below this threshold, it could be a determinant in age-related bone loss in a large number of males [48,53,60,61]. A recent cross-sectional study, in which volumetric BMD and bone geometry at different sites were assessed by QCT, further extended these observations, indicating that in men the relationship between bioavailable estradiol and volumetric BMD at cortical versus trabecular sites appears to be different [62]. The supposed threshold level for estrogen deficiency appeared to be lower for cortical than for trabecular bone. In other words, trabecular bone seems to be more sensitive to small declines in estrogen levels with aging, while cortical bone appears to be more insensitive. The same associations were confirmed in a similar QCT study in women [62].

Since only a small fraction of circulating estradiol (below 15%) is derived directly from the testes, it is likely that peripheral aromatization of testicular and adrenal androgen precursors into estrogen exert a key role in maintaining estradiol levels above the threshold with aging [63]. The experiments of nature, in which aromatase activity or estrogen response are absent or inhibited, have shown clearly that estrogen production from androgen precursors represents an important mechanism to preserve skeletal health in the male. Men who are born with a defect in the aromatase gene and are completely estrogen deficient are severely osteoporotic. This raises the possibility that significant differences in aromatase activity per se might be present among males [64,65] due to variability in aromatase activity and/or estrogen sensitivity and that this variability may be important for skeletal homeostasis [63,66,67]. The expression of this variability might become particularly important in elderly males in whom age-related declines in testicular and adrenal androgen precursors are common. It may, however, be even more relevant in postmenopausal women, where availability of androgen precursors for aromatization to estrogen is much lower than in men [68,69]. Thus, it is likely that individual differences in aromatase activity with aging may help to distinguish among men and their rates of bone loss. Recent studies on aromatase *CYP19* gene suggest that polymorphic variation of this gene may account at least in part for these differences in aromatase activity [42,43]. Males with a high number of TTTA repeat sequences in intron 4 of the CYP19 gene showed higher 17β-estradiol levels and decreased rates of bone loss than those with a lower number of repeats irrespective of sex hormone binding globulin (SHBG) or androgen levels. Consistent with these clinical observations, higher in vitro aromatase efficiency and greater estrogen production were observed in fibroblasts from a high TTTA repeat sequence genotype in comparison to fibroblasts from a low TTTA repeat sequence genotype [42]. Importantly, the observations correlating the (TTTA)$_n$ polymorphism of the CYP19 gene to estrogen levels and to bone density in males appear to be dependent on fat mass. When analyses are restricted to subjects with a normal body mass index, the differences in BMD between *CYP19* genotypes were greater, while such differences progressively decreased in magnitude when overweight and obese men were considered among these polymorphic distribution profiles [42]. This point suggests that fat mass may be a mitigating factor in the expression of *CYP19* genotypes on bone. It is possible that with more adipose tissue, the associated overall increase in adipose aromatase activity dominates any effect of the gene polymorphisms on intrinsic aromatase activity. Indeed, weight reduction has been associated with bone loss in elderly males, and particularly in those with lower baseline bioavailable sex steroids or in those with greater declines in these hormones [70,71]. In addition to genetic considerations, several additional mechanisms have been proposed in which aromatase activity and estrogen production could be modulated under certain circumstances in different tissues [63].

An interaction among androgens, estrogen, growth hormone (GH), and insulin-like growth factor I (IGF-I) has also been hypothesized. Declining concentrations of GH and IGF-I have been observed with advancing age [72] and could contribute to reduced bone formation. Decreasing IGF-I levels may explain, at least in part, the age-related increase in SHBG. In fact, serum SHBG levels are inversely correlated with IGF-I levels [73] and IGF-I has been shown to inhibit SHBG production by hepatocytes in vitro [74]. Moreover, declining GH and IGF-I levels may also contribute to an impairment in periosteal apposition [75]. Several reports have shown a significant reduction in IGF-I values in men with idiopathic osteoporosis and have correlated these reductions with reduced bone density of the spine and forearm [76,77]. GH deficiency does not easily explain these reductions, because these men respond normally to GH stimulation tests [78]; however, it remains possible that subtle abnormalities in GH dynamics exist in terms of either pulsatility or circadian rhythm. Interestingly, the reduction in IGF-I levels seems to be associated with a particular allelic configuration of the polymorphic microsatellite region of the IGF-I gene composed of variable cytosine-adenosine repeats 1 kb upstream from the transcription start site. The frequency of homozygosity for the allele in question, designated 192, in a group of men with idiopathic osteoporosis was 64%, twice as high as that in a number of control populations [45]. The gene frequency for this allele was greater than 90%. The mean IGF-I level for those with the 192/192 genotype was significantly lower than that for subjects with any other genotype. A recent population-based cross-sectional study using high-resolution three-dimensional pQCT described age effects on bone microstructure as well as its relationship with hormonal variables [79,80]. In young men, the conversion of thick trabeculae into more numerous, thinner trabeculae observed between young adulthood and mid-life was most closely associated with declining IGF-I levels. Conversely, sex steroids, and particularly bioavailable estradiol, appeared as the major hormonal determinants of trabecular microstructure in elderly men.

Prospective, longitudinal studies are needed to verify these findings and to determine the relationships between sex steroids and other hormones to health outcomes in older men. In particular, the independent and codependent effects of sex hormones and the growth hormone/IGF-I axis on periosteal and endosteal modeling and remodeling during growth as well as aging remains to be defined [21]. Even though it was assumed that androgen is the main regulator of periosteal apposition, with experimental evidence showing a suppressive effect of estrogen at the periosteum, more recent clinical investigations by pQCT clearly indicate that estrogen could indeed promote periosteal growth and increase bone size in humans [62,81]. Moreover, the exact mechanisms of action of estrogen and androgen on bone cells still remain poorly understood. Even though ERα seems to be predominantly involved in mediating estrogen action in bone, the exact role of ERβ, the contribution of genomic versus nongenomic pathways as well as the possibility of mechanisms of estrogen and androgen on bone not specific to gender or gnome [82,83] still remain to be investigated.

Clinical approach and management

Since BMD measurement is obtained uncommonly in men (even in the presence of clear risk factors), height loss, kyphosis, fracture, or symptomatic back pain are the most characteristic initial clinical presentations of male osteoporosis. This presentation is quite different from the typical postmenopausal woman with osteoporosis, in whom it is now much more likely for the diagnosis to be made by BMD. Actually, the BMD criteria (thresholds) that should be used to identify osteoporotic men in need of therapeutic intervention are controversial. Until additional data are available, it is reasonable to use gender-specific criteria to make a diagnosis of osteoporosis in men (that is a T score −2.5 SD below the young male reference mean) [84,85]. Consensus concerning which men would benefit from BMD measures still needs to be developed. However, there are some populations of men for whom BMD measures are unequivocally indicated. Those include men who have suffered low trauma fractures (including prevalent vertebral deformity), have radiographic low bone mass, or have secondary conditions recognized to increase bone loss and fracture risk. A positive family history, smoking, and low weight/weight loss, have been linked to low bone mass and fractures in different studies and could represent additional indications for BMD measurement. In addition, the International Society for Clinical Densitometry recommends bone measurement in all men over 70 years of age.

After DXA measurement has indicated the presence of osteoporosis, all reasonable potential causes of bone loss should be considered. Routine measurements of serum and urinary calcium and phosphorus, serum alkaline phosphatase, and serum proteins as well as liver, renal, adrenal, pituitary, and thyroid function tests are indicated. Sex steroid measurements are useful, including total testosterone, estrone, estradiol, and SHBG. Tests of the calciotropic axis should include parathyroid hormone (PTH), 25-hydroxyvitamin D, and, perhaps also, 1,25-dihydroxyvitamin D levels. Specific markers of bone formation (ie, serum bone-specific alkaline phosphatase activity or osteocalcin) and of bone resorption (collagen crosslinks, C- or N-telopeptides or deoxypyridinoline) are also indicated. Clues to a possible occult gastrointestinal disorder are low 25-hydroxyvitamin D levels, high PTH levels, and low urinary calcium excretion. In this setting, gluten enteropathy needs to be considered in particular. A percutaneous bone biopsy can be helpful in some circumstances to evaluate more definitively the histomorphometric and dynamic parameters as well as to rule out potential secondary causes such as occult forms of osteomalacia, osteogenesis imperfecta, mastocytosis, and malignancy.

Patients can be monitored with sequential BMD measurements, as they are useful surrogate indexes of therapeutic efficacy. The use of bone formation and resorption markers may also be helpful, as has been shown in a number of large-scale studies in postmenopausal women [86,87]. Since an association between markers of bone turnover and bone loss has been reported in elderly men [88], it is likely that a reduction in bone markers after antiresorptive therapy in men will provide the same predictive information about therapeutic results that have been shown in postmenopausal women; however, this area has been poorly investigated in men.

Treatment of male osteoporosis

Pharmacological agents have been less well studied in men than in women with osteoporosis. Many of the clinical trials, even those that have led to drug approval in men, have been conducted with many fewer subjects and much more uncertain outcome results. Moreover, osteoporosis in men is rarely recognized and treated, even after a fracture has occurred [89–91]. A recent retrospective cohort study in 1171 men aged 65 or older demonstrated that only 7.1% of osteoporotic subjects and 16% of those with a hip or vertebral fracture received medication for osteoporosis [91]. Preventive interventions in males are similar to the approach used for women. Dietary calcium intake should be 1200 to 1500 mg, consistent with the National Institutes of Health (NIH) and Food and Nutrition Board recommendations for optimal calcium intake [92,93]. Vitamin D intake must also be adequate and individuals should receive 400 to 600 IU per day. In men over 70, a general recommendation of 600 to 800 IU per day is made by many experts. Adequate exercise should also be strongly advised. However, drug therapy is almost always indicated in men at high risk for fracture.

Bisphosphonate therapy is becoming a mainstay in the treatment of male osteoporosis [94]. Initially, their use in men was based on several uncontrolled observational studies by assuming that therapeutic results were similar to favorable findings from previous, much larger trials in women.

Orwoll and colleagues [95] conducted a large, randomized, placebo-controlled trial reporting an increase in BMD in a subgroup of men with osteoporosis treated with alendronate. The extent was very similar to that seen previously in studies of postmenopausal women. BMD increases were independent of baseline free testosterone, age (less or more than 65 yrs), BMD T-score and presence or absence of prevalent vertebral fractures. Height loss was also reduced in the alendronate-treated group, as was the incidence of vertebral fractures. The number of nonvertebral fractures was too low to evaluate the effect of alendronate treatment in their prevention. More recently, reports of additional trials of alendronate have become available, showing similar positive effects on BMD and prevention of vertebral fractures in men with primary osteoporosis [96–99]. Comparable incremental effects on BMD in men and women with primary and secondary osteoporosis within 12 months of treatment were observed in two different studies [100,101]. A recent health economic study from Sweden indicated that treating osteoporotic men with alendronate would be cost-effective, assuming the same fracture-risk–reducing effect of alendronate for men as for women [102]. Indeed, a meta-analysis evaluating cumulative antifracture efficacy of randomized controlled trials in men has indicated that alendronate treatment efficiently decreases the risk of vertebral fractures in men with low bone mass or fractures, but there is currently insufficient evidence to prove a significant effect on nonvertebral fractures [103]. Of note, the relative risk of vertebral fracture in alendronate-treated men was similar to that previously observed in a meta-analysis of data from postmenopausal women [104]. Weekly administration of alendronate (70 mg) appears to be equivalent to once daily alendronate (10 mg) in men as well [105,106].

Risedronate has also been shown to increase BMD and to reduce vertebral fractures [107], and has recently been approved in the United States for osteoporosis in men. Both alendronate and risedronate are also effective in men with secondary causes of osteoporosis including glucocorticoid excess, hypogonadism, or transplantation [108–118], and have been approved for treatment of glucocorticoid-induced osteoporosis in men in a variety of countries [119].

Recently, several different randomized controlled trials demonstrated that human recombinant PTH(1-34)—teriparatide—is effective in men at high fracture risk (either in primary or secondary osteoporosis, such as hypogonadal osteoporosis), but the drug's cost, complex administration schedule, and potential risks have caused it to be restricted to men at highest risk for fracture [120–124]. When administered at a daily dose of 20 μg, teriparatide exerts anabolic effects on bone with rapid increases in lumbar BMD and bone formation markers [125]. Similar but less marked increases in hip BMD occur. To date there are no conclusive data for the efficacy of PTH therapy to reduce fractures in men, perhaps because the size of the trials has been small and/or the trials have not been performed long enough. However, an observational study has demonstrated that teraparatide

reduced the risk of moderate or severe vertebral fracture with respect to placebo after PTH treatment was discontinued [123]. When these results are
compared with those from similar studies in women, the reductions in vertebral fracture risk are essentially the same. In men as in women, concurrent
therapy with bisphosphonates does not appear to confer any benefits over
teriparatide alone. Sequential therapy with alendronate once teriparatide
is discontinued is associated with maintenance or further enhancement of
bone mass. In individuals who have been treated previously with a potent
antiresorptive agent, like alendronate, the subsequent actions of PTH on
bone density may be transiently delayed, particularly if bone turnover is
markedly suppressed [126–128]. There are currently no data available concerning the combination of PTH with other bisphosphonates or testosterone
replacement.

Other treatment options are reserved for selected patients. In hypogonadism, a number of studies have demonstrated that testosterone replacement
in men is associated with an increase in BMD, even though the effects of
fracture risk remain unknown [129,130]. Alendronate treatment was also effective in hypogonadal men given alone or in combination with androgen
replacement [95,110]. In a 2-year study, the increase in bone loss following
acute hypogonadism induced by GnRH agonist therapy for prostate cancer
was completely abrogated by periodic intravenous pamidronate treatment
(60 mg intravenously every 12 weeks) [131]. An unresolved clinical issue is
the management of older men with low BMD who have moderately low
testosterone levels, as a consequence of age-related declines in gonadal function. A meta-analysis of placebo-controlled trials of testosterone treatment
in men with any degree of androgen deficiency (most of them showing low
normal or normal testosterone levels at baseline) suggested a beneficial effect
on lumbar spine BMD, but equivocal findings at the femoral neck [132].
Generally, trials of intramuscular testosterone report significantly larger
effects on bone density than trials of transdermal testosterone. Of interest,
in a study on androgen supplementation in eugonadal men with osteoporosis, the increase in BMD and the reduction in bone turnover positively correlated with change in estradiol, but not in testosterone levels, further
indicating that the skeletal effects of androgens in men are mainly attributable to their conversion to estrogens [133]. Major concerns of androgen
treatment in eugonadal men relate to their possible associated negative
implications in other target organs, such as the gonads, the prostate, and
the cardiovascular system. In particular, trials of testosterone treatment enrolled men without evidence of significant prostate disease and have been of
short duration. Thus, the effects of long-term treatment with testosterone on
prostate health remain unknown.

Given their preliminary in vitro inhibitory effects in human prostate cancer
cell lines [134] and the lack of feminizing effects, selective estrogen receptor
modulators (SERMs) such as raloxifene, have been recently regarded for potential application in men, including the prevention of bone loss. Indeed,

another first-generation SERM, tamoxifene, has been administered to men as a fertility-promoting drug, without relevant adverse side events [135]. More recently, two studies investigated the skeletal effects of raloxifene in healthy men. In a study of 50 elderly men, raloxifene treatment (60 mg per day) for 6 months was no different from placebo in terms of its effects on urinary cross-linked N-telopeptide of type I collagen (NTX) [136]. However, consistent with the threshold estradiol hypothesis, changes in urinary NTX were related directly to baseline serum estradiol levels. Subjects with serum estradiol levels below 96 pmol/L (26 pg/mL, corresponding approximately to serum bioavailable levels of 9 pg/mL) responded to raloxifene with a decrease in bone resorption markers. In this group, raloxifene was serving as an agonist. Above this estrogen value, raloxifene caused an increase in bone resorption. In this group with higher estrogen levels, raloxifene was acting as an estrogen antagonist. This seems to be remarkably comparable to the findings of a similar study in which raloxifene was given at a greater dose (120 mg per day) for 6 weeks in middle-aged eugonadal men [137]. In fact no major relevant effect on bone resorption and formation markers was observed in the overall raloxifene-treated group, while in the group of subjects with estradiol levels below a threshold value of 101.8 pmol/L, raloxifene treatment was associated with a significant decrease in bone turnover markers. In this study, as well as in a somewhat longer study, 120 mg daily doses of raloxifene significantly increased serum concentrations of luteinizing hormone, follicle-stimulating hormone, estradiol, and total or bioavailable testosterone [137–139]. The increase in estradiol after raloxifene treatment was more pronounced in those subjects with a low baseline serum estradiol level [137]. No major treatment-related adverse events or feminizing effects were observed in these studies. Thus, in men, raloxifene treatment might exert beneficial effects on bone metabolism only if serum concentrations of estradiol are low. Additional studies on raloxifene and other SERMs under development are needed to determine whether these compounds can be useful in the treatment of osteoporosis in hypogonadal men.

References

[1] Cummings SR, Melton LJ 3rd. Epidemiology and outcomes of osteoporotic fractures. Lancet 2002;359:1761–7.

[2] Genant HK, Cooper C, Poor G, et al. Interim report and recommendations of the World Health Organization Task-Force for Osteoporosis. Osteoporos Int 1999;10:259–64.

[3] Cooper C, Campion G, Melton LJ. Hip fractures in the elderly: a worldwide projection. Osteoporos Int 1992;2:285–9.

[4] Melton LJ III, Khosla S, Achenbach SJ, et al. Effects of body size and skeletal site on the estimated prevalence of osteoporosis in women and men. Osteoporos Int 2000;11: 977–83.

[5] Schuitt SC, van der Klift M, Weel AE, et al. Fracture incidence and association with bone mineral density in elderly men and women: the Rotterdam Study. Bone 2004;34:195–202.

[6] Johnell O, Kanis JA, Oden A, et al. Predictive value of BMD for hip and other fractures. J Bone Miner Res 2005;20:1185–94.

[7] Cummings SR, Cawthon PM, Ensrud KE, et al. Osteoporotic Fractures in Men (MrOS) Research Groups; Study of Osteoporotic Fractures Research Groups. BMD and risk of hip and nonvertebral fractures in older men: a prospective study and comparison with older women. J Bone Miner Res 2006;21(10):1550–6.

[8] Melton LJ. Epidemiology of fractures. In: Riggs BL, Melton LJ, editors. Osteoporosis: etiology, diagnosis and management. 2nd edition. Philadelphia: Lippincott-Raven Publishers; 1995. p. 225–47.

[9] Melton LJ, Chrischilles EA, Cooper C, et al. How many women have osteoporosis? J Bone Miner Res 1992;7:1005–10.

[10] Kanis JA, Johnell O, Oden A, et al. Long-term risk of osteoporotic fracture in Malmö. Osteoporos Int 2000;11:669–74.

[11] Melton LJ, Atkinson EJ, O'Conner MK, et al. Bone density and fracture risk in men. J Bone Miner Res 1998;13(12):1915–23.

[12] Osteoporosis and men, leaflet from Osteoporosis Australia. Med J Aust 1997;167:51–5.

[13] Melton LJ, O'Fallon WM, Riggs BL. Secular trends in the incidence of hip fractures. Calcif Tissue Int 1987;41:57–64.

[14] Seeman E. Osteoporosis in men. Am J Med 1993;30:S22–8.

[15] Cooper C, Atkinson EJ, O'Fallon WM, et al. Incidence of clinically diagnosed vertebral fractures: a population-based study in Rochester, Minnesota 1985–89. J Bone Miner Res 1992;7:221–7.

[16] Agnusdei D, Gerardi D, Camporeale A, et al. The European vertebral osteoporosis study in Siena, Italy. Bone 1994;16(1S):118S.

[17] Kanis JA, Pitt FA. Epidemiology of osteoporosis. Bone 1992;13:S7–15.

[18] Alffram PA, Bauer CGH. Epidemiology of fractures of the forearm. J Bone Joint Surg Am 1962;44:105–14.

[19] Duan Y, Beck TJ, Wang X-F, et al. Structural and biomechanical basis of sexual dimorphism in femoral neck fragility has its origins in growth and aging. J Bone Miner Res 2003;18:1766–74.

[20] Wang XF, Duan Y, Beck T, et al. Varying contributions of growth and ageing to racial and sex differences in femoral neck structure and strength in old age. Bone 2005;36:978–86.

[21] Seeman E, Bianchi G, Khosla S, et al. Bone fragility in men—where are we? Osteoporos Int 2006;17(11):1577–83.

[22] Riggs BL, Melton LJ III, Robb RA, et al. A population-based study of age and sex differences in bone volumetric density, size, geometry and structure at different skeletal sites. J Bone Miner Res 2004;19:1945–54.

[23] Chavassieux P, Meunier PJ. Histomorphometric approach of bone loss in men. Calcif Tissue Int 2001;69:209–13.

[24] Khosla S. Editorial: Idiopathic osteoporosis—is the osteoblast to blame? J Clin Endocrinol Metab 1997;82:2792–4.

[25] Pernow Y, Granberg B, Saaf M, et al. Osteoblast dysfunction in male idiopathic osteoporosis. Calcif Tissue Int 2006;78:90–7.

[26] Heshmati HM, Khosla S. Idiopathic osteoporosis: a heterogeneous entity. Ann Med Interne (Paris) 1998;149(2):77–81.

[27] Perry HM III, Fallon MD, Bergfeld M, et al. Osteoporosis in young men. Arch Intern Med 1982;142:1295–8.

[28] Resch H, Pietschmann P, Woloszczuk W, et al. Bone mass with biochemical parameters of bone metabolism in men with spinal osteoporosis. J Clin Invest 1992;22:542–5.

[29] Bilezikian JP. Osteoporosis in men. J Clin Endocrinol Metab 1999;84(10):3431–4.

[30] Orwoll ES. Osteoporosis in men. Endocr Rev 1995;16:87–116.

[31] Seeman E. Osteoporosis in men: epidemiology, pathophysiology, and treatment possibilities. Am J Med 1993;95(Suppl 5A):22–8.

[32] Cauley JA, Fullman RL, Stone KL, et al. Mr. OS Research Group. Factors associated with the lumbar spine and proximal femur bone mineral density in older men. Osteoporos Int 2005;16(12):1525–37.

[33] Lau EM, Leung PC, Kwok T, et al. The determinants of bone mineral density in Chinese men—results from Mr. Os (Hong Kong), the first cohort study on osteoporosis in Asian men. Osteoporos Int 2006;17(2):297–303.

[34] Seeman E, Melton LJ III, O'Fallon WM, et al. Risk factors for spinal osteoporosis in men. Am J Med 1983;75:977–82.

[35] Looker AC, Orwoll ES, Johnston CC, et al. Prevalence of low femoral bone density in older US adults from NHANES III. J Bone Miner Res 1997;12:1761–8.

[36] Smith DM, Nance WE, Kang KW, et al. Genetic factors in determining bone mass. J Clin Invest 1973;52:2800–8.

[37] Gennari L, Brandi ML. Genetics of male osteoporosis. Calcif Tissue Int 2001;69(4): 200–4.

[38] Eisman JA. Genetics of osteoporosis. Endocr Rev 1999;20:788–804.

[39] Cohen-Solal ME, Baudoin C, Omouri M, et al. Bone mass in middle-aged osteoporotic men and their relatives: familial effect. J Bone Miner Res 1998;13:1909–14.

[40] Soroko SB, Barrett-Connor E, Edelstein SL, et al. Family history of osteoporosis and bone mineral density at the axial skeleton: the Rancho-Bernardo Study. J Bone Miner Res 1994; 9:761–9.

[41] Diaz MN, O'Neill WO, Silman AJ. European Vertebral Osteoporosis Study Group. The influence of family history of hip fracture on the risk of vertebral deformity in men and women: the European Vertebral Osteoporosis Study. Bone 1997;20:145–9.

[42] Gennari L, Masi L, Merlotti D, et al. A polymorphic CYP19 TTTA repeat influences aromatase activity and estrogen levels in elderly men: effects on bone metabolism. J Clin Endocrinol Metab 2004;89(6):2803–10.

[43] Van Pottelbergh I, Goemaere S, Kaufman JM. Bioavailable estradiol and aromatase gene polymorphism are determinants of bone mineral density changes in men over 70 years of age. J Clin Endocrinol Metab 2003;88(7):3075–81.

[44] Ferrari SL, Deutsch S, Baudoin C, et al. LRP5 gene polymorphisms and idiopathic osteoporosis in men. Bone 2005;37(6):770–5.

[45] Rosen CJ, Kurland ES, Vereault D, et al. An association between serum IGF-1 and a simple sequence repeat in the IGF-1 gene: implications for genetic studies of bone mineral density. J Clin Endocrinol Metab 1998;83:2286–90.

[46] Riggs BL, Khosla S, Melton LJ III. Sex steroids and the construction and conservation of the adult skeleton. Endocr Rev 2002;23(3):279–302.

[47] Harman SM, Metter JF, Tobin JD, et al. Longitudinal effects of aging on serum total and free testosterone levels in healthy men. J Clin Endocrinol Metab 2001;86(2):724–31.

[48] Khosla S, Melton LJ III, Atkinson EJ, et al. Relationship of serum sex steroid levels to longitudinal changes in bone density in young versus elderly men. J Clin Endocrinol Metab 2001;86(8):3555–61.

[49] Gennari L, Merlotti D, Martini G, et al. Longitudinal association between sex hormone levels, bone loss, and bone turnover in elderly men. J Clin Endocrinol Metab 2003; 88(11):5327–33.

[50] Lamberts SWJ, van den Beld AW, van der Lely A. The endocrinology of aging. Science 1997;278:419–24.

[51] Gray A, Feldman HA, McKinlay JB, et al. Age, disease and changing sex hormone levels in middle-aged men: results of the Massachusetts male aging study. J Clin Endocrinol Metab 1991;73:1016–25.

[52] Kaufman JM, Vermeulen A. Declining gonadal function in elderly men. Baillieres Clin Endocrinol Metab 1997;11:289–309.

[53] Orwoll E, Lambert LC, Marshall LM, et al. Testosterone and estradiol among older men. J Clin Endocrinol Metab 2006;91(4):1336–44.

[54] Slemenda CW, Longcope C, Zhou L, et al. Sex steroids and bone mass in older men: positive associations with serum estrogens and negative associations with androgens. J Clin Invest 1997;100(7):1755–9.

[55] Szulc P, Munoz B, Claustrat B, et al. Bioavailable estradiol may be an important determinant of osteoporosis in men. The MINOS Study. J Clin Endocrinol Metab 2001;86(1): 192–9.

[56] Greendale GA, Edelstein S, Barrett-Connor E. Endogenous sex steroids and bone mineral density in older women and men: the Rancho Bernardo Study. J Bone Miner Res 1997; 12(11):1833–43.

[57] Khosla S, Melton LJ III, Atkinson EJ, et al. Relationship of serum sex steroid levels and bone turnover markers with bone mineral density in men and women: a key role for bioavailable estrogen. J Clin Endocrinol Metab 1998;83(7):2266–74.

[58] Ongphiphadhanakul B, Rajatanavin R, Chanprasertyothin S, et al. Serum estradiol and oestrogen-receptor gene polymorphism are associated with bone mineral density independently of serum testosterone in normal males. Clin Endocrinol (Oxf) 1998; 49(6):803–9.

[59] Amin S, Zhang Y, Sawin CT, et al. Association of hypogonadism and estradiol levels with bone mineral density in elderly men from the Framingham study. Ann Intern Med 2000; 133(12):951–63.

[60] Barrett-Connor E, Mueller JE, von Muhlen DG, et al. Low levels of estradiol are associated with vertebral fractures in older men, but not women: the Rancho Bernardo Study. J Clin Endocrinol Metab 2000;85(1):219–23.

[61] Khosla S, Melton LJ 3rd, Riggs BL. Clinical review 144: estrogen and the male skeleton. J Clin Endocrinol Metab 2002;87(4):1443–50.

[62] Khosla S, Melton LJ III, Robb RA, et al. Relationship of volumetric BMD and structural parameters at different skeletal sites to sex steroid levels in men. J Bone Miner Res 2005; 20(5):730–40.

[63] Gennari L, Nuti R, Bilezikian JP. Aromatase activity and bone homeostasis in men. J Clin Endocrinol Metab 2004;89(12):5898–907.

[64] Purohit A, Flanagan AM, Reed MJ. Estrogen synthesis by osteoblast cell lines. Endocrinology 1992;131(4):2027–9.

[65] Tanaka S, Haji M, Nishi Y, et al. Aromatase activity in human osteoblast-like osteosarcoma cell. Calcif Tissue Int 1993;52(2):107–9.

[66] Sasano H, Uzuki M, Sawai T, et al. Aromatase in human bone tissue. J Bone Miner Res 1997;12(9):1416–23.

[67] Schweikert HU, Wolf L, Romalo G. Oestrogen formation from androstenedione in human bone. Clin Endocrinol (Oxf) 1995;43(1):37–42.

[68] Simpson EV, Davis SR. Minireview: aromatase and the regulation of estrogen biosynthesis—some new perspectives. Endocrinology 2001;142(11):4589–94.

[69] Labrie F, Belanger A, Luu-The V, et al. DHEA and the intracrine formation of androgens and estrogens in peripheral target tissue: its role during aging. Steroids 1998; 63(5–6):322–8.

[70] Ensrud KE, Fullman RL, Barrett-Connor E, et al. Osteoporotic Fractures in Men Study Research Group. Voluntary weight reduction in older men increases hip bone loss: the osteoporotic fractures in men study. J Clin Endocrinol Metab 2005;90(4):1998–2004.

[71] Ensrud KE, Lewis CE, Lambert LC, et al. Osteoporotic Fractures in Men MrOS Study Research Group. Endogenous sex steroids, weight change and rates of hip bone loss in older men: the MrOS study. Osteoporos Int 2006;17(9):1329–36.

[72] Rosen CJ, Donahue LR, Hunter SJ. Insulin-like growth factors and bone: the osteoporosis connection. Proc Soc Exp Biol Med 1994;206:83–102.

[73] Pfeilshifter J, Scheidt-Nave C, Leidig-Bruckner G, et al. Relationship between circulating insulin-like growth factor components and sex hormones in a population-based sample of 50- to 80-year-old men and women. J Clin Endocrinol Metab 1996;81:2534–40.

[74] Crave JC, Lejeune H, Brebant C, et al. Differential effects of insulin-like growth factor I on the production of plasma steroid-binding globulins by human hepatoblastoma-derived (HepG2) cells. J Clin Endocrinol Metab 1995;80:1283–9.

[75] Bateman TA, Zimmerman RJ, Ayers RA, et al. Histomorphometric, physical, and mechanical effects of spaceflight and insulin-like growth factor-I on rat long bones. Bone 1998;23: 527–35.

[76] Kurland ES, Roson CJ, Cosman F, et al. Insulin-like growth factor-1 men with idiopathic osteoporosis. J Clin Endocrinol Metab 1997;82:2799–805.

[77] Ljunghall S, Johansson AG, Burman P, et al. Low plasma levels of insulin-like growth factor 1 (IGF-1) in male patients with idiopathic osteoporosis. J Intern Med 1992;232:59–64.

[78] Kurland ES, Chan FKW, Rosen CJ, et al. Normal growth hormone secretory reserve in men with idiopathic osteoporosis and reduced circulating levels of insulin-like growth factor-1. J Clin Endocrinol Metab 1998;83:2576–9.

[79] Khosla S, Riggs BL, Atkinson EJ, et al. Effects of sex and age on bone microstructure at the ultradistal radius: a population-based noninvasive in vivo assessment. J Bone Miner Res 2006;21:124–31.

[80] Khosla S, Melton LJ 3rd, Achenbach SJ, et al. Hormonal and biochemical determinants of trabecular microstructure at the ultradistal radius in women and men. J Clin Endocrinol Metab 2006;91:885–91.

[81] Boullion R, Bex M, Vanderschueren D, et al. Estrogen are essential for male pubertal periosteal expansion. J Clin Endocrinol Metab 2004;89(12):6025–9.

[82] Manolagas SC, Kousteni S, Jilka RL. Sex steroids and bone. Recent Prog Horm Res 2002; 57:385–409.

[83] Kousteni S, Chen JR, Bellido T, et al. Reversal of bone loss in mice by nongenotropic signaling of sex steroids. Science 2002;298(5594):843–6.

[84] Orwoll E. Assessing bone density in men. J Bone Miner Res 2000;15:1867–70.

[85] Lewiecki EM, Watts NB, McClung MR, et al. International Society for Clinical Densitometry. Official positions of the international society for clinical densitometry. J Clin Endocrinol Metab 2004;89:3651–5.

[86] Greenspan SL, Parker RA, Ferguson L, et al. Early changes in biochemical markers of bone turnover predict the long-term response to alendronate therapy in representative elderly women: a randomized clinical trial. J Bone Miner Res 1998;13:1431–8.

[87] Ravn P, Clemmesen B, Christiansen C. Biochemical markers can predict the response in bone mass during alendronate treatment in early postmenopausal women. Bone 1999;24: 237–44.

[88] Szulc P, Garnero P, Marchand F, et al. Biochemical markers of bone formation reflect endosteal bone loss in elderly men-MINOS study. Bone 2005;36(1):13–21.

[89] Kiebzak GM, Beinart GA, Perser K, et al. Undertreatment of osteoporosis in men with hip fracture. Arch Intern Med 2002;162:2217–22.

[90] Feldstein AF, Elmer PJ, Orwoll E, et al. Bone mineral density measurement and treatment for osteoporosis in older individuals with fractures: A gap in evidence-based practice guideline. Arch Intern Med 2003;163:2165–72.

[91] Feldstein AC, Nichols G, Orwoll E, et al. The near absence of osteoporosis treatment in older men with fractures. Osteoporos Int 2005;16(8):953–62.

[92] Bilezikian JP. Panel Members. Optimal calcium intake: statement of the consensus development panel on optimal calcium intake. JAMA 1994;272:1942–8.

[93] Food and Nutrition Board, Institute of Medicine, National Research Council. Dietary reference intakes. Washington, DC: National Academy Press; 1998.

[94] Orwoll ES. Treatment of osteoporosis in men. Calcif Tissue Int 2004;75:114–9.

[95] Orwoll E, Ettinger M, Weiss S, et al. Alendronate for the treatment of osteoporosis in men. N Engl J Med 2000;43:604–10.

[96] Ringe ID, Faber H, Dorst A. Alendronate treatment of established primary osteoporosis in men: results of a 2-year prospective study. J Clin Endocrinol Metab 2001;86:5252–5.

[97] Weber TJ, Drezner MK. Effect of alendronate on bone mineral density in male idiopathic osteoporosis. Metabolism 2001;50:912–5.

[98] Gonnelli S, Cepollaro C, Montagnani A, et al. Alendronate treatment in men with primary osteoporosis: a three-year longitudinal study. Calcif Tissue Int 2003;73:133–9.

[99] Ringe JD, Dorst A, Faber H, et al. Alendronate treatment of established primary osteoporosis in men: 3-year results of a prospective, comparative, two-arm study. Rheumatol Int 2004;24(2):110–3.

[100] Ho YV, Frauman AG, Thomson W, et al. Effects of alendronate on bone density in men with primary and secondary osteoporosis. Osteoporos Int 2000;11:98–101.

[101] Iwamoto J, Takeda T, Sato Y, et al. Comparison of the effect of alendronate on lumbar bone mineral density and bone turnover in men and postmenopausal women with osteoporosis. Clin Rheumatol 2006;26:161–7.

[102] Borgstrom F, Johnell O, Jonsson B, et al. Cost effectiveness of alendronate for the treatment of male osteoporosis in Sweden. Bone 2004;4(6):1064–71.

[103] Sawka AM, Papaioannou A, Adachi JD, et al. Does alendronate reduce the risk of fracture in men? A meta-analysis incorporating prior knowledge of anti-fracture efficacy in women. BMC Musculoskelet Disord 2005;6:39.

[104] Cranney A, Wells G, Willan A, et al. Meta-analyses of therapies for postmenopausal osteoporosis. II. Meta-analysis of alendronate for the treatment of postmenopausal women. Endocr Rev 2002;23(4):508–16.

[105] Miller P, Orwoll E, MacIntyre B, et al. Treatment with alendronate 70 mg once weekly for 12 months increases BMD and decreases biochemical markers of bone turnover in men with osteoporosis. Presented at the Second International Conference on Osteoporosis in Men. Genoa (Italy), October 4, 2003.

[106] Greenspan S, Field–Munves E, Tonino R, et al. Tolerability of once-weekly alendronate in patients with osteoporosis: a randomized, double-blind, placebocontrolled study. Mayo Clin Proc 2002;77:1044–52.

[107] Ringe JD, Faber H, Farahmand P, et al. Efficacy of risedronate in men with primary and secondary osteoporosis: results of a 1-year study. Rheumatol Int 2006;26(5):427–31.

[108] de Nijs RN, Jacobs JW, Lems WF, et al. Alendronate or alfacalcidol in glucocorticoid-induced osteoporosis. N Engl J Med 2006;355(7):675–84.

[109] Eshed V, Benbassat CA, Laron Z. Effect of alendronate on bone mineral density in adult patients with Laron syndrome (primary growth hormone insensitivity). Growth Horm IGF Res 2006;16(2):119–24.

[110] Shimon I, Eshed V, Doolman R, et al. Alendronate for osteoporosis in men with androgen-repleted hypogonadism. Osteoporos Int 2005;16(12):1591–6.

[111] Smith BJ, Laslett LL, Pile KD, et al. Randomized controlled trial of alendronate in airways disease and low bone mineral density. Chron Respir Dis 2004;1(3):131–7.

[112] Millonig G, Graziadei IW, Eichler D, et al. Alendronate in combination with calcium and vitamin D prevents bone loss after orthotopic liver transplantation: a prospective single-center study. Liver Transpl 2005;11(8):960–6.

[113] Shane E, Addesso V, Namerow PB, et al. Alendronate versus calcitriol for the prevention of bone loss after cardiac transplantation. N Engl J Med 2004;350(8):767–76.

[114] Smith MR. Management of treatment-related osteoporosis in men with prostate cancer. Cancer Treat Rev 2003;29(3):211–8.

[115] Sato Y, Iwamoto J, Kanoko T, et al. Risedronate sodium therapy for prevention of hip fracture in men 65 years or older after stroke. Arch Intern Med 2005;165(15):1743–8.

[116] Lange U, Illgner U, Teichmann J, et al. Skeletal benefit after one year of risedronate therapy in patients with rheumatoid arthritis and glucocorticoid-induced osteoporosis: a prospective study. Int J Clin Pharmacol Res 2004;24(2–3):33–8.

[117] Reid DM, Adami S, Devogelaer JP, et al. Risedronate increases bone density and reduces vertebral fracture risk within one year in men on corticosteroid therapy. Calcif Tissue Int 2001;69(4):242–7.

[118] Reid DM, Hughes RA, Laan RF, et al. Efficacy and safety of daily risedronate in the treatment of corticosteroid-induced osteoporosis in men and women: a randomized trial. European Corticosteroid-Induced Osteoporosis Treatment Study. J Bone Miner Res 2000;15(6): 1006–13.

[119] Physicians' desk reference: PDR. 57th edition. Montvale (NJ): Thomson PDR; 2003. p. 3550.

[120] Kurland ES, Cosman F, McMahon DJ, et al. Parathyroid hormone as a therapy for idiopathic osteoporosis in men: effects on bone mineral density and bone markers. J Clin Endocrinol Metab 2000;85(9):3069–76.

[121] Orwoll ES, Scheele WH, Paul S, et al. The effect of teriparatide [human parathyroid hormone (1-34)] therapy on bone density in men with osteoporosis. J Bone Miner Res 2003; 18(1):9–17.

[122] Misof BM, Roschger P, Cosman F, et al. Effects of intermittent parathyroid hormone administration on bone mineralization density in iliac crest biopsies from patients with osteoporosis: a paired study before and after treatment. J Clin Endocrinol Metab 2003;88(3): 1150–6.

[123] Kaufman JM, Orwoll E, Goemaere S, et al. Teriparatide effects on vertebral fractures and bone mineral density in men with osteoporosis: treatment and discontinuation of therapy. Osteoporos Int 2005;16(5):510–6.

[124] Bilezikian JP, Kurland ES. Therapy of male osteoporosis with parathyroid hormone. Calcif Tissue Int 2001;69(4):248–51.

[125] Hodsman AB, Bauer DC, Dempster DW, et al. Parathyroid hormone and teriparatide for the treatment of osteoporosis: a review of the evidence and suggested guidelines for its use. Endocr Rev 2005;26(5):688–703.

[126] Finkelstein JS, Hayes A, Hunzelman JL, et al. The effects of parathyroid hormone, alendronate, or both in men with osteoporosis. N Engl J Med 2003;349:1216–26.

[127] Kurland ES, Heller SL, Diamond B, et al. The importance of bisphosphonate therapy in maintaining bone mass in men after therapy with teriparatide [human parathyroid hormone(1-34)]. Osteoporos Int 2004;15(12):992–7.

[128] Bilezikian JP, Rubin MR. Combination/sequential therapies for anabolic and antiresorptive skeletal agents for osteoporosis. Curr Osteoporos Rep 2006;4(1):5–13.

[129] Behre HM, Kliesch S, Leifke E, et al. Long-term effect of testosterone therapy on bone mineral density in hypogonadal men. J Clin Endocrinol Metab 1997;82:2386–90.

[130] Snyder PJ, Peachey H, Berlin JA, et al. Effects of testosterone replacement in hypogonadal men. J Clin Endocrinol Metab 2000;85(8):2670–7.

[131] Nair KS, Rizza RA, O'Brien P. DHEA in elderly women and DHEA or testosterone in elderly men. N Engl J Med 2006;355(16):1647–59.

[132] Smith MR, McGovern FJ, Zietman AL, et al. Pamidronate to prevent bone loss during androgen deprivation therapy for prostate cancer. N Engl J Med 2001;345:948–55.

[133] Tracz MJ, Sideras K, Bolona ER, et al. Testosterone use in men and its effects on bone health. A systematic review and meta-analysis of randomized placebo-controlled trials. J Clin Endocrinol Metab 2006;91(6):2011–6.

[134] Anderson FH, Francis RM, Peaston RT, et al. Androgen supplementation in eugonadal men with osteoporosis: effects of six months' treatment on markers of bone formation and resorption. J Bone Miner Res 1997;12(3):472–8.

[135] Kim IY, Seong DH, Kim BC, et al. Raloxifene, a selective estrogen receptor modulator, induces apoptosis in androgen-responsive human prostate cancer cell line LNCaP through an androgen-independent pathway. Cancer Res 2002;62(18):3649–53.

[136] Vandekerckhove P, Lilford R, Vail A, et al. Clomiphene or tamoxifen for idiopathic oligo/asthenospermia. Cochrane Database Syst Rev 2000;2:CD000151.

[137] Doran PM, Riggs BL, Atkinson EJ, et al. Effects of raloxifene, a selective estrogen receptor modulator, on bone turnover markers and serum sex steroid and lipid levels in elderly men. J Bone Miner Res 2001;16(11):2118–25.

[138] Uebelhart B, Herrmann F, Pavo I, et al. Raloxifene treatment is associated with increased serum estradiol and decreased bone remodeling in healthy middle-aged men with low sex hormone levels. J Bone Miner Res 2004;19(9):1518–24.
[139] Duschek EJ, Gooren LJ, Netelenbos C. Effects of raloxifene on gonadotrophins, sex hormones, bone turnover and lipids in healthy elderly men. Eur J Endocrinol 2004;150(4): 539–46.

ELSEVIER
SAUNDERS

Endocrinol Metab Clin N Am
36 (2007) 421–434

ENDOCRINOLOGY
AND METABOLISM
CLINICS
OF NORTH AMERICA

Hormonal Implications in the Development and Treatment of Prostate Cancer

Christopher Ip, MD[a], Simon J. Hall, MD[a,b],*

[a]Department of Urology, Mount Sinai School of Medicine, Box 1272,
1 Gustave L. Levy Place, New York, NY 10029, USA
[b]Deane Prostate Health & Research Center, Mount Sinai School of Medicine,
1 Gustave L. Levy Place, New York, NY 10029, USA

The prostate, an accessory sex organ, is a walnut-sized gland located just below the bladder neck. A passageway through it encompasses the first part of the posterior urethra. It secretes approximately 30% of the ejaculate, supplying nutrients and enzymes that are believed to aid in liquefying the thicker secretions of the seminal vesicles. The normal development of the prostate is dependent on the production and recognition of androgens, particularly dihydrotestosterone (DHT). Testosterone is taken up by cells within the gland and converted by 5α-reductase to DHT; this activity is more apparent in stromal than epithelial cells [1]. Disturbances in this pathway through loss-of-function mutations in the androgen receptor (AR) or 5α-reductase result in the lack of prostate development. Furthermore, it has long been known that eunuchs (surgically castrated men) have small prostates and do not develop prostatic enlargement or benign prostatic hypertrophy (BPH), which are generally observed with aging [2].

It has been known since the 1940s that prostate cancer retains a dependence on the androgen pathway after the successful use of surgical castration and estrogens to treat metastatic prostate cancer. The exact role of androgens in promoting the malignant pathway remains unknown and controversial. In this article, the conflicting data concerning the androgen axis and prostate cancer development are reviewed in addition to how this pathway may be exploited to prevent the development of prostate cancer. The expanding role of hormone ablative therapy alone or in conjunction

---

* Corresponding author. Department of Urology, Box 1272, Mount Sinai School of Medicine, 1 Gustave L. Levy Place, New York, NY 10029.
E-mail address: Simon.Hall@mssm.edu (S.J. Hall).

0889-8529/07/$ - see front matter © 2007 Elsevier Inc. All rights reserved.
doi:10.1016/j.ecl.2007.03.009

with standard therapies is reviewed, and the controversies of timing of therapy and the completeness of ablation and its use on an intermittent basis are discussed.

Androgenic pathway and prostate cancer risk

The role of serum androgens

The concept that androgenic stimulation is a significant factor in the development of prostate cancer has been studied for many years with disparate outcomes. Numerous older studies have not demonstrated any difference between levels of testosterone in men who have prostate cancer versus control subjects [3–6]. Likewise, more recent studies have not found any increased risk of prostate cancer based on levels of testosterone, free testosterone, DHT, or sex-hormone–binding globulin [7–9]. In contrast, several other studies have noted positive correlations between levels of androgens and prostate cancer risk. In these studies, elevated androstenedione, higher testosterone conversion rates, elevated plasma testosterone levels, and elevated free testosterone levels increased the risk of cancer [10–13]. These seemingly contradictory data may be partly due to small sample size in some instances, the diurnal fluctuations of androgen levels, and adequate screening of control groups for cancer by prostate-specific antigen (PSA) testing or biopsies. Therefore, it is hard to correlate cancer risk with elevated levels of androgen.

The possibility that androgens can promote carcinogenesis is a clinically relevant discussion when treating hypogonadal men with testosterone replacement. It remains a concern that testosterone supplementation may "cause" prostate cancer versus unmasking a cancer already in existence. Because PSA production is dependent on androgens, it would be expected that PSAs rise in response to replacement. Because the vast majority of cancers are diagnosed by changes in PSA, it is not surprising that this therapy results in higher numbers of cancers being diagnosed. Although a large–scale, prospective study addressing this question has not been performed, results of small and relatively short-term studies have not noted any enhanced diagnosis of prostate cancer with treatment, even in higher-risk patients, such as those who have prostatic intraepithelial neoplasia [14–16]. PSA levels increase after therapy, although these are small incremental rises seen over the first 3 to 6 months of less than 0.5 ng/ml [17]; elevations of more than this level should result in a prostate biopsy to rule out an underlying malignancy.

The role of androgen receptor function

Studies have been exploring the potential role of mutations of the AR in the initiation of prostate cancers. Within exon A of the AR gene, there exists a highly conserved CAG (glutamine) repeat, the length of which seems to be variable based on racial backgrounds [18]. The average length is longest in Asian Americans (22.4) and shortest for African Americans (20.1), with Caucasians in between (22.0). Because it has been demonstrated that ARs containing shorter repeats have higher transactivating potentials [19], this ethnic difference in AR genetics may explain the same differences in prostate cancer incidence between the races. Early studies indicated that shorter CAG repeats predicted higher incidence of cancers [20], but recent studies have not shown any link between CAG repeat length and cancer risk [9,21]. Therefore, there is no strong link between the activity of the androgenic pathway, as measured by AR activity, and enhanced or inhibited prostate cancer development.

Inhibition of the androgenic pathway as preventative therapy for prostate cancer

Only recently has the concept of exploiting the dependence of prostate cancer on androgens been applied as prevention. This is due in large part to the significant side effects of androgen ablative therapy as outlined later in this article, which preclude its acceptance in this setting. In its place, studies have focused on a lesser form of androgen deprivation, the inhibition of 5α-reductase, which is more commonly used as a treatment for symptomatic BPH. The objective of the Prostate Cancer Prevention Trial was to determine whether finasteride (Proscar) could reduce the prevalence of prostate cancer among healthy men. Over 18,000 men were randomly assigned to treatment with finasteride or placebo for 7 years. Men were biopsied for changes in PSA or rectal examination or at the end of the trial. The study found that 24.4% (1147/5142) of men who received placebo were diagnosed with prostate cancer compared with 18.4% (803/4368) who received finasteride, a 25% overall reduction in diagnoses [22]. While reducing the number of positive diagnoses, finasteride therapy increased the likelihood of being diagnosed with higher-grade cancers; 37% (280/757) were Gleason score 7, 8, 9, or 10, compared with 22.2% (237/1068) of the placebo group. The central question concerns whether this difference was the result of higher incidence of more aggressive, difficult-to-treat cancer caused by finasteride therapy or an effective decrease in the risk of low-grade cancers with 5α-reductase inhibition. Another theory is that finasteride changes the morphologic appearance of the glandular architecture, resulting in an artificial high-grade appearance of cancers. There is a body of literature indicating that this is not the case [23]. Due to this controversy, the use of finasteride as preventative therapy for prostate cancer is not being advocated, but this concept is under investigation. There is an ongoing study (the REDUCE trial) that will compare dutasteride, a dual 5α-reductase inhibitor, with placebo in preventing the development of prostate cancer in men who have a history of an elevated PSA and a negative prostate biopsy over a course of 4 years [24].

Androgen ablative therapy for prostate cancer

Hormonal ablative therapy has traditionally been used as palliative therapy in patients who have clinically manifest metastatic disease, usually to the bone. Some of the earliest debates about the timing of therapy have yet to be resolved. Furthermore, the widespread use of PSA has resulted in two important influences on the use of hormonal therapy. First, it has resulted in a dramatic stage migration; the finding of metastases at initial diagnosis is uncommon [25]. Second, its ability to detect recurrent disease after definitive therapy and before there is clinical evidence of disease has resulted in a new target for therapy—rising PSA posttreatment—which has added pressure from physician and patient to institute therapy earlier.

Historical overview

Huggins and Hodges [26] are credited with first exploiting the dependence of prostate cancer on testosterone through studies of orchiectomy and estrogen in patients who had metastatic disease 45 years after it had been reported that symptomatic BPH could be successfully treated with orchiectomy [27]. Much of our understanding and teaching of the use of hormonal manipulations for the treatment of advanced prostate cancer came from the Veterans Administration Cooperative Urological Research Group's randomized studies performed from 1960 to 1975 [28]. The largest of these studies, VACURG I, randomized 1105 men who had locally advanced or metastatic disease to placebo, orchiectomy, 5 mg diethylstilbestrol (DES), and orchiectomy plus DES. Patients in the placebo arm were crossed over to hormonal therapy when progression was detected. This study demonstrated equal survival for placebo and orchiectomy, with reduced survival for those treated with DES due to significant cardiovascular toxicities [28]. These findings have been the bedrock supporting the widely held view that hormonal therapy does not enhance survival. Furthermore, with equal survival in patients receiving immediate therapy and those in the placebo arm who later crossed over to therapy with disease progression, the concept that earlier intervention holds no benefits was born.

Methods of hormonal therapy

Orchiectomy

The use of estrogens fell out of favor due the effects of their significant toxicity, especially cardiovascular disease. This is true for the 5-mg dose of DES; in contrast, the 1-mg dose demonstrated efficacy without significant toxicity in a smaller VACURG study [28] and is often discussed as a potential therapy in many circles, although it is difficult to obtain in the United States and thus is rarely used. Orchiectomy became the standard approach to treating advanced prostate cancer. It is a safe procedure, performed under local anesthesia via a transscrotal incision, which results in rapid reduction of testosterone to castrate levels. A major drawback to this approach is the profound adverse psychologic impact it has on the patient, which is a significant reason underlying the subsequent adoption of medical castration. Furthermore, orchiectomy has none of the flexibility required of hormonal therapy in the modern era necessary for the neoadjuvant/adjuvant or intermittent approach.

Gonadotropin-releasing hormone agonists

The most popular method of androgen ablation in the United States is the use of gonadotropin-releasing hormone (GnRH) agonists leuprolide acetate (Lupron) or goserelin acetate (Zoladex). These drugs bind to receptors in the pituitary gland, resulting in a rise of luteinizing hormone and follicle-stimulating hormone production, which results in a surge of testosterone production. The constant stimulation by the agonist depletes stocks of luteinizing hormone and downregulates expression of GnRH receptors to shut down production of testosterone by the Leydig cells. The surge of testosterone occurs at 10 to 14 days, and castrate levels of testosterone are achieved by 4 weeks [29]. The main side effects of treatment are hot flashes, lethargy, loss of libido, impotence, redistribution of body fat to the abdomen, weight gain, and gynecomastia. More recent attention has noted the induction of osteoporosis with even short courses of therapy amenable to treatment with bisphosphonate therapy [30]. Furthermore, there is an emerging body of evidence indicating that hormone ablative therapy induces insulin resistance [31] and may predispose patients to developing diabetes and cardiovascular disease [32].

Antiandrogens

Although GnRH agonists and orchiectomy result in castrate levels of testosterone, detectable levels of androgen produced by the adrenal glands remain that could support survival of androgen-sensitive cells under conditions of androgen ablation. The commonly used nonsteroidal antiandrogens are flutamide (Eulexin), nilutamide (Nilandron), and bicalutamide (Casodex). Each has unique side effects that have limited their use for flutamide (diarrhea) and nilutamide (ocular effects). Bicalutamide is a once-a-day drug with an acceptable side-effect profile. Most commonly, an antiandrogen is used to cover the surge of testosterone induced during the first 2 weeks of therapy. This is especially important for men who have symptomatic locally advanced or metastatic cancers who could experience symptoms without antiandrogen blockade.

Controversies in the use of androgen ablative therapy

Use of antiandrogens

Complete androgen ablation

There are differing viewpoints as to the duration of use of antiandrogens in combination with GnRH agonists. The controversy lies in how long to maintain complete androgen blockade. The landmark study in support of combined therapy randomized over 600 men to leuprolide plus flutamide to leuprolide plus placebo. Combination therapy proved superior in terms of time to progression (median 16.5 versus 13.9 months) and survival (median 35.6 versus 28.3 months) over monotherapy [33]. A large confirmatory study comparing orchiectomy versus orchiectomy plus flutamide failed to demonstrate a statistically significant enhancement of survival with complete androgen blockade [34]. The major difference between these two studies lies in the mechanism of androgen ablation. With orchiectomy, there is no flare phenomenon, so the comparison involving flutamide is a true study of complete androgen ablation. In contrast in the leuprolide study, the flare response was not blocked in patients receiving placebo. Therefore, the difference in outcome for patients receiving antiandrogen may not have been due to positive benefits of total androgen blockade but may have been due to disease progression through a few weeks of unblocked testosterone surge resulting in a poorer outcome for patients receiving placebo. The study noted a trend for seeing the effect of flutamide in protecting against disease progression and pain within the first 4 to 12 weeks of therapy, supporting this interpretation.

Meta-analyses of studies of complete androgen ablation have indicated a small benefit of the combined approach. Denis and Murphy [35] reported on phase III studies involving over 5000 patients, demonstrating a 7% survival enhancement in favor of combined therapy. However, a meta-analysis from the Prostate Cancer Trialist's Collaborative Group indicated a modest but not statistically improvement in survival in favor of combined therapy [36]. The slight improvement in survival in favor of combined androgen ablation must be balanced against the additional side effects (gynecomastia and hepatic toxicity) and cost associated with therapy. The lack of definitive convincing data has yielded two options for patients who have advanced disease: total androgen blockade from the initiation of therapy versus adding the antiandrogen when the PSA begins to rise.

Antiandrogen monotherapy

The use of antiandrogens alone has been explored as an alternate choice because it does not decrease testosterone levels and therefore spares the intensity and number of side effects experienced. All of these studies have focused on bicalutamide because of its easy dosing and relatively benign side-effect profile. An important initial question should address a comparison of outcome between castration and antiandrogen monotherapy. A group of European investigators has studied this issue in 480 patients who had locally advanced, nonmetastatic prostate cancer. The most recent publication reported on 6-year follow-up, noting no difference in time to progression or survival between the two treatment conditions [37]. The side effect profile favored bicalutamide, especially in terms of maintaining libido and sexual functioning and an overall sense of physical capacity. The major side effect of bicalutamide is gynecomastia and breast pain, which can be reduced with a short course of radiation therapy. A second study compared total androgen blockade with bicalutamide in 220 patients, approximately half of whom had metastatic disease [38]. The study design also included a cross-over arm to castration for patients taking bicalutamide who experienced disease progression. The study was underpowered due to poor accrual but indicated no difference in overall time to progression or survival between the treatments, although subgroup analysis suggested that monotherapy was inferior to castration in patients who had high-grade disease. Although these studies suggest equal efficacy between castration and antiandrogen monotherapy in the absence of metastatic disease, there is insufficient experience in patients who have metastatic disease to endorse its use instead of traditional hormone ablative therapy.

Antiandrogen monotherapy has also been explored in conjunction with standard therapies in higher-risk patients, much like tamoxifen has been used in patients who have localized breast cancer. The largest experience has been reported by the Early Prostate Cancer trial program, enrolling over 8000 men divided into three different studies numbered 23, 24, and 25. Trial 23 was performed in the United States and randomized patients to 2 years of bicalutamide or placebo after radical prostatectomy (80%) or radiation therapy (20%). At median follow-up of 7.4 years, there was no difference in time to progression or survival between the two groups [39]. Only 15% of placebo patients had any degree of progression in this time frame, indicating that in this is a low-risk group a short course of therapy is unlikely to yield any benefit. Trial 25 enrolled mostly patients who opted for watchful waiting; bicalutamide after 7 years of follow-up prolonged time to progression but had no impact on survival [40]. Trial 24 was similar to 23 but included more higher-risk patients who had locally advanced disease; it demonstrated overall the same result. Subgroup analyses by stage and type of standard therapy noted enhancements in survival for patients treated with radiotherapy only, especially those who had locally advanced disease; the trend observed for radical prostatectomy was the opposite [40]. No information on tumor grade or PSA levels was recorded to further substratify which patients this therapy may help.

Given the large amount of data that has not shown any survival benefit, antiandrogen monotherapy must be prescribed with caution. In clinical practice, its use is limited to patients who have rising PSA after surgery or radiation therapy without evidence of metastasis who want to spare libido and maintain a better sense of physical well-being, with the understanding that it may not have an impact on survival.

Timing of hormone ablative therapy

One of the longest discussion points in using hormone therapy in prostate cancer has centered on the timing of treatment initiation. The original VA studies had included a crossover arm in men treated with placebo, demonstrating no decreased survival with delayed therapy compared with immediate therapy [28]. For years, therefore, dogma had dictated that hormone therapy could be held until patients experienced symptoms from advanced disease. Several studies have challenged this concept. The Medical Research Council in the United Kingdom randomized 934 patients who had locally advanced or asymptomatic metastatic prostate cancer to immediate hormone therapy or delayed treatment until patients became symptomatic or clearly progressed by radiographs or later rapid PSA rise. In the deferred group, treatment was initiated for local progression almost as frequently as for the development of metastatic disease. Disease progression from M0 to M1 disease occurred more rapidly in deferred patients [41]. Furthermore, complications of disease progression, including pathologic fracture, spinal cord compression, ureteric obstruction, and urinary retention, were twice as common in deferred patients. Patients were more likely to die from prostate cancer in the deferred arm, although the difference in survival was apparent only for patients who began in the M0 group [41]. These conclusions have been challenged due to the lack of consistency in instituting treatment of patients in the delayed group; in some cases, they were never treated before they died. A second study randomized men found to have lymph-node–positive disease at the time of radical prostatectomy to immediate hormone therapy versus delayed therapy [42]. At a median follow-up of nearly 12 years, immediate therapy strongly influenced progression-free survival, cancer-specific survival, and overall survival. Death from prostate cancer occurred in seven (15%) of the patients treated with immediate androgen deprivation therapy and 25 (49%) of the patients in the observed group. The researchers noticed an increase in the number of deaths not related to prostate cancer in the immediately treated group (10 patients) relative to the observed group (three patients). Although this study shows a benefit from early therapy, it has been criticized for being underpowered; the original study was to enroll 350 patients but was closed at 98 due to poor accrual. A subgroup analysis of patients who had node positive prostate cancer in RTOG 85-31 was treated with radiation therapy plus continuous hormone ablation versus radiation therapy followed by hormonal ablation at progression. Patients maintained on hormone therapy versus those who started treatment upon disease progression experienced improvements in biochemical control, progression to metastasis, and absolute survival (9 years follow-up: 62% versus 38% alive) [43]. Advocates for the early use of hormone therapy point to this evidence as supporting its use, especially before evidence of visceral or bone metastases. However, other studies have not shown such strong progression-free or cancer-specific survival that would favor early treatment in similar patient groups [44]. Furthermore, these studies focused on men who had locally advanced or lymph-node positive disease; it is unclear how this debate affects men who have rising PSAs as the only evidence of disease after radical prostatectomy or radiation therapy and who have significantly lower tumor burden and may have years before clinical manifestation of metastasis appears [45].

Neoadjuvant-adjuvant hormonal therapy

To enhance the outcomes of local therapy, hormone therapy has been combined with radiation therapy and radical prostatectomy. When combined with surgery, 3 months of neoadjuvant androgen deprivation decreases the rate of positive surgical margins, normally an indicator predictive of PSA recurrence, from 48% to 18% [46]. This had no impact on the likelihood of PSA recurrence at 5 years [47]. The lengthening of hormone therapy to 8 months did not have any further impact on PSA recurrence rates beyond those seen with 3 months of treatment, indicating that adding hormone therapy in the setting of radical prostatectomy seems to have no benefit on disease recurrence [48].

In contrast, numerous studies have noted a strong benefit of combining hormone therapy with radiation therapy in moderate- and high-risk patients. In a randomized study, 70 Gy of external radiation therapy was compared with radiation therapy plus 6 months of hormone ablative therapy in moderate-risk patients. After relatively short follow-up, the estimated overall 5-year survival was 88% for the combined treatment group versus 78% for the treatment group receiving radiation alone [49]. The likelihood of receiving salvage therapy for recurrence at 5 years was 18% in the combination group versus 43% in the group treated with radiation alone. Similar positive findings have been noted in high-risk patients in large United States and European studies. The most widely quoted data stem from Bolla [50], who reported a European Organisation for Research and Treatment of Cancer study comparing radiation therapy alone versus radiation plus 3 years of hormone ablative therapy in high-risk patients [50]. At median follow-up of 5.5 years, combination therapy resulted in better outcomes in terms of disease progression (13% versus 43%), development of metastases (9.8% versus 29.2%), clinical disease-free survival (74% versus 40%), and overall survival (78% versus 62%). In the United States, there have been two large studies, RTOG 86-10 and RTOG 85-31; the major differences between these studies is the duration of hormone ablative therapy and the inclusion of patients who had metastatic disease in RTOG 85-31. In RTOG 86-10, patients who had moderate- to high-risk features were randomized to hormone ablative therapy beginning 2 months before starting radiation therapy and continuing during the radiation treatment versus radiation therapy alone. With median follow-up of 6.7 years, androgen ablation has been associated with a reduction in the incidence of distant metastases (34% versus 45%), disease-free survival (33% versus 21%), and cause-specific mortality (23% versus 31%) [51]. Subset analysis indicates that the beneficial effect of short-term androgen ablation appears only in patients who have well differentiated disease with significant improvement in all endpoints, including survival (70% versus 52%). In RTOG 85-31, high-risk patients were randomized to radiation therapy plus continuous hormone therapy versus radiation alone with crossover to hormonal ablative therapy at progression [52]. Among the patients were those who had lymph node involvement (28%) and elevated prostatic acid phosphatase (35%), an indicator of metastatic disease. At a median follow-up of 7.6 years, the calculated rate of disease recurrence, development of metastases, and disease-specific and overall survival favored combination therapy, although the improvement was not as great as reported by Bolla. This is due to the inclusion of patients who had overt systemic disease. There is clear evidence that neoadjuvant hormone therapy has benefits for patients who have higher-risk disease when combined with radiation therapy but not surgery. The critical questions are what is the duration of hormone therapy needed to achieve the enhanced outcomes and who needs the treatment among low-, moderate-, and high-risk patients.

Intermittent androgen deprivation therapy

Although the vast majority of patients respond to hormone ablative therapy, the emergence of the androgen-independent phenotype begins on average within 3 to 4 years of treatment. The specific steps by which this occurs are unknown, but it seems that the AR is central to this process via several mechanisms. These include AR gene amplification, resulting in AR being responsive to subphysiologic levels of androgens. Mutations in the androgen-binding domain may allow other steroids, such as estrogens, glucocorticoids, or antiandrogens, to activate the AR. Finally, the AR might be converted to an "outlaw" receptor, whereby the AR remains phosphorylated in the unbound state, activating downstream targets to maintain growth [53]. Upregulation of the AR is the most common finding in gene arrays of human androgen-independent xenografts [54]. The concept of intermittent hormonal therapy has emerged as a possible way of delaying this evolution. In the Shionogi androgen-dependent mouse mammary carcinoma model [55], castration induces an increase in the proportion of stem cells that are androgen independent; if androgen suppression is stopped earlier, this transformation is delayed, and the cells remain androgen sensitive.

Several phase II clinical trials have explored this concept in patients, most of whom were experiencing relapse solely indicated by PSA recurrence after definitive therapy [56]. Patients are maintained on therapy during the first cycle for 6 to 9 months and are restarted when the PSA rises to 10 ng/mL. The time off therapy averages 12 months, a portion of which patients have a normal testosterone level and regain normal quality of life. In subsequent cycles, the time off therapy becomes shorter, with most patients completing three or four cycles before becoming refractory. These studies are relatively small (fewer than 100 patients) and are heterogeneous in the disease states treated and the timing of therapy and trigger points for reinstituting therapy. There are no survival data comparing outcomes with continuous therapy, so this treatment cannot be recommended for patients who have metastatic disease and as such is generally reserved for PSA-only relapse patients until phase III trials comparing intermittent with continuous therapy are completed.

Summary

Hormonal ablative therapy remains an important weapon in treating men who have prostate cancer. Its use as adjuvant treatment with radiation therapy has yielded positive results in patients who have high-risk disease. Some of the oldest questions concerning who should be treated, when they should be treated, and for how long remain unanswered. Furthermore, the use of PSA has increased the number and time line of men diagnosed with disease recurrence to define a new category of patients who may be treated. The design and execution of appropriate clinical trials to answer these questions are crucial to further improve outcomes for men who have high-risk and metastatic disease.

References

[1] Silver RI, Wiley EL, Thigpen AE, et al. Cell type specific expression of steroid 5 alpha-reductase 2. J Urol 1994;152(2 Pt 1):438–42.
[2] Wilson JD, Roehrborn C. Long-term consequences of castration in men: lessons from the Skoptzy and the eunuchs of the Chinese and Ottoman courts. J Clin Endocrinol Metab 1999;84(12):4324–31.
[3] Meikle AW, Stanish WM. Familial prostatic cancer risk and low testosterone. J Clin Endocrinol Metab 1982;54(6):1104–8.
[4] Ghanadian R, Puah CM, O'Donoghue EP. Serum testosterone and dihydrotestosterone in carcinoma of the prostate. Br J Cancer 1979;39(6):696–9.
[5] Hammond GL, Kontturi M, Vihko P, et al. Serum steroids in normal males and patients with prostatic diseases. Clin Endocrinol 1978;9(2):113–21.
[6] Comstock GW, Gordon GB, Hsing AW. The relationship of serum dehydroepiandrosterone and its sulfate to subsequent cancer of the prostate. Cancer Epidemiol Biomarkers Prev 1993;2(3):219–21.
[7] Chen C, Weiss NS, Stanczyk FZ, et al. Endogenous sex hormones and prostate cancer risk: a case-control study nested within the Carotene and Retinol Efficacy Trial. Cancer Epidemiol Biomarkers Prev 2003;12(12):1410–6.
[8] Stattin P, Lumme S, Tenkanen L, et al. High levels of circulating testosterone are not associated with increased prostate cancer risk: a pooled prospective study. Int J Cancer 2004; 108(3):418–24.

[9] Platz EA, Leitzmann MF, Rifai N, et al. Sex steroid hormones and the androgen receptor gene CAG repeat and subsequent risk of prostate cancer in the prostate-specific antigen era. Cancer Epidemiol Biomarkers Prev 2005;14(5):1262–9.

[10] Barrett-Connor E, Garland C, McPhillips JB, et al. A prospective, population-based study of androstenedione, estrogens, and prostatic cancer. Cancer Res 1990;50(1):169–73.

[11] Meikle AW, Smith JA, Stringham JD. Production, clearance, and metabolism of testosterone in men with prostatic cancer. Prostate 1987;10(1):25–31.

[12] Gann PH, Hennekens CH, Ma J, et al. Prospective study of sex hormone levels and risk of prostate cancer. J Natl Cancer Inst 1996;88(16):1118–26.

[13] Parsons JK, Carter HB, Platz EA, et al. Serum testosterone and the risk of prostate cancer: potential implications for testosterone therapy. Cancer Epidemiol Biomarkers Prev 2005; 14(9):2257–60.

[14] Thorpe JF, Jain S, Marczylo TH, et al. A review of phase III clinical trials of prostate cancer chemoprevention. Ann R Coll Surg Engl 2007;89(3):207–11.

[15] Rhoden EL, Morgentaler A. Testosterone replacement therapy in hypogonadal men at high risk for prostate cancer: results of 1 year of treatment in men with prostatic intraepithelial neoplasia. J Urol 2003;170(6 Pt 1):2348–51.

[16] Wang C, Cunningham G, Dobs A, et al. Long-term testosterone gel (AndroGel) treatment maintains beneficial effects on sexual function and mood, lean and fat mass, and bone mineral density in hypogonadal men. J Clin Endocrinol Metab 2004;89(5):2085–98.

[17] Rhoden EL, Morgentaler A. Risks of testosterone-replacement therapy and recommendations for monitoring. N Engl J Med 2004;350(5):482–92.

[18] Edwards A, Hammond HA, Jin L, et al. Genetic variation at five trimeric and tetrameric tandem repeat loci in four human population groups. Genomics 1992;12(2):241–53.

[19] Chamberlain NL, Driver ED, Miesfeld RL. The length and location of CAG trinucleotide repeats in the androgen receptor N-terminal domain affect transactivation function. Nucleic Acids Res 1994;22(15):3181–6.

[20] Irvine RA, Yu MC, Ross RK, et al. The CAG and GGC microsatellites of the androgen receptor gene are in linkage disequilibrium in men with prostate cancer. Cancer Res 1995; 55(9):1937–40.

[21] Gilligan T, Manola J, Sartor O, et al. Absence of a correlation of androgen receptor gene CAG repeat length and prostate cancer risk in an African-American population. Clin Prostate Cancer 2004;3(2):98–103.

[22] Thompson IM, Goodman PJ, Tangen CM, et al. The influence of finasteride on the development of prostate cancer. N Engl J Med 2003;349(3):215–24.

[23] Rubin MA, Allory Y, Molinie V, et al. Effects of long-term finasteride treatment on prostate cancer morphology and clinical outcome. Urology 2005;66(5):930–4.

[24] Thorpe JF, Jain S, Marczylo TH, et al. A review of phase III clinical trials of prostate cancer chemoprevention. Ann R Coll Surg Engl 2007;89(3):207–11.

[25] Chu KC, Tarone RE, Freeman HP. Trends in prostate cancer mortality among black men and white men in the United States. Cancer 2003;97(6):1507–16.

[26] Huggins C, Hodges CV. Studies on prostatic cancer. I: the effect of castration, of estrogen and androgen injection on serum phosphatases in metastatic carcinoma of the prostate. Cancer Res 1941;1:293.

[27] White JW. The results of double castration in hypertrophy of the prostate. Ann Surg 1895; 22:1.

[28] Byar DP, Corle DK. Hormone therapy for prostate cancer: results of the Veterans Administration Cooperative Urological Research Group studies. NCI Monogr 1988;7: 165–70.

[29] The Leuprolide Study Group. Leuprolide versus diethylstilbestrol for metastatic prostate cancer. The Leuprolide Study Group. N Engl J Med 1984;311(20):1281–6.

[30] Smith MR, McGovern FJ, Zietman AL, et al. Pamidronate to prevent bone loss during androgen-deprivation therapy for prostate cancer. N Engl J Med 2001;345(13):948–55.

[31] Smith MR, Lee H, Nathan DM. Insulin sensitivity during combined androgen blockade for prostate cancer. J Clin Endocrinol Metab 2006;91(4):1305–8.

[32] Keating NL, O'Malley AJ, Smith MR. Diabetes and cardiovascular disease during androgen deprivation therapy for prostate cancer. J Clin Oncol 2006;24(27):4448–56.

[33] Crawford ED, Eisenberger MA, McLeod DG, et al. A controlled trial of leuprolide with and without flutamide in prostatic carcinoma. N Engl J Med 1989;321:419–24.

[34] Eisenberger MA, Blumenstein BA, Crawford ED, et al. Bilateral orchiectomy with or without flutamide for metastatic prostate cancer. N Engl J Med 1998;339:1036–42.

[35] Denis L, Murphy GP. Overview of phase III trials on combined androgen treatment in patients with metastatic prostate cancer. Cancer 1993;72:3888–95.

[36] Schmitt B, Wilt TJ, Schellhammer PF, et al. Combined androgen blockade with nonsteroidal antiandrogens for advanced prostate cancer: a systematic review. Urology 2001;57:727–32.

[37] Iversen P, Tyrrell CJ, Kaisary AV, et al. Bicalutamide monotherapy compared with castration in patients with nonmetastatic locally advanced prostate cancer: 6.3 years of followup. J Urol 2000;164:1579–82.

[38] Boccardo F, Barichello M, Battaglia M, et al, Italian Prostate Cancer Group. Bicalutamide monotherapy versus flutamide plus goserelin in prostate cancer: updated results of a multicentric trial. Eur Urol 2002;42(5):481–90.

[39] McLeod DG, See WA, Klimberg I, et al. The bicalutamide 150 mg early prostate cancer program: findings of the North American trial at 7.7-year median followup. J Urol 2006;176:75–80.

[40] McLeod DG, Iversen P, See WA, et al, Casodex Early Prostate Cancer Trialists' Group. Bicalutamide 150 mg plus standard care vs standard care alone for early prostate cancer. BJU Int 2006;97(2):247–54.

[41] The Medical Research Council Prostate Cancer Working Party Investigators Group. Immediate versus deferred treatment for advanced prostatic cancer: initial results of the Medical Research Council Trial. The Medical Research Council Prostate Cancer Working Party Investigators Group. Br J Urol 1997;79(2):235–46.

[42] Messing EM, Manola J, Yao J, et al. Eastern Cooperative Oncology Group study EST 3886. Immediate versus deferred androgen deprivation treatment in patients with node-positive prostate cancer after radical prostatectomy and pelvic lymphadenectomy. Lancet Oncol 2006;7(6):472–9.

[43] Lawton CA, Winter K, Grignon D, et al. Androgen suppression plus radiation versus radiation alone for patients with stage D1/pathologic node-positive adenocarcinoma of the prostate: updated results based on national prospective randomized trial Radiation Therapy Oncology Group 85-31. J Clin Oncol 2005;23(4):800–7.

[44] Studer UE, Whelan P, Albrecht W, et al. Immediate or deferred androgen deprivation for patients with prostate cancer not suitable for local treatment with curative intent: European Organisation for Research and Treatment of Cancer (EORTC) Trial 30891. J Clin Oncol 2006;24(12):1868–76.

[45] Pound CR, Partin AW, Eisenberger MA, et al. Natural history of progression after PSA elevation following radical prostatectomy. JAMA 1999;281(17):1591–7.

[46] Soloway MS, Pareek K, Sharifi R, et al, Lupron Depot Neoadjuvant Prostate Cancer Study Group. Neoadjuvant androgen ablation before radical prostatectomy in cT2bNxMo prostate cancer: 5-year results. J Urol 2002;167(1):112–6.

[47] Schulman CC, Debruyne FM, Forster G, et al. 4-Year follow-up results of a European prospective randomized study on neoadjuvant hormonal therapy prior to radical prostatectomy in T2-3N0M0 prostate cancer. European Study Group on Neoadjuvant Treatment of Prostate Cancer. Eur Urol 2000;38(6):706–13.

[48] Gleave ME, Goldenberg L, Chin JL, et al. Randomized comparative study of 3 vs 8 months of neoadjuvant hormonal therapy prior to radical prostatectomy: 3 year PSA recurrence rates. J Urol 2003;169(4):Abstract 690.

[49] D'Amico AV, Manola J, Loffredo M, et al. 6-month androgen suppression plus radiation therapy vs radiation therapy alone for patients with clinically localized prostate cancer: a randomized controlled trial. JAMA 2004;292(7):821–7.

[50] Bolla M, Collette L, Blank L, et al. Long-term results with immediate androgen suppression and external irradiation in patients with locally advanced prostate cancer (an EORTC study): a phase III randomised trial. Lancet 2002;360(9327):103–6.

[51] Pilepich MV, Winter K, John MJ, et al. Phase III radiation therapy oncology group (RTOG) trial 86–10 of androgen deprivation adjuvant to definitive radiotherapy in locally advanced carcinoma of the prostate. Int J Radiat Oncol Biol Phys 2001;50(5):1243–52.

[52] Pilepich MV, Winter K, Lawton CA, et al. Androgen suppression adjuvant to definitive radiotherapy in prostate carcinoma–long-term results of phase III RTOG 85–31. Int J Radiat Oncol Biol Phys 2005;61(5):1285–90.

[53] Feldman BJ, Feldman D. The development of androgen-independent prostate cancer. Nat Rev Cancer 2001;1:34–45.

[54] Chen CD, Welsbie DS, Tran C, et al. Molecular determinants of resistance to antiandrogen therapy. Nat Med 2004;10:33–9.

[55] Bruchovsky N, Rennie PS, Coldman AJ, et al. Effects of androgen withdrawal on the stem cell composition of the Shionogi carcinoma. Cancer Res 1990;50(8):2275–82.

[56] Bhandari MS, Crook J. Hussain. Should intermittent androgen deprivation be used in routine clinical practice? J Clin Oncol 2005;23(32):8212–8.

ELSEVIER
SAUNDERS

Endocrinol Metab Clin N Am
36 (2007) 435–452

ENDOCRINOLOGY
AND METABOLISM
CLINICS
OF NORTH AMERICA

A Clinical Paradigm for the Combined Management of Androgen Insufficiency and Erectile Dysfunction

Irwin Goldstein, MD[a,b],*

[a]Sexual Medicine, Alvarado Hospital, 5555 Reservoir Drive, Suite 203,
San Diego, CA 92120, USA
[b]The Journal of Sexual Medicine, 85 Old Farm Road, Milton, MA 02186, USA

Androgen insufficiency and erectile dysfunction (ED) have historically been considered separate and distinctly different conditions affecting the aging man. Men who had ED were historically treated with a psychologic focus [1]. Current data from basic science laboratories and clinical investigations have shown that the most frequent biologic pathophysiologies of ED are endothelial dysfunction and vasculopathy [2,3].

Hormonal pathophysiologies of ED were considered rare [1]. New information on the cellular mechanisms of erectile physiology has led to the consistent observation that erectile physiology, especially vascular and endothelial function, is strongly dependent on sex steroid hormonal integrity [4,5]. Clinical interest in androgen insufficiency and ED has increased [6–9].

Since the isolation and synthesis of testosterone in the mid-1930s [10], testosterone has been clinically available for use in aging men. Edwards and colleagues first reported the effects of testosterone on the vasculature in 1939 [11]. In the 1940s, several investigators used testosterone to treat angina in men who had coronary artery disease [12,13]. Androgens have not been popular therapies for sexual dysfunction, in part due to fear of prostate cancer facilitation [7,9]. Another problem was the lack of basic science to support a direct relationship between testosterone and sexual dysfunction. In addition, testosterone delivery systems were not user friendly and were associated with side effects or marked variations in blood levels. The recent advent of the hydroalcoholic testosterone gels [14,15] has enabled, for the first time, patient-friendly drug delivery of stable, eugonadal testosterone

* The Journal of Sexual Medicine, 85 Old Farm Road, Milton, MA 02186.
E-mail address: irwingoldstein@comcast.net

0889-8529/07/$ - see front matter © 2007 Elsevier Inc. All rights reserved.
doi:10.1016/j.ecl.2007.02.002

endo.theclinics.com

values, and the prostate-specific antigen (PSA) blood test [16] has simplified the clinical strategy to monitor for prostate cancer.

Contemporary basic science laboratory and clinical research data consistently show synergy between androgen insufficiency and ED. There are shared physiologic and pathophysiologic mechanisms [17,18]. Published prevalence rates of androgen insufficiency in men who have ED vary but are as high as 35% [19]. Increased numbers of patients (and partners) [20–22] are seeking combined health care management of androgen insufficiency and ED. A general approach to the management of ED related to other etiologies is discussed by Brant and colleagues elsewhere in this issue. This article focuses on a rational, evidence-based clinical management paradigm (Fig. 1) that combines the diagnosis and treatment of men who have androgen insufficiency and ED [6,23–30]. There is close interplay with hormonal, sexual, medical, and lifestyle variables in aging men, and appropriate clinical management needs to engage all these contributing variables [31].

Identification of androgen insufficiency and erectile dysfunction

A comprehensive sexual, psychosocial, medical, and medication history [23], physical examination, and laboratory testing are essential for the diagnosis and management of androgen insufficiency and ED (Fig. 1A, B). Androgen insufficiency [32,33] is a syndrome in which there are signs and symptoms in conjunction with a biochemical blood test. The signs and symptoms are nonspecific and not sufficient for the diagnosis of androgen insufficiency.

History

The medical history should include focused questions on the patient's medical history, including possible risk factors and associated medical conditions of androgen insufficiency and ED, such as diabetes, cardiovascular disease, and depression [32,33]. Androgen insufficiency is associated with an increase in visceral fat and a decrease in lean body mass with associated diminution in muscle volume and strength. Androgen insufficiency is also related to a decrease in body hair, skin alterations, and decreased bone mineral density, resulting in osteoporosis [32–36].

The sexual history should include past and present characteristics of the patient's erectile qualities and other aspects of sexual function, such as sexual interest, sexual orgasm and ejaculatory function, penile sensation capabilities, and sexual pleasure and satisfaction. Some symptoms of androgen insufficiency exist in several other syndromes, such as depression and hypothyroidism, and may have broad variation in patients. The sexual symptoms of androgen insufficiency include decreased sexual interest; diminished erectile quality (particularly of nocturnal erections); muted, delayed, or absent orgasms; decreased genital sensation; and reduced sexual pleasure [32,33].

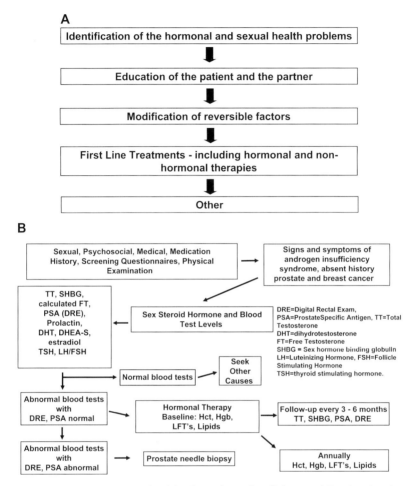

Fig. 1. Diagnosis and treatment algorithm for androgen insufficiency and ED. A rational, cost-effective, evidence-based clinical management paradigm that combines diagnosis and treatment of men who have androgen insufficiency and ED. This clinical paradigm is stepwise and advances from simple, low-cost, reversible, and minimally invasive strategies to more complicated invasiveness, costly, and irreversible strategies. The first step is critical and should include a careful clinical history, a focused physical examination, and select laboratory tests. Modification of reversible causes of androgen insufficiency and ED is recommended before initiation of therapeutic interventions. Mandatory blood tests include total testosterone, SHBG (albumen if the patient has a chronic medical condition), a calculated free testosterone based on the use of the free testosterone calculator (www.issam.ch/freetesto.htm), and PSA. Optional tests include DHEA-S, DHT, prolactin, LH, FSH, estradiol, and TSH. Mandatory follow-up at 3 months is a DRE and PSA, along with a calculated free testosterone value. Various treatments can be offered to the patient who has androgen insufficiency and ED. Safe and effective management requires a detailed follow-up strategy. (Fig. 1B *Adapted from* Morales A, Heaton JP, Carson CC III. Andropause: a misnomer for a true clinical entity. J Urol 2000;163:705–12; with permission.)

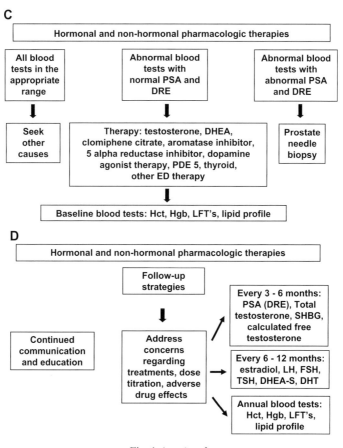

Fig. 1 (*continued*)

A psychosocial assessment is valuable because sexual dysfunction may affect the patient's self-esteem and coping ability. Androgen insufficiency is associated with changes in mood, diminished well-being, blunted motivation, changes in spatial orientation, reduced intellectual ability, fatigue, depression, and anger or irritability [32,33].

Medication use is relevant when the diagnosis of androgen insufficiency is suspected. Failure to respond to a maximum dose of oral phosphodiesterase type 5 (PDE5) inhibitor is a premonitory sign of androgen insufficiency [27,29]. Amar and colleagues reported that when patients who have ED cannot successfully benefit from PDE5 inhibitors, prescribing testosterone may improve the response [24]. Shabsigh stated that the combination of testosterone with PDE5 inhibitors may be considered for the treatment of ED in men who have low to low-normal testosterone levels and inadequate response to prior treatment with PDE5 inhibitors alone [26]. Greenstein and colleagues noted that combined treatment with a PDE5 inhibitor and testosterone gel had a beneficial effect on patients who had ED and androgen insufficiency in whom treatment with testosterone supplement alone failed [37]. Rosenthal and colleagues showed successful use of testosterone gel with a PDE5 inhibitor in men who had low-normal serum testosterone levels in whom the PDE5 inhibitors alone failed [38]. They further stated that this underscores the large numbers of men with low to low-normal testosterone levels who would benefit from testosterone screening when evaluated for ED [38].

Aversa and colleagues were among the initial investigators to note the association between testosterone and androgen insufficiency and ED. They reported that aging men who have androgen insufficiency who fail first-line oral treatments should be considered for treatment with a combination of testosterone and PDE5 inhibitors to improve erectile function and quality of life, unless androgens are contraindicated [27,28]. In men who have ED, low free testosterone correlated independently of age with the impaired relaxation of the cavernous smooth muscle cells. These findings gave clinical support to the experimental knowledge of the importance of androgens in regulating smooth muscle function [28]. Androgen insufficiency seems to reduce the cavernosal expression of nitric oxide synthase (NOS) mRNA and protein and enzyme activity, whereas testosterone supplementation restores NOS expression and activity. The clinical responsiveness of PDE5 inhibitor seems to be strongly linked to NOS activity in vascular endothelial tissues [27,28].

The clinical diagnosis of androgen insufficiency may be aided by the use of screening questionnaires. These include the Androgen Deficiency of the Aging Male, which is widely used but has poor specificity in aging men [39]; the Aging Male Scale [40]; the low testosterone screener by Smith and colleagues, which reliably detects men at risk of androgen insufficiency [41]; and the ANDROTEST [42], which is a structured interview for the screening of androgen insufficiency in men who have sexual dysfunction. Although all of these questionnaires are useful to varying degrees, validated questionnaires cannot replace a detailed history and physical examination [23].

Physical examination

The physical examination may corroborate aspects of the medical history and may reveal unsuspected physical findings [23]. It should emphasize the endocrinologic examination, especially if the response to a PDE5 inhibitor is not robust. Androgen insufficiency is associated with small, less firm testes; a decrease in beard and body hair growth; skin thinning alterations; a decrease in lean body mass; an increase in body fat and a decrease in muscle mass and strength; and the development of breast tissue [32,33].

The diagnosis of androgen insufficiency in men should be based on a suggestive clinical picture and on the biochemical demonstration of androgen deficiency [23,32,33]. Low androgen levels are not sufficient reason for instituting therapy. The most sophisticated biochemical measures of serum androgens can be at best an approximation of the androgen status. Such a measure does not take into account the intracrinologic role of the metabolism of androgens into bioactive metabolites or individual differences in androgen sensitivity based on endocrine disruptors. Based on these issues, there will be a variable response by the target organs to the levels of androgens in different individuals [23,32,33].

Laboratory testing

There is no universally accepted cut-off value of total testosterone that defines the state of androgen insufficiency [32,33]. Total testosterone values fall with age and at various times throughout the day. The ideal time to clinically measure total testosterone is in the early morning, except in aging men, in whom testosterone values can be measured at any time of the day because of the flattening of the circadian rhythm [23].

Total testosterone measurements can be misleading. Unbound testosterone is the major form entering the cells and initiating critical protein synthesis (growth factors, sex hormone receptors, enzymes, etc.) via genomic effects. In normal men, 2% of testosterone is free (unbound), 30% is bound to sex hormone–binding globulin (SHBG) with high affinity, and the remainder is bound with much lower avidity to albumin and other proteins. Thus, the sex hormone binding protein, in part, regulates androgen function. Conditions associated with high values of SHBG lower the unbound, physiologically available form of testosterone [32].

Rather than relying on total testosterone exclusively, the health care provider has the option of assessing free testosterone values. The confusion arises on the methodologies used to measure free testosterone. Antibody-based, free testosterone assays using a testosterone analogue are not accurate. Reliable assays for free testosterone are based on equilibrium dialysis, a test that is usually difficult and time consuming to perform and not widely used clinically. Bioavailable testosterone measures free and albumin-bound fractions of testosterone and is more commonly accessible, more reliable, and less expensive than free testosterone values measured via equilibrium dialysis [30]. A contemporary management strategy for the health care provider is to record the total testosterone and the SHBG and to use the free testosterone calculator [23] from the International Society for the Study of the Aging Male (www.issam.ch/freetesto.htm). The calculated free testosterone, based on the total testosterone and SHBG values, has been shown to correlate to the free testosterone by equilibrium dialysis.

A calculated free testosterone value of less than 5 ng/dl is consistent with an abnormal calculated free testosterone. Morris and colleagues stated that when total testosterone is borderline, calculated free testosterone values are useful to help confirm androgen insufficiency [43]. The calculated free testosterone is reliable in most clinical situations but should not be relied upon in situations with potential massive interference by steroids binding to SHBG, such as in men during treatment inducing high levels of dihydro-testosterone (DHT). Hwang and colleagues reported that calculated free testosterone declined and SHBG rose with age in normal patients and in patients who had ED [44]. Martinez-Jabaloyas and colleagues investigated the frequency of hypogonadism in men who had ED and the factors associated with low testosterone levels [45]. Using the calculated free testosterone levels, 17.6% of the men had criteria for androgen insufficiency. Hypertension, aging, absence of nocturnal erections, and a low erectile function score were associated with lower free testosterone levels.

Androgen administration is contraindicated in men who have been diagnosed with or are suspected of having carcinoma of the prostate [32,33]. Determination of serum PSA and digital rectal examination (DRE) are mandatory as baseline measurements of prostate health before therapy with androgens [46–48]. Many health care providers consider PSA levels of 0 to 2.5 ng/ml as low and values greater than 2.6 to 10 ng/ml as slightly to moderately elevated. PSA screening and DRE should be repeated every 3 to 6 months for the first 12 months and annually thereafter. When in doubt with the assessment of the prostate by PSA or DRE, the health care clinician should consider recommending a prostate biopsy [46]. If the PSA increases during androgen therapy and the biopsy is negative for prostate cancer, androgen therapy can continue with the PSA and DRE, repeated every 3 to 6 months. There is no evidence that androgen therapy causes prostate cancer. The risk that androgen therapy may accelerate an existing underlying prostate cancer must be clearly understood by the patient, and the regular and routine follow-up prostate check is thus particularly important.

Hyperprolactinemia is an uncommon cause of ED and androgen insufficiency [49,50]. If a patient presents with signs and symptoms of androgen insufficiency, such as diminished sexual interest by history and gynecomastia on physical examination, and has biochemical evidence of androgen insufficiency, determination of serum prolactin is recommended [50].

For some androgen-dependent functions, testosterone is a prohormone peripherally converted to DHT via the enzyme 5-alpha reductase. Physiologically, the most active androgen acting on the androgen receptors seems to be DHT [51].

Nonphysiologically high levels of DHT may be observed after topical testosterone gel administration, presumably related to the presence of high concentrations of 5-alpha reductase enzyme in skin and the much greater skin surface area of testosterone application using the gels compared with the patch [52]. These high values of DHT may be associated with the side effects of acne and scalp hair loss [53]. Successful management of elevated DHT-associated side effects may be achieved with low doses of 5-alpha reductase enzyme inhibitors [51].

Nonphysiologically low levels of DHT may occur with the medical treatment for lower urinary tract symptoms (LUTS) using 5-alpha reductase inhibitors that block the conversion of testosterone to DHT. This results in a circulating level of DHT that can be reduced by as much as 70% [51]. The 5-alpha reductase inhibitors finasteride and dutasteride have been associated with a greater risk of ED, ejaculatory dysfunction, and decreased libido compared with placebo [54,55].

Animals treated with finasteride had significantly lower DHT levels and had significant ultrastructural changes, including marked irregularities in the tunica albuginea consistent with thick and irregular-arranged collagenous fibers and in the trabeculae of the corpus cavernosum [56]. Mantzoros and colleagues found serum DHT to be an independent hormonal predictor of increased frequency of orgasms [57].

Estradiol is synthesized in men peripherally by metabolism of testosterone via the enzyme aromatase. In aging men, estradiol values increase over time [58,59]. Elevated estradiol increases the liver synthesis of SHBG, which lowers unbound physiologically available testosterone. Mancini and colleagues found that estradiol values were significantly higher in patients who had venous leak compared with control subjects, supporting the hypothesis that estradiol level can influence penile smooth muscle function [60]. Estradiol levels were greater in the men who had aging male symptoms [61].

Dihydroepiandrosterone (DHEA) is an androgen precursor produced by the adrenal glands that has been shown to exert its effects via downstream conversion to testosterone and estradiol. DHEA values steadily decrease from age 40 [62]. It may be involved in multiple biologic effects, including cognitive, memory, metabolic, vascular, immune, and sexual functions [63]. Deficiencies of DHEA in men have been reported to be associated with various drugs and with endocrine, nonhormonal, and age-related disorders.

Dihydroepiandrosterone sulfate (DHEA-S) levels were significantly lower in the men who had aging male symptoms and in men who had sexual dysfunction as determined by the International Index of Erectile Function score [61]. Alexopoulou and colleagues reported that patients who had ED and type 1 diabetes had lower levels of DHEA and DHEA-S compared with men who had diabetes but no ED [64]. DHEA-S showed an inverse correlation with age and a positive correlation with testosterone [65].

No well designed clinical trials have definitively substantiated the role of DHEA in these functions in humans or the safety and efficacy of DHEA therapy [66]. In a small study, Reiter and colleagues evaluated the efficacy of DHEA replacement in the treatment of ED and determined that it was associated with higher mean scores for all five domains of the International Index of Erectile Function but had no impact on PSA and testosterone [67].

The thyroid gland promotes tissue growth and development, regulates energy metabolism, and indirectly plays a role in sexual health. Bodie and colleagues evaluated the prevalence of laboratory abnormalities in men presenting for initial evaluation and therapy of ED and found that a total of 4% had increased thyroid-stimulating hormone [68].

Serum luteinizing hormone (LH) and follicle-stimulating hormone (FSH) determination may be of value in men who have ED and androgen insufficiency, especially in those who are being considered for therapy by clomiphene citrate because this agent is effective only in hypogonadotropic hypogonadism [69]. In patients who have ED and androgen insufficiency, hypogonadotropic hypogonadism, and a LH level of less than 13 mIU/ml, Bunch and colleagues found that 10% had hypothalamic-pituitary structural abnormalities [70].

Patient/partner education

An essential component in the management of androgen insufficiency and erectile dysfunction is patient and partner education (Fig. 1) that is uniquely matched to individual needs [23]. Educational subjects include an overview of pertinent anatomy and physiology, relevant pathophysiology, full disclosure of risks and benefits, and appropriate discussion of expectations with treatment. Efforts are made to translate the results of the history taking, physical examination, and laboratory testing into understandable management strategies in the presence of the patient and his partner, if possible. The education process is ongoing through regular follow-up visits. During the education process, patient's and partner's preferences for management should be respected and taken into consideration [23].

Modifying reversible causes

ED and androgen insufficiency are potentially reversible if specific etiologic factors can be addressed (Fig. 1). This may apply to altering or modifying prescription or nonprescription drug use, such as LUTS treatment with a 5-alpha reductase inhibitor, or altering psychosocial factors, such as stress and anger from poor partner relationship and communication.

Many patients have a history of prescription or nonprescription drug use. Of the drugs that may induce sexual dysfunction or androgen insufficiency, the most common are antihypertensives, antiarrhythmics, antidepressant agents, and antipsychotic agents. Drugs commonly used in the treatment of prostate disease typically lead to ED and diminished sexual interest. Recreational drug use should be considered as a potential negative influence.

Partner relationship factors should be appropriately addressed by a certified trained mental health care professional who provides psychosexual or couples therapy. Therapy can be conducted with the patient alone, but it is preferable to include the partner. For patients being treated concomitantly with medical therapy, a modified sex therapy approach can address psychologic reactions to the medical treatment. If there has been an extended period of abstinence, brief sex therapy may facilitate resumption of sexual activity for the couple [71,72].

First-line therapies

Pharmacologic treatment (Fig. 1C) is delivered with reference to ease of medication administration and cost. Hormonal agents include testosterone, DHEA, clomiphene citrate, aromatase inhibitors, 5-alpha reductase inhibitors, dopamine agonists, and thyroid therapies. Nonhormonal treatments include vasodilators, such as PDE5 inhibitors, and intracavernosal agents. Before testosterone, DHEA, clomiphene citrate, or aromatase inhibitor therapy is considered, a patient should have signs and symptoms and biochemical confirmation of androgen insufficiency, a PSA and DRE not consistent with prostate cancer or a negative prostate biopsy, and an absent history of breast cancer [32,33].

Hormonal pharmacologic treatment

Although testosterone has a recognized physiologic role in erections, its importance in ED treatment has been controversial. Relative contraindications include elevated hematocrit, abnormal liver function studies, LUTS, and sleep apnea. Testosterone therapy used selectively and carefully may be administered by topical (gel, patch, or cream) or parenteral (intramuscular) administration. Oral administration with methyltestosterone is discouraged due to limited efficacy data and potential associated hepatic side effects. There is a critical need for large-scale, long-term, randomized controlled trials to investigate the efficacy of testosterone therapy in men who have androgen insufficiency and ED [32,33].

Isidori and colleagues conducted a systematic review and meta-analysis of randomized, placebo-controlled studies to assess the effects of testosterone on the different domains of the sexual response. In men who had an average testosterone level at baseline below 12 nmol/l, testosterone treatment improved the number of nocturnal erections and successful intercourses, sexual thoughts, scores of erectile function, and overall sexual satisfaction but had no effect on in eugonadal men. The effect of testosterone tended to decline over time and was progressively smaller with increasing baseline T levels. Long-term safety data were not available [73].

Because DHEA is available over the counter, men can take it without physician supervision. Saad and colleagues reviewed clinical studies evaluating DHEA treatment for decreased DHEA values [62]. DHEA supplementation had positive effects on the cardiovascular system, body composition, bone mineral density, skin, central nervous system, the immune system, and sexual function. DHEA use may be justified in aging men when the diagnosis is based on the clinical picture and biochemical evidence, when there are periodic evaluations, and when individual dose adjustments are performed to maintain serum concentrations in the physiologic range [74].

Exogenous testosterone suppresses gonadotropins from the hypothalamic-pituitary axis as a result of elevation of the circulating values of testosterone. This may be deleterious in men who have relative infertility [32,33]. An alternative treatment is clomiphene citrate, particularly when the androgen insufficiency is due to hypogonadotropic hypogonadism, because this therapy increases gonadotropins [69]. Guay and colleagues found significant increases in LH and free testosterone and improved sexual function. Erectile improvement was lower in aging men and in men who had diabetes, hypertension, coronary artery disease, and multiple medication use [75]. In another study, results showed a significant increase in LH, FSH, and total and free testosterone levels versus placebo. Sexual function improved in limited parameters in younger and healthier men [76].

Because androgens are the precursors of estrogens, the administration of exogenous testosterone results in a suspicion of an increase in estradiol values by virtue of aromatization. Anastrozole is a potent and highly selective aromatase inhibitor, with no intrinsic estrogenic, antiestrogenic, androgenic, antiandrogenic, progestogenic, glucocorticoid, antiglucocorticoid, or mineralocorticoid activities [77]. Leder and colleagues investigated anastrozole's ability to increase endogenous testosterone production in men who had hypogonadism. Aromatase inhibition increased serum bioavailable and total testosterone levels in older men who had mild hypogonadism [78]. Serum estradiol levels decreased modestly but remained within the normal male range. The sexual benefits of aromatase inhibitor therapy were reported in a case report [79]. The use of an aromatase inhibitor normalized the testosterone level and improved sexual functioning. Greco and colleagues showed that sustained improvement in sexual function after 12 months of PDE5 inhibitor administration is associated with increased testosterone to estradiol ratio mainly related to reduction of estradiol levels. These investigators hypothesized that androgen–estrogen cross-talk and possible inhibition of aromatase activity during chronic exposure to PDE5 inhibitor use might play a role in the regulation of erectile function [80].

Hirsutism and acne are common and can be distressing complaints in individuals who have high values of androgens, in particular DHT. The most efficacious pharmacologic therapy to reduce DHT is by 5-alpha reductase inhibitors [81]. Mechanical therapies for hirsutism include laser photothermolysis and electrolysis. Other acne therapies include topical and systemic retinoids and antibiotics and topical antibacterial agents.

Nonhormonal pharmacologic treatment

Clinical use of dopamine agonists has been reported to improve sexual function based on research showing that sexual motivation is modulated by a number of central nervous system neurotransmitter and receptor changes [82]. These changes are induced, in part, by the action of sex steroids and by the central neurotransmitter dopamine, which may play a critical intermediary role in the central regulation of sexual arousal and excitation, mood, and incentive-related sexual behavior and, in particular, in the motivational responses to conditioned external stimuli [83–85]. Androgens may be central in this by allowing more estradiol to be distributed to central nervous system target tissues via aromatase.

Treatment with a dopamine agonist such as bromocriptine or with cabergoline, a more potent and long-lasting ergoline-derived dopamine agonist, is beneficial in the presence of documented hyperprolactinemia. Six months of treatment with cabergoline normalized testosterone levels in most cases, thus restoring and maintaining during treatment the capability of normal sexual activity in hyperprolactinemic men [86]. In another study, De Rosa and colleagues compared the effects of chronic treatment with cabergoline and bromocriptine on sexual function in hyperprolactinemic men and found that in men who had prolactinomas, cabergoline normalized prolactin levels and improved sexual function earlier than bromocriptine treatment [87]. In men who had psychogenic ED and no prolactinoma, cabergoline treatment resulted in improvement in erectile function, sexual desire, orgasmic function, and in the patient's and the partner's sexual satisfaction [82]. Safarinejad reported that cabergoline is effective in salvage therapy for sildenafil nonresponders [88].

Bupropion is a dopamine agonist antidepressant with fewer reported adverse sexual effects than traditional selective serotonin reuptake inhibitors and therefore is clinically useful as an antidote to antidepressant-associated sexual dysfunction. Taylor and colleagues assessed the effectiveness of management strategies for sexual dysfunction caused by antidepressant medication [89]. Compared with serotonin reuptake inhibitors, the dopamine agonist bupropion revealed less desire dysfunction and less orgasm dysfunction and superior overall satisfaction with sexual functioning. No differences were found in self-reported sexual function, number of erections, total erection time, or penile rigidity in healthy subjects taking bupropion compared with those taking placebo or baseline [89,90].

In summary, dopamine agonist pharmacologic agents such as bupropion, bromocriptine, cabergoline, apomorphine, and Parkinson-type drugs such as L-dopa, pergolide, pramipexole, and ropinirole may be helpful in men who have sexual dysfunction [91,92].

If a patient who has androgen insufficiency and ED has a concomitant thyroid abnormality, it is likely that androgen therapy would not be successful until the thyroid status has been normalized. Carani and colleagues studied 34 men who had hyperthyroidism treated with methimazole and 14 who had hypothyroidism treated with thyroxine [93]. A total of 50% and 64%, respectively, had some abnormality in sexual function (decreased sexual desire, ED, or premature or delayed ejaculation) that improved with thyroid treatment without concomitant PDE5-inhibitor therapy. Based on an animal model of hypothyroidism, Kilicarslan and colleagues concluded that hypothyroidism results in an autonomic neuropathy and endothelial dysfunction adversely influencing the release or synthesis of NO from nitrergic nerves and endothelium [94].

Follow-up strategies

Patients undergoing hormonal treatment for androgen insufficiency and ED should undergo reassessment and follow-up at regular and routine intervals (Fig. 1D). The major goals of reassessment and follow-up are to ensure optimum patient–physician communication and to assess the progress of therapy and the sexual, general medical, and psychosocial status of the patient and partner [23].

Strategies for safe blood test monitoring during testosterone therapy should include blood tests every 3 to 6 months for total testosterone, SHBG (albumin if appropriate), PSA screening, and DRE. Strategies for medical health monitoring during testosterone therapy should engage hematocrit and hemoglobulin, liver function tests, and lipid profile evaluations annually. Follow-up blood tests for LH, FSH, thyroid-stimulating hormone, DHEA-S, prolactin, DHT, and estradiol should be obtained as indicated in each individual [32,33].

During follow-up visits, the health care provider may address any relevant patient concerns regarding the treatments. There may be a need for dosage titration or substitution of another treatment intervention. Patients may change treatment preferences, seek new information, or wish to re-evaluate their current treatment choices. Patients may change medication strategies for these and other health problems. Adverse drug reactions or drug interaction effects should be carefully monitored [23].

Other treatments

Men who have androgen insufficiency and ED may not respond to the interventions described in this article and may need to consider such options as a vacuum erection device, intraurethral or intracavernosal administration of alprostadil or other vasoactive agents, surgical intervention with penile prostheses, or reconstructive surgery, such as penile revascularization [23] (Fig. 1).

Summary

Androgen insufficiency and ED are highly prevalent medical disorders in aging men who have associated multiple risk factors. Good clinical practice requires the use of appropriate strategies for patient- and goal-directed diagnosis and treatment. In the future, we will likely see new basic science investigations that may lead to new treatment strategies. In this fashion, management can be delivered in a more safe and effective manner for the majority of afflicted patients (and partners). New basic science laboratory and clinical research studies will provide a new awareness of the significance of sexual health medicine because sexual health is an important element in the physical health and psychologic well-being of most patients. The contemporary health care provider must be aware of these issues to provide good medical practice.

References

[1] Spark RF, White RA, Connolly PB. Impotence is not always psychogenic: newer insights into hypothalamic-pituitary-gonadal dysfunction. JAMA 1980;243(8):750–5.
[2] Burnett AL. Nitric oxide in the penis: science and therapeutic implications from erectile dysfunction to priapism. J Sex Med 2006;3(4):578–82.
[3] Latini DM, Penson DF, Wallace KL, et al. Longitudinal differences in psychological outcomes for men with erectile dysfunction: results from ExCEED. J Sex Med 2006;3(6): 1068–76.
[4] Latini DM, Penson DF, Wallace KL, et al. Clinical and psychosocial characteristics of men with erectile dysfunction: baseline data from ExCEED. J Sex Med 2006;3(6): 1059–67.
[5] Traish AM, Guay AT. Are androgens critical for penile erections in humans? Examining the clinical and preclinical evidence. J Sex Med 2006;3(3):382–404.
[6] Lazarou S, Reyes-Vallejo L, Morgentaler A. Wide variability in laboratory reference values for serum testosterone. J Sex Med 2006;3(6):1085–9.
[7] Rhoden EL, Morgentaler A. Risks of testosterone-replacement therapy and recommendations for monitoring. N Engl J Med 2004;350(5):482–92.
[8] Wald M, Meacham RB, Ross LS, Niederberger CS. Testosterone replacement therapy for older men. J Androl 2006;27(2):126–32.
[9] Nieschlag E, Swerdloff R, Behre HM, et al. Investigation, treatment, and monitoring of late-onset hypogonadism in males: ISA, ISSAM, and EAU Recommendations: 2006. J Androl 2006;27(2):135–7.
[10] David K, Dingemanse E, Freud J, et al. Uber krystallinisches mannliches Hormon aus Hoden (Testosteron) wirksamer als aus harn oder aus Cholesterin bereitetes Androsteron. Hoppe Seyler Z Physiol Chem 1935;233:281–2.
[11] Edwards E, Hamilton J, Duntley S. Testosterone propionate as a therapeutic agent in patients with organic disease of peripheral vessels. N Engl J Med 1939;220:865–9.
[12] Hamm L. Testosterone propionate in the treatment of angina pectoris. J Clin Endocrinol 1942;2:325–8.
[13] Lesser MA. Testosterone propionate therapy in one hundred cases of angina pectoris. J Clin Endocrinol 1946;6:549–57.
[14] Steidle CP. New advances in the treatment of hypogonadism in the aging male. Rev Urol 2003;5(Suppl 1):S34–40.
[15] Wang C, Cunningham G, Dobs A, et al. Long-term testosterone gel (AndroGel) treatment maintains beneficial effects on sexual function and mood, lean and fat mass, and bone mineral density in hypogonadal men. J Clin Endocrinol Metab 2004;89(5):2085–98.
[16] El-Sakka AI, Hassoba HM, Elbakry AM, et al. Prostatic specific antigen in patients with hypogonadism: effect of testosterone replacement. J Sex Med 2005;2(2):235–40.
[17] Yassin AA, EdD F, Saad F, et al. Testosterone undecanoate restores erectile function in a subset of patients with venous leakage: a series of case reports. J Sex Med 2006; 3(4):727–35.
[18] Zhang XH, Filippi S, Morelli A, et al. Testosterone restores diabetes-induced erectile dysfunction and sildenafil responsiveness in two distinct animal models of chemical diabetes. J Sex Med 2006;3:253–64.
[19] El-Sakka AI. Association of risk factors and medical comorbidities with male sexual dysfunctions. J Sex Med 2006; [epub ahead of print].

[20] Shindel A, Quayle S, Yan Y, et al. Sexual dysfunction in female partners of men who have undergone radical prostatectomy correlates with sexual dysfunction of the male partner. J Sex Med 2005;2(6):833–41.

[21] Fisher W, Rosen R, Mollen M, et al. Improving the sexual quality of life of couples affected by erectile dysfunction: a double-blind, randomized, placebo-controlled trial of vardenafil. J Sex Med 2005;2(5):699–708.

[22] Goldstein I, Fisher WA, Sand M, et al. Women's sexual function improves when partners are administered vardenafil for erectile dysfunction: a prospective, randomized, double-blind placebo-controlled trial. J Sex Med 2005;2(6):819–32.

[23] Moreira ED Jr, Kim SC, Glasser D, et al. Sexual activity, prevalence of sexual problems, and associated help-seeking patterns in men and women aged 40-80 years in Korea: data from the Global Study of Sexual Attitudes and Behaviors (GSSAB). J Sex Med 2006;3(2):201–11.

[24] Sharlip ID. Guidelines for the diagnosis and management of premature ejaculation. J Sex Med 2006;3(Suppl 4):309–17.

[25] Edwards D, Hackett G, Collins O, et al. Vardenafil improves sexual function and treatment satisfaction in couples affected by erectile dysfunction (ED): a randomized, double-blind, placebo-controlled trial in PDE5 inhibitor-naive men with ED and their partners. J Sex Med 2006;3(6):1028–36.

[26] Sadovsky R, Nusbaum M. Sexual health inquiry and support is a primary care priority. J Sex Med 2006;3(1):3–11.

[27] Klotz T, Mathers M, Klotz R, et al. Patients responding to phosphodiesterase type 5 inhibitor therapy: what do their sexual partners know? J Sex Med 2007;4(1):162–5.

[28] Aversa A, Isidori AM, Spera G, et al. Androgens improve cavernous vasodilation and response to sildenafil in patients with erectile dysfunction. Clin Endocrinol 2003;58(5):632–8.

[29] Shamloul R, Ghanem H, Fahmy I, et al. Testosterone therapy can enhance erectile function response to sildenafil in patients with PADAM: a pilot study. J Sex Med 2005;2:559–64.

[30] Reyes-Vallejo L, Lazarou S, Morgentaler A. Subjective sexual response to testosterone replacement therapy based on initial serum levels of total testosterone. J Sex Med 2006; [epub ahead of print].

[31] Beutel ME, Wiltink J, Hauck EW, et al. Correlations between hormones, physical, and affective parameters in aging urologic outpatients. Eur Urol 2005;47(6):749–55.

[32] Morales A, Buvat J, Gooren LJ, et al. Endocrine aspects of sexual dysfunction in men. J Sex Med 2004;1(1):69–81.

[33] Morales A, Heaton JPW. Hypogonadism and erectile dysfunction: pathophysiological observations and therapeutic outcomes. BJU Int 2003;92(9):896–9.

[34] Jockenhövel F. Testosterone therapy: what, when and to whom? Aging Male 2004;7(4):319–24.

[35] Yassin AA, Saad F, Traish A. Testosterone undecanoate restores erectile function in a subset of patients with venous leakage: a series of case reports. J Sex Med 2006;3(4):727–35.

[36] Schulman C, Lunenfeld B. The ageing male. World J Urol 2002;20(1):4–10.

[37] Greenstein A, Mabjeesh NJ, Sofer M, et al. Does sildenafil combined with testosterone gel improve erectile dysfunction in hypogonadal men in whom testosterone supplement therapy alone failed. J Urol 2005;173(2):530–2.

[38] Rosenthal BD, May NR, Metro MJ, et al. Adjunctive use of AndroGel (testosterone gel) with sildenafil to treat erectile dysfunction in men with acquired androgen deficiency syndrome after failure using sildenafil alone. Urology 2006;67(3):571–4.

[39] Tancredi A, Reginster JY, Schleich F, et al. Interest of the androgen deficiency in aging males (ADAM) questionnaire for the identification of hypogonadism in elderly community-dwelling male volunteers. Eur J Endocrinol 2004;151(3):355–60.

[40] Heinemann LA, Saad F, Heinemann K, et al. Can results of the Aging Males' Symptoms (AMS) scale predict those of screening scales for androgen deficiency? Aging Male 2004;7(3):211–8.

[41] Smith KW, Feldman HA, McKinlay JB. Construction and field validation of a self-administered screener for testosterone deficiency (hypogonadism) in ageing men. Clin Endocrinol (Oxf) 2000;53(6):703–11.

[42] Corona G, Mannucci E, Petrone L, et al. ANDROTEST©: a structured interview for the screening of hypogonadism in patients with sexual dysfunction. J Sex Med 2006;3(4):706–15.

[43] Morris PD, Malkin CJ, Channer KS, et al. A mathematical comparison of techniques to predict biologically available testosterone in a cohort of 1072 men. Eur J Endocrinol 2004; 151(2):241–9.

[44] Hwang TIS, Juang GD, Yeh CH, et al. Hormone levels in middle-aged and elderly men with and without erectile dysfunction in Taiwan. Int J Impot Res 2006;18:160–3.

[45] MartÍNez-Jabaloyas JM, Queipo-ZaragozÁ A, Pastor-HernÁNdez F, et al. Testosterone levels in men with erectile dysfunction. BJU Int 2006;97(6):1278.

[46] Wilt TJ. Prostate cancer: epidemiology and screening. Rev Urol 2003;5(6):S3–9.

[47] Guay Md Face AT, Perez Md JB, Fitaihi Md WA, et al. Testosterone treatment in hypogonadal men: prostate-specific antigen level and risk of prostate cancer. Endocr Pract 2000; 6(2):132–8.

[48] Svetec DA, Canby ED, Thompson IM, et al. The effect of parenteral testosterone replacement on prostate specific antigen in hypogonadal men with erectile dysfunction. J Urol 1997;158(5):1775–7.

[49] Zeitlin S, Rajfer J. Hyperprolactinemia and erectile dysfunction. Rev Urol 2000;2:39–42.

[50] Buvat J, Lemaire A. Endocrine screening in 1,022 men with erectile dysfunction: clinical significance and cost-effective strategy. J Urol 1997;158(5):1764–7.

[51] Clark RV, Hermann DJ, Cunningham GR, et al. Marked suppression of dihydrotestosterone in men with benign prostatic hyperplasia by dutasteride, a dual 5alpha-reductase inhibitor. J Clin Endocrinol Metab 2004;89(5):2179–84.

[52] Mazer N, Bell D, Wu J, et al. Comparison of the steady-state pharmacokinetics, metabolism, and variability of a transdermal testosterone patch versus a transdermal testosterone gel in hypogonadal men. J Sex Med 2005;2(2):213–26.

[53] Libecco JF, Bergfeld WF. Finasteride in the treatment of alopecia. Expert Opin Pharmacother 2004;5(4):933–40.

[54] Giuliano F. Impact of medical treatments for benign prostatic hyperplasia on sexual function. BJU Int 2006;97(2):34–8.

[55] Miner M, Rosenberg MT, Perelman MA. Treatment of lower urinary tract symptoms in benign prostatic hyperplasia and its impact on sexual function. Clin Ther 2001;2006:13–25.

[56] Shen ZJ, Zhou XL, Lu YL, et al. Effect of androgen deprivation on penile ultrastructure. Asian J Androl 2003;5(1):33–6.

[57] Mantzoros CS, Georgiadis EI, Trichopoulos D. Contribution of dihydrotestosterone to male sexual behaviour. Br Med J 1995;310(6990):1289–91.

[58] Oettel M. Is there a role for estrogens in the maintenance of men's health? Aging Male 2002; 5(4):248–57.

[59] Cohen PG. The role of estradiol in the maintenance of secondary hypogonadism in males in erectile dysfunction. Med Hypotheses 1998;50(4):331–3.

[60] Mancini A, Milardi D, Bianchi A, et al. Increased estradiol levels in venous occlusive disorder: a possible functional mechanism of venous leakage. Int J Impot Res 2005;17:239–42.

[61] Basar MM, Aydin G, Mert HC, et al. Relationship between serum sex steroids and Aging Male Symptoms score and International Index of Erectile Function. Urology 2005;66(3): 597–601.

[62] Saad F, Hoesl CE, Oettel M, et al. Dehydroepiandrosterone treatment in the aging male: what should the urologist know? Eur Urol 2005;48(5):724–33.

[63] Webb SJ, Geoghegan TE, Prough RA, et al. The biological actions of dehydroepiandrosterone involves multiple receptors. Drug Metab Rev 2006;38(1):89–116.

[64] Alexopoulou O, Jamart J, Maiter D, et al. Erectile dysfunction and lower androgenicity in type 1 diabetic patients. Diabetes Metab 2001;27(3):329–36.

[65] Tomova A, Kumanov P. Are dehydroepiandrosterone sulphate and lipids associated with erectile dysfunction? Maturitas 2005;50(4):294–9.

[66] Lunenfeld B. Androgen therapy in the aging male. World J Urol 2003;21(5):292–305.

[67] Reiter WJ, Schatzl G, Märk I, et al. Dehydroepiandrosterone in the treatment of erectile dysfunction in patients with different organic etiologies. Urol Res 2001;29(4):278–81.

[68] Bodie J, Lewis J, Schow D, et al. Laboratory evaluations of erectile dysfunction: an evidence based approach. J Urol 2003;169(6):2262–4.

[69] Hayes FJ, DeCruz S, Seminara SB, et al. Differential regulation of gonadotropin secretion by testosterone in the human male: absence of a negative feedback effect of testosterone on follicle-stimulating hormone secretion1. J Clin Endocrinol Metab 2001;86(1):53–8.

[70] Bunch TJ. Pituitary radiographic abnormalities and clinical correlates of hypogonadism in elderly males presenting with erectile dysfunction. Aging Male 2002;5(1):38–46.

[71] Shamloul R. Management of honeymoon impotence. J Sex Med 2005;3(2):361–6.

[72] Titta M, Tavolini IM, Fabrizio Dal Moro MD, et al. Psychology sexual counseling improved erectile rehabilitation after non-nerve-sparing radical retropubic prostatectomy or cystectomy: results of a randomized prospective study. J Sex Med 2006;3:267–73.

[73] Isidori AM, Giannetta E, Gianfrilli D, et al. Effects of testosterone on sexual function in men: results of a meta-analysis. Clin Endocrinol (Oxf) 2005;63(4):381–94.

[74] Buvat J. Androgen therapy with dehydroepiandrosterone. World J Urol 2003;21(5): 346–55.

[75] Guay AT, Jacobson J, Perez JB, et al. Clomiphene increases free testosterone levels in men with both secondary hypogonadism and erectile dysfunction: who does and does not benefit? Int J Impot Res 2003;15:156–65.

[76] Guay AT. Effect of raising endogenous testosterone levels in impotent men with secondary hypogonadism: double blind placebo-controlled trial with clomiphene citrate. J Clin Endocrinol Metab 1995;80(12):3546–52.

[77] Dukes M, Edwards PN, Large M, et al. The preclinical pharmacology of "Arimidex" (anastrozole; ZD1033): a potent, selective aromatase inhibitor. J Steroid Biochem Mol Biol 1996; 58(4):439–45.

[78] Leder BZ, Rohrer JL, Rubin SD, et al. Effects of aromatase inhibition in elderly men with low or borderline-low serum testosterone levels. J Clin Endocrinol Metab 2004;89(3): 1174–80.

[79] Harden C, MacLusky NJ. Aromatase inhibition, testosterone, and seizures. Epilepsy Behav 2004;5(2):260–3.

[80] Greco EA, Pili M, Bruzziches R, et al. Testosterone:estradiol ratio changes associated with long-term tadalafil administration: a pilot study. J Sex Med 2006;3(4):716–22.

[81] Moghetti P, Toscano V. Treatment of hirsutism and acne in hyperandrogenism. Baillieres Best Pract Res Clin Endocrinol Metab 2006;20(2):221–34.

[82] Nickel M, Moleda D, Loew T, et al. Cabergoline treatment in men with psychogenic erectile dysfunction: a randomized, double-blind, placebo-controlled study. Int J Impot Res 2006; 19(1):104–7.

[83] Giuliano F, Allard J. Dopamine and male sexual function. European Urology 2001;40(6): 601–8.

[84] Pfaus JG. Revisiting the concept of sexual motivation. Annu Rev Sex Res 1999;10:120–56.

[85] Pfaus JG, Shadiack A, Van Soest T, et al. Selective facilitation of sexual solicitation in the female rat by a melanocortin receptor agonist. Proc Natl Acad Sci U S A 2004;101(27): 10201–4.

[86] De Rosa M, Zarrilli S, Vitale G, et al. Six months of treatment with cabergoline restores sexual potency in hyperprolactinemic males: an open longitudinal study monitoring nocturnal penile tumescence. J Clin Endocrinol Metab 2004;89(2):621–5.

[87] De Rosa M, Colao A, Di Sarno A, et al. Cabergoline treatment rapidly improves gonadal function in hyperprolactinemic males: a comparison with bromocriptine. Eur J Endocrinol 1998;138(3):286–93.

[88] Safarinejad MR. Salvage of sildenafil failures with cabergoline: a randomized, double-blind, placebo-controlled study. Int J Impot Res 2006;8(6):550–8.

[89] Taylor JT, Rudkin L, Hawton K. Strategies for managing antidepressant-induced sexual dysfunction: systematic review of randomised controlled trials. J Affect Disord 2005;88: 241–54.

[90] Kukkonen TM, Binik YM, Amsel R, et al. Thermography as a physiological measure of sexual arousal in both men and women. J Sex Med 2007;4(1):93–105.

[91] Pohanka M, Kanovsky' P, Bareš M, et al. The long-lasting improvement of sexual dysfunction in patients with advanced, fluctuating Parkinson's disease induced by pergolide: evidence from the results of an open, prospective, one-year trial. Parkinsonism and Relat Disord 2005;11(8):509–12.

[92] Klos KJ, Bower JH, Josephs KA, et al. Pathological hypersexuality predominantly linked to adjuvant dopamine agonist therapy in Parkinson's disease and multiple system atrophy. Parkinsonism Relat Disord 2005;11(6):381–6.

[93] Carani C, Isidori AM, Granata A, et al. Multicenter study on the prevalence of sexual symptoms in male hypo- and hyperthyroid patients. J Clin Endocrinol Metab 2005;90(12):6472–9.

[94] Kilicarslan H, Bagcivan I, Yildirim MK, et al. Effect of hypothyroidism on the NO/cGMP pathway of corpus cavernosum in rabbits. J Sex Med 2006;3(5):830–7.

ELSEVIER
SAUNDERS

Endocrinol Metab Clin N Am
36 (2007) 453–463

ENDOCRINOLOGY
AND METABOLISM
CLINICS
OF NORTH AMERICA

ED²: Erectile Dysfunction = Endothelial Dysfunction

André T. Guay, MD, FACP, FACE[a,b,*]

[a]*Center for Sexual Function/Endocrinology, Lahey Clinic Northshore, Peabody,
One Essex Center Drive, Peabody, MA 01960, USA*
[b]*Harvard Medical School, Boston, MA, USA*

Erectile dysfunction (ED), defined as a persistent inability to achieve and/ or maintain an erection adequate for satisfactory sexual activity, occurs in nearly 30 million men in the United States [1]. The Massachusetts Male Aging Study has shown that 52% of men between the ages of 40 and 70 years have some degree of ED, and suggests that there is a significant correlation with coronary artery disease (CAD) [2]. In fact, the authors stated that men with cardiovascular disease (CVD) have four times the risk of ED. Another longitudinal study, the Rancho Bernardo Study, showed that men with multiple cardiac risks had a 2.2-fold increased risk of ED many years later [3].

CVD has been recognized as the leading cause of mortality in men, especially in their advancing years [4], and so the link between the two conditions is not surprising. Indeed, it has been confirmed that that 65% to 75% of men with CAD have symptoms of ED [5,6]. Solomon and colleagues [6] not only showed that 65% of 137 men with angiographically proven CAD had ED, but that most had the coronary problem diagnosed or confirmed after symptoms of ED had been evident for some time.

The converse, that there is a high incidence of CAD in men with ED, was initially demonstrated by Dr Pritzker in 1999 [7]. Pritzker studied 50 men who had ED but no history or symptoms of CVD, yet 80% of these men had multiple cardiac risk factors by questionnaire analysis. Further, 56% failed a treadmill stress test, and when 20 of these 28 men had coronary angiography, they all had one- to three-vessel disease. This high incidence of silent ischemia prompted the suggestion that ED might be a precursor of more serious cardiac manifestations in the future. He further suggested that ED may be

---
* Center For Sexual Function/Endocrinology, Lahey Clinic Northshore, Peabody, One Essex Center Drive, Peabody, MA 01960.
E-mail address: andre.t.guay@lahey.org

0889-8529/07/$ - see front matter © 2007 Elsevier Inc. All rights reserved.
doi:10.1016/j.ecl.2007.03.007
endo.theclinics.com

a useful marker of a future cardiac event. Not surprisingly, Blumentals and investigators [8] showed that men with ED had twice the risk of having a myocardial infraction. Shamoul and colleagues [9] was further able to correlate decreased penile blood flow as measured by corpus duplex ultrasound with abnormal stress electrocardiography. Vlachopoulos and colleagues [10] documented that up to 19% of patients with vascular ED have documented silent CAD.

Erectile dysfunction and cardiovascular disease share many risk factors

The fact that diabetes, hypertension, hyperlipidemia, and smoking are major factors for heart disease has been long known, and that these risks directly act on vascular function [11]. Even obesity has now been shown to be an independent risk factor for CAD because of decreased coronary blood flow [12]. A number of studies have shown that these same risk factors also cause ED [2,13–16]. It should be noted that various disciplines consistently show the same major risk factors of hypertension and diabetes. Table 1 shows these similarities between a large epidemiological database and a much smaller clinical study in one sexual function clinic. The prevalences of diabetes and hypertension are quite similar and reflect what many internists and general practitioners would see in their clinical practices. The difference in prevalence for hyperlipidemia is explained because the smaller clinical study by Walczak and colleagues [16] defined hyperlipidemia narrowly as a low-density lipoprotein (LDL) cholesterol level above 120 mg/dL, consistent with most cardiology practices. Seftel and colleagues [17], in a large database study, used International Classification of Diseases, Ninth Revision (ICD9), codes that are nonspecific and are left to varied interpretation by practicing physicians. Cardiologists feel that an LDL cholesterol above 120 mg/dL confers vascular risk, and so probably reflects a truer prevalence of cardiac risk in men with symptomatic ED.

Table 1
Comparison of the prevalences of the major erectile dysfunction and cardiovascular disease risk factors in a large epidemiological database versus that of a smaller clinical study

Risk factor	Epidemiological study, %[a]	Clinical study, %[b]
Hypertension	42	44
Diabetes mellitus	20	23
Hyperlipidemia	42	74

For the epidemiological study, n = 272,325; for the clinical study, n = 154.

[a] *Data from* Seftel AD, Sun P, Swindle R. The prevalence of hypertension, hyperlipidemia, diabetes mellitus and depression in men with erectile dysfunction. J Urol 2004;171:2341–5.

[b] *Data from* Walczak MK, Lokhandwala N, Hodge MB, et al. Prevalence of cardiovascular risk factors in erectile dysfunction. J Gend Specif Med 2002;5:19–24.

The link between erectile dysfunction and cardiovascular disease is endothelial dysfunction

The common denominator underlying the pathophysiology of both ED and CVD is vascular insufficiency promoted by atherosclerosis [18]. The basic pathology in these conditions, as characterized in Fig. 1, is endothelial dysfunction, promoted by oxidative stress from the various medical conditions listed [19–21]. Endothelial dysfunction is the basic initiator in the formation of atherosclerotic plaques [22]. Lekakis and investigators [23] demonstrated endothelial dysfunction by brachial arm blood flow testing after smoking a cigarette, and Baron [24] demonstrated decreased endothelium function by insulin resistance, seen in both obesity and type 2 diabetes mellitus. Suwaidi and colleagues [12] demonstrated increased endothelial dysfunction in coronary artery blood flow with increasing levels of increased weight above a normal body mass index (BMI) of 25. Endothelial dysfunction and decreased nitric oxide formation has been shown in hypertension, the most common cause of ED in many series (see Table 1) [25]. In hyperlipidemia, oxidized LDL cholesterol impairs endothelial relaxation, and the free radicals that are formed inactivate the most important vasodilator, nitric oxide [22]. The pathophysiological mechanisms regulating nitric oxide metabolism affecting both ED and CVD have been outlined clearly and succinctly by Ganz [26].

Numerous studies have been reported that demonstrate endothelial dysfunction and decreased nitric oxide formation (or activity) in ED, both on the basic science level and on the clinical level [27]. The idea that ED was an early manifestation of endothelial dysfunction was clinically shown by

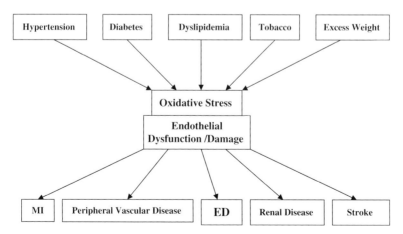

Fig. 1. The relation of erectile dysfunction (ED) to cardiovascular disease as seen through their common pathophysiological mechanism, endothelial dysfunction. MI indicates myocardial infarction. (*Data from* Guay AT. Relation of endothelial cell function to erectile dysfunction: implications for treatment. Am J Cardiol 2005;96(suppl 12B):52M–56M.)

Kaiser and colleagues [28]. They compared 30 men who had ED but no overt manifestations or risk factors of vascular disease with a similar control group who did not have ED. No differences were found between groups as far as intima-medial thickness, coronary calcification, pulse wave velocity, or aortic distension. There was, however, a significant decrease in endothelial-dependent flow-mediated brachial artery vasodilatation in the men with ED, suggesting that ED may be the first manifestation of vascular flow abnormalities. Bocchio and colleagues [29] have even elucidated this in a more basic biochemical model. They studied three groups of men with ED. One group had diabetes, another had hypertension, and one had no cardiovascular risk factors. The groups with diabetes and hypertension had decreased penile blood flow while the men with cardiac risks had normal blood flow. All groups, however, had increased inflammatory cytokines, known factors in early manifestations of endothelial dysfunction and atherosclerosis. The conclusion suggested is that ED is an extremely early manifestation of future vascular insufficiency, manifested even before actual decrease in blood flow. ED may indeed be the early factor that cardiologists have been looking for to alert them to practice primary cardiac prevention. For the clinician, this may mean that when men are seen for ED, a search of cardiac risk factors should be undertaken, and then appropriate treatment suggested.

Another early marker of atherosclerosis is a deficiency of progenitor cells from the bone marrow, whose job it is to repair damaged endothelial cells. The number of these cells is reduced in overt cardiovascular disease and has been shown to correlate with the presence of various cardiac risk factors, even in the preclinical stages [30]. It is interesting that even healthy subjects with endothelial dysfunction have a reduced number of these cells [31]. Foresta and colleagues [32] has further demonstrated that men with ED have a reduced number of progenitor cells in their peripheral blood, and even that the level of decreased cells was no different in men with or without cardiovascular risk factors. This is further proof of ED as probably the earliest clinical manifestation of cardiovascular risk.

Metabolic syndrome and insulin resistance as markers of endothelial dysfunction

Metabolic syndrome and insulin resistance are well known markers of cardiovascular risk, especially diabetes, hypertension, hyperlipidemia, and obesity [33,34]. Insulin resistance is felt by some to be at the core of the metabolic syndrome, and to be important in endothelial dysfunction [35,36]. A recent review has confirmed that endothelial dysfunction occurs early in the insulin-resistant state [37]. The relationship can be seen if one considers the components of the metabolic syndrome: elevated blood pressure, high triglycerides, low high-density lipoprotein (HDL) cholesterol, elevated waist circumference (or elevated BMI), and other aspects of insulin resistance manifested as diabetes or glucose intolerance. Three of the five criteria qualify as having the metabolic syndrome. These components are quite interrelated as obesity has been found to be a strong determinant of insulin resistance and the subsequent rise in glucose in the metabolic syndrome [38].

We have previously shown that in a group of men evaluated for ED from a medical-endocrine clinic, one or more cardiovascular risk factors were seen in 91% of the population [16]. In a further study (of this same group of men with organic ED), we demonstrated that there is a higher proportion of men with metabolic syndrome and insulin resistance than would be found in the general population [39]. The incidence of metabolic syndrome, using the National Education Program Adult Treatment Panel III criteria, was 43%, compared with 25% in a general population study. The incidence of insulin resistance, as measured by the Quantitative Insulin Sensitivity Check Index (QUICKI) [40] was 79%, versus 26% in a general population study. Even eliminating the men who had diabetes, as these men have insulin resistance by definition, the incidence of insulin resistance was 73%, still much higher than in the general population.

This is just another way of emphasizing that there is a strong link between ED and potential, or present, cardiovascular disease. Another finding (as outlined in Table 2) is that the more serious the ED, as manifested by lower scores in the five-item version of the International Index of Erectile Function (IIEF-5) questionnaire [41], the higher the percentage of men with metabolic syndrome and with insulin resistance, as well as the number of men with glucose intolerance, a precursor of both diabetes and cardiovascular disease. It is already known that the severity of ED has been related to the number and severity of the atherosclerotic involvement of the coronary arteries [18].

Is there a relationship between endothelial dysfunction and hypogonadism?

The topic of testosterone and hypogonadism will be discussed in more detail elsewhere but a few pertinent comments to this discussion are in order.

Table 2
Relationship between the severity of erectile dysfunction and the incidence of metabolic syndrome and insulin resistance, as well as glucose intolerance, in a population of men with organic erectile dysfunction (N = 154)

Severity of IIEF-5 score	The metabolic syndrome, %	Insulin resistance, %	FBS >110 mg/dL, %
Mild ED (17–21)	14.5	14.8	19.1
Moderate ED (11–16)	35.5	32.8	25.5
Severe ED (1–10)	50.0	44.2	46.8

Abbreviations: FBS, fasting blood sugar; IIEF-5, International Index of Erectile Function five-question shortened version (normal is score of 22 of 25 out of max possible score of 25).
Data from Bansal TC, Guay AT, Jacobson J, et al. Incidence of metabolic syndrome and insulin resistance in a population with organic erectile dysfunction. J Sex Med 2005;2:96–103.

The definite role of testosterone in penile development and erectile physiology has recently been reviewed [27]. In animal experiments, Lugg and colleagues [42] showed that testosterone, and especially its active conversion product dihydrotestosterone, was the active androgen that maintained nitric oxide–mediated penile erection. This clearly showed that androgens were necessary for penile artery endothelial function by comparing the level of nitric oxide activity after castration versus a control group. Aversa and colleagues [43] confirmed the role of testosterone in penile blood flow in humans. They highlighted a direct relationship between plasma free testosterone levels and cavernous dilatation and blood flow in men with ED.

Hypogonadism is intertwined with the cardiac risks that we have been discussing, including metabolic syndrome and insulin resistance. Hypogonadism has found to have an inverse relationship with obesity and a direct relationship to CAD [44]. A number of studies have demonstrated a strong relationship between hypogonadism and the metabolic syndrome [45,46] as well as insulin resistance [47,48]. Traish and colleagues [49] also showed adipocyte accumulation in the corpora cavernosum of castrated animals, suggesting an animal parallel to human adipocyte accumulation in men with metabolic syndrome. Laaksonen and colleagues [50] suggest that hypogonadism actually predicts the metabolic syndrome, and thus may be an early marker for disturbed insulin and glucose metabolism. Tsai and colleagues [51] confirmed this by pointing out a significant inverse relationship between testosterone levels and markers of insulin resistance. It is becoming clear that testosterone levels should be checked in men with ED and also in men who have the chronic illnesses found in the metabolic syndrome.

Implications of treatment of erectile dysfunction risks on endothelial dysfunction

In treating ED, a growing number of physicians have been promoting the concept of modifying lifestyle measures, and modifying the medical risk factors for ED, rather than just treating the symptom of ED with the PDE5 inhibitors, sildenafil, vardenafil, tardalafil, or any other treatment modalities [19,52]. Although the PDE5 inhibitors do ameliorate endothelial dysfunction as well as correcting the ED [53], directing therapy to the cause(s) of the endothelial dysfunction conceivably will decrease the progress of atherosclerosis in its early stages. Modification of risk factors common to ED and to CVD has been shown to decrease cardiovascular events. Weight loss in obesity has been shown to decrease insulin resistance and improve endothelial function [54]. Esposito and colleagues [55] demonstrated that decreasing weight in obese men had a positive effect in improving sexual function as shown by an improvement in erectile questionnaire parameters.

Cigarette smoking has been shown to decrease blood flow in atherosclerotic penile arteries causing vascular ED as well as causing generalized atherosclerosis [56,57]. We have previously shown that smoking cessation rapidly improves multiple erectile parameters, as monitored by nocturnal penile tumescence and rigidity testing [58]. Although the Massachusetts Male Aging Study did not find that smoking cessation decreased the development of future ED [59], Mannino and colleagues [60], in a study of 4500 veterans, found that the prevalence of ED was significantly lowered in former compared with active smokers. There is still controversy as to the exact extent of involvement of tobacco abuse in vascular ED.

Diabetes is one of the most difficult causes of ED to treat for a number of reasons. Many diabetic men have subclinical neuropathy, decreasing the effectiveness of the oral PDE5 inhibitors. Also, diabetic men have multiple concurrent risk factors, especially obesity, hyperlipidemia, and hypertension. In the literature, 40% to 60% of diabetic men have hypertension, and the combination of diabetes and hypertension occurs in 10% of the men presenting to our ED clinic [61]. Controlling blood sugar is important and does help erectile function. Romeo and colleagues [62] observed a positive correlation between glycemic control and sexual function. It has now been shown that in diabetic patients, controlling blood pressure and lowering lipids, in addition to controlling the blood sugar, significantly reduced the risk of cardiovascular events [63].

There are no controlled studies that have shown that lowering lipids improves ED, as opposed to the known effects on reducing cardiovascular events in large cardiology series. A small, case-controlled study did show evidence, using nocturnal penile tumescence and rigidity monitoring, that lowering total and LDL cholesterol led to improved erections in men whose only identifiable risk for ED was hypercholesterolemia [64]. Testosterone treatment of hypogonadal men seems, in early studies, to improve many of the risks mentioned above, especially obesity, insulin resistance, glycemic control, and hyperlipidemia [65]. The study of the relationship between hypogonadism and cardiac risk is only in its infancy, and therefore is still controversial.

More studies in the area of ED and endothelial function are definitely needed. The fact that the PDE5 inhibitors will improve erectile function by reversing the decreased vascular flow caused by endothelial dysfunction from a variety of cardiovascular risk factors may have some far-reaching implications. It is possible that the chronic use of the PDE5 inhibitors might lead to decreased cardiac risk by helping to heal or retard the progression of endothelial disease. A hint of this might be gleaned from the work of Rosano and colleagues [66]. They showed that after just 4 weeks of tadalafil, 20 mg every other day, endothelial function, as measured by brachial artery flow-mediated dilatation, was significantly improved over placebo. The benefit was also sustained for at least 2 weeks after discontinuation of therapy.

Summary

It has been shown that ED and CVD share multiple risk factors. The common denominator is decreased vascular flow from endothelial dysfunction. This is why the PDE5 inhibitors have been so successful, as they increase blood flow by counteracting the pathophysiological etiology of ED common to many conditions, endothelial dysfunction. A philosophy of modifying risk factors of ED has been gaining popularity in the past few years, rather than just treating the symptoms of ED nonspecifically. This is because ED is being recognized more and more as a symptom of underlying disease, and not just as a specific disease by itself. Modifying the risk factors has been shown to greatly increase the effectiveness of one of the PDE5 inhibitors, sildenafil [67]. A logical conclusion is that when a man appears with the symptom of ED, a thorough search should be done for cardiovascular risk factors, and recommendations for correction of these factors should be undertaken. In this way, clinicians may be able to practice primary cardiac prevention. Thus, ED^2 may be upgraded to ED^3: erectile dysfunction = endothelial dysfunction = early detection (of cardiac disease).

References

[1] Cohan P, Korenman SG. Erectile dysfunction. J Clin Endocrinol Metab 2001;86:2191–4.
[2] Feldman HA, Goldstein I, Hatzichristou DG, et al. Impotence and its medical and psychosocial correlates: results of the Massachusetts Male Aging Study. J Urol 1994;151:54–61.
[3] Barrett-Connor E. Heart disease risk factors predict erectile dysfunction 25 years later (The Rancho Bernardo Study). Am J Cardiol 2005;96(Suppl 12B):3M–7M.
[4] Bhatt DL, Steg PG, Ohman EM, et al. International prevalence, recognition, and treatment of cardiovascular risk factors in outpatients with atherothrombosis. JAMA 2006;295:180–9.
[5] Kloner RA, Mullin SH, Shook T, et al. Erectile dysfunction in the cardiac patient: how common and should we treat? J Urol 2003;170:S46–50.
[6] Solomon H, Man JW, Wierzbicki AS, et al. Relation of erectile dysfunction to angiographic coronary artery disease. Am J Cardiol 2003;91:230–1.
[7] Pritzker M. The penile stress test: a window to the hearts of man? Circulation 1999;100(Suppl 1):350–3.
[8] Blumentals WA, Gomez-Caminero A, Joo S, et al. Should erectile dysfunction be considered a marker for acute myocardial infarction? Results from a retrospective cohort study. Int J Impot Res 2004;16:1–4.
[9] Shamoul R, Ghanem HM, Salem A, et al. Correlation between penile duplex findings and stress electrocardiography in men with erectile dysfunction. Int J Impot Res 2004;16:235–7.
[10] Vlachopoulos C, Rokkas K, Iokeimides N, et al. Prevalence of asymptomatic coronary artery disease in men with vasculogenic erectile dysfunction: a prospective angiographic study. Eur Urol 2005;48:996–1003.
[11] Maas R, Schwedhelm E, Albsmeier J, et al. The pathophysiology of erectile dysfunction related to endothelial dysfunction and mediators of vascular function. Vasc Med 2001;7: 213–25.
[12] Suwaidi JA, Higano ST, Holmes DR, et al. Obesity is independently associated with coronary endothelial dysfunction in patients with normal or mildly diseased coronary arteries. J Am Coll Cardiol 2001;37:1523–8.
[13] Virag R, Bouilly P, Frydman D. Is impotence an arterial disorder? A study of arterial risk factors in 440 impotent men. Lancet 1985;1:181–4.
[14] Martin-Morales A, Sanchez-Cruz JJ, Saenz de Tejada I, et al. Prevalence and independent risk factors for erectile dysfunction in Spain: results of the Epidemiologia de la Disfuncion Erectil Masculina Study. J Urol 2001;166:569–74.

[15] Blanker MH, Bohnen AM, Groeneveld FP, et al. Correlates for erectile and ejaculatory dysfunction in older Dutch men: a community-based study. J Am Geriatr Soc 2001;49: 436–42.
[16] Walczak MK, Lokhandwala N, Hodge MB, et al. Prevalence of cardiovascular risk factors in erectile dysfunction. J Gend Specif Med 2002;5:19–24.
[17] Seftel AD, Sun P, Swindle R. The prevalence of hypertension, hyperlipidemia, diabetes mellitus and depression in men with erectile dysfunction. J Urol 2004;171:2341–5.
[18] Jackson G. Sex, the heart and erectile dysfunction. London: Taylor & Francis; 2004. p. 10.
[19] Guay AT. Relation of endothelial cell function to erectile dysfunction: implications for treatment. Am J Cardiol 2005;96(Suppl 12B):52M–6M.
[20] Solomon H, Man JW, Jackson G. Erectile dysfunction and the cardiovascular patient: endothelial dysfunction is the common denominator. Heart 2003;89:251–3.
[21] Bivalaqua TJ, Usta MF, Champion HC, et al. Endothelial dysfunction in erectile dysfunction: role of the endothelium in erectile physiology and disease. J Androl 2003;24: S17–37.
[22] Cooke JP. The endothelium: a new target for therapy. Vasc Med 2000;5:49–53.
[23] Lekakis J, Papamichael C, Vemmos C, et al. Effects of acute cigarette smoking on endothelium-dependent arterial dilatation in normal subjects. Am J Cardiol 1998;81: 1225–8.
[24] Baron AD. Hemodynamic actions of insulin. Am J Physiol 2004;267:187–202.
[25] Higashi Y, Sasaki S, Nakagawa K, et al. Effects of obesity on endothelium-dependent nitric oxide mediated vasodilatation in normotensive individuals and patients with essential hypertension. Am J Hypertens 2001;14:1038–45.
[26] Ganz P. Erectile dysfunction: pathophysiologic mechanisms pointing to underlying cardiovascular disease. Am J Cardiol 2005;96(Suppl 12 B):8M–12M.
[27] Traish AM, Guay AT. Are androgens critical for penile erections in humans? Examining the clinical and preclinical evidence. J Sex Med 2006;3:382–407.
[28] Kaiser DR, Billups K, Mason C, et al. Impaired brachial artery endothelium-dependent and -independent vasodilation in men with erectile dysfunction and no other clinical cardiovascular disease. J Am Coll Cardiol 2004;43:179–84.
[29] Bocchio M, Desideri G, Scarpelli P, et al. Endothelial cell activation in men with erectile dysfunction without cardiovascular risk factors and overt vascular damage. J Urol 2004;171: 1601–4.
[30] Asahara T, Murohara T, Sullivan A, et al. Isolation of putative progenitor endothelial cells for angiogenesis. Science 1997;275:964–7.
[31] Dimmeler S, Zeiher AM. Vascular repair by circulating endothelial progenitor cells: the missing link in atherosclerosis? J Mol Med 2004;82:671–7.
[32] Foresta C, Caretta N, Lana A, et al. Circulating endothelial progenitor cells in subjects with erectile dysfunction. Int J Impot Res 2005;17:288–90.
[33] Hu G, Qiao Q, Tuomilehto J, et al. Prevalence of the metabolic syndrome and its relation to all-cause and cardiovascular mortality in non-diabetic European men and women. Arch Intern Med 2004;164:1066–76.
[34] Hanley AJG, Stern MP, Williams K, et al. Homeostasis model assessment of insulin resistance in relation to the incidence of cardiovascular disease: the San Antonio Heart Study. Diabetes Care 2002;25:1177–84.
[35] Pinkey JH, Stehouwer CDA, Coppack SW, et al. Endothelial dysfunction: cause of the insulin resistance syndrome. Diabetes 1997;46(Suppl 2):S9–13.
[36] Jackson G. The metabolic syndrome and erectile dysfunction; multiple vascular risk factors and hypogonadsim. Eur Urol 2006;50:426–7.
[37] Hsueh WA, Lyon CJ, Quinones MJ. Insulin resistance and the endothelium. Am J Med 2004; 117:109–17.
[38] Carnethon MR, Palaniappan LP, Burchfiel CM, et al. Serum insulin, obesity, and the incidence of type 2 diabetes in black and white adults. Diabetes Care 2002;25:1358–64.

[39] Bansal TC, Guay AT, Jacobson J, et al. Incidence of metabolic syndrome and insulin resistance in a population with organic erectile dysfunction. J Sex Med 2005;2:96–103.

[40] Katz A, Nambi SS, Mather K, et al. Quantitative Insulin Sensitivity Check Index: a simple, accurate method for assessing insulin sensitivity in humans. J Clin Endocrinol Metab 2000; 85:2402–10.

[41] Rosen RC, Cappelleri JC, Smith MD, et al. Developement and evaluation of an abridged, 5-item version of the International Index of Erectile function (IIEF-5) as a diagnostic tool for erectile dysfunction. Int J Impot Res 1999;11:319–26.

[42] Lugg JA, Rajfer J, Gonzalez-Cadavid NF. Dihydrotestosterone is the active androgen in the maintenance of nitric oxide-mediated penile erection in the rat. Endocrinology 1995;136: 1495–501.

[43] Aversa A, Isidori AM, De Martino MU, et al. Androgens and penile erection: evidence for a direct relationship between free testosterone and cavernous dilatation in men with erectile dysfunction. Clin Endocrinol (Oxf) 2000;53:517–22.

[44] Shapsigh R, Katz M, Yan G, et al. Cardiovascular issues in hypogonadism and testosterone therapy. Am J Cardiol 2005;96(Suppl 12B):67M–72M.

[45] Kupelian V, Page ST, Aruajo AB, et al. Low sex hormone-binding globulin, total testosterone, and symptomatic androgen deficiency are associated with development of the metabolic syndrome in non-obese men. J Clin Endocrinol Metab 2006;91:843–50.

[46] Muller M, Grobbee DE, den Tonkelar I, et al. Endogenous sex hormones and the metabolic syndrome in aging men. J Clin Endocrinol Metab 2005;90:2618–23.

[47] Kapoor D, Malkin CJ, Channer KS, et al. Androgens, insulin resistance and vascular disease in men. Clin Endocrinol (Oxf) 2005;63:239–50.

[48] Pittleloud N, Hardin M, Dwyer AA, et al. Increasing insulin resistance is associated with a decrease in Leydig cell testosterone secretion in men. J Clin Endocrinol Metab 2005;90: 2636–41.

[49] Traish AM, Toselli P, Jeong SJ, et al. Adipocyte accumulation in penile corpus cavernosum of the orchiectomized rabbit: a potential mechanism for venoocclusive dysfunction in androgen deficiency. J Androl 2005;26:242–8.

[50] Laaksonen DE, Niskanen L, Punnonen K, et al. Testosterone and sex hormone-binding globulin predict the metabolic syndrome and diabetes in middle-aged men. Diabetes Care 2004;27:1036–41.

[51] Tsai EC, Matsumoto AM, Fujimoto WY, et al. Association of bioavailable, free, and total testosterone with insulin resistance. Diabetes Care 2004;27:861–8.

[52] Billups KL. Sexual dysfunction and cardiovascular disease: integrative concepts and strategies. Am J Cardiol 2005;96(suppl 12B):57M–61M.

[53] DeBusk RF. Erectile dysfunction therapy in special populations and applications: coronary artery disease. Am J Cardiol 2005;96(Suppl 12B):62M–6M.

[54] Hamdy O, Mousa A, Ledbury S, et al. Lifestyle modification improves endothelial function in obese subjects with the insulin resistance syndrome. Diabetes Care 2003;26:2119–25.

[55] Esposito K, Giugliano F, DiPalo C, et al. Effect of lifestyle changes on erectile dysfunction in obese men: a randomized controlled trial. JAMA 2004;291:2978–84.

[56] Rosen MP, Greenfield AJ, Walker TJ, et al. Cigarette smoking: an independent risk factor for atherosclerosis in the hypogastric-cavernous arterial bed of men with arteriogenic impotence. J Urol 1991;145:759–63.

[57] McVary KT, Carrier S, Wessles H, for the Subcommittee on Smoking and Erectile Dysfunction Socioeconomic Committee, Sexual Medicine Society of North America. Smoking and erectile function: evidence-based analysis. J Urol 2001;166:1624–32.

[58] Guay AT, Perez JB, Heatley GJ. Cessation of smoking rapidly decreases erectile dysfunction. Endocr Pract 1998;4:23–6.

[59] Derby CA, Mohr BA, Goldstein I, et al. Modifiable risk factors and erectile dysfunction: can lifestyle changes modify risk? Urology 2000;56:302–6.

[60] Mannino DM, Klevans RM, Flanders WD. Cigarette smoking: an independent risk factor for impotence? Am J Epidemiol 1994;140:1003–8.

[61] Guay AT, Velasquez E, Perez JB. Characterization of patients in a medical endocrine-based center for male sexual dysfunction. Endocr Pract 1999;5:314–21.

[62] Romeo JH, Seftel AD, Madhun ZT, et al. Sexual function in men with diabetes type 2: association with glycemic control. J Urol 2000;163:788–91.

[63] Beckman JA, Creager MA, Libbly P. Diabetes and atherosclerosis: epidemiology, pathophysiology, and management. JAMA 2002;287:2570–81.

[64] Saltzman EA, Guay AT, Jacobson J. Improvement in erectile function in men with organic erectile dysfunction by correlation of elevated cholesterol levels: a clinical observation. J Urol 2004;172:255–8.

[65] Kapoor D, Goodwin E, Cahnner KS, et al. Testosterone replacement therapy improves insulin resistance, glycemic control, visceral adiposity and hypercholesterolemia in hypogonadal men with type 2 diabetes. Eur J Endocrinol 2006;154:899–906.

[66] Rosano GM, Aversa A, Vitale C, et al. Chronic treatment with tadalafil improves endothelial function in men with increased cardiovascular risk. Eur Urol 2005;47:214–20.

[67] Guay AT, Perez JB, Jacobson J, et al. Efficacy and safety of sildenafil citrate for treatment of erectile dysfunction in a population with associated organic risk factors. J Androl 2001;22:793–7.

ELSEVIER
SAUNDERS

Endocrinol Metab Clin N Am
36 (2007) 465–479

ENDOCRINOLOGY
AND METABOLISM
CLINICS
OF NORTH AMERICA

Treatment Options for Erectile Dysfunction

William O. Brant, MD[a],*, Anthony J. Bella, MD[b],
Tom F. Lue, MD[b]

[a]University of Colorado School of Medicine, P.O. Box 40,000, Vail, CO 81658, USA
[b]Department of Urology, University of California,
Box A633, 400 Parnassus Avenue, San Francisco, CA 94143, USA

Oral therapies

In a normal erection, nitric oxide activates guanylate cyclase, which facilitates the conversion of guanosine triphosphate to cyclic GMP (cGMP) and leads to a cascade of events culminating in decreased intracellular calcium and resultant smooth muscle relaxation. At the same time, cGMP is broken down to GMP by the enzyme phosphodiesterase (PDE), the type 5 isoform of which is found in relatively high concentrations in the corpora cavernosa. PDE type 5 inhibitors (PDE5is) act at this step, slowing the breakdown of cGMP. The higher cGMP levels, therefore, act as amplifiers of the normal erectile physiology and are dependent on intact libido, sexual stimulation, sensory pathways, and a multitude of other factors that must be present in normal erectile function [1]. There are three such PDE5is commercially available: sildenafil (Viagra, Pfizer, New York, New York), tadalafil (Cialis, Lilly, Indianapolis, Indiana), and vardenafil (Levitra, Bayer, West Haven, Connecticut). U.S. Food and Drug Administration (FDA) approval was granted for sildenafil in 1998 and 2003 for tadalafil and vardenafil. Although each medication is relatively specific for PDE 5, there are cross-over effects on other PDE isoforms; these effects are partially responsible for the individual side effects seen with the individual medications. For example, sildenafil and, to a lesser extent, vardenafil, have cross-reactivity with PDE 6, found in the eye, which is responsible for the sensitivity to light and other ocular disturbances (eg, blue vision) that are seen with these medications. Tadalafil does not demonstrate significant cross-reactivity to PDE 6 but

---

* Corresponding author.
E-mail address: dr.w.brant@gmail.com (W.O. Brant).

does affect PDE 11, which is found in disparate organs such as testis and heart, although the clinical implications of this are not clear [2].

Although the PDE5is act via a common pathway and thus share many similarities, there are pharmacologic and therapeutic differences, particularly with regard to timing of the clinical effect.

Onset and duration

Sildenafil, as assessed by Rigiscan measurements, has an onset of action within 30 to 60 minutes and lasts up to 4 hours [3], although its action may begin as quickly as within 14 minutes in over one third of users [4]. Vardenafil acts somewhat more rapidly at 25 minutes and also lasts for 4 hours [5,6]. In contrast, tadalafil acts relatively quickly (45 minutes as assessed by Rigiscan or as little as 16 minutes as assessed by patient-controlled stopwatch) but lasts much longer, with efficacy continuing to 36 hours [7]. The subtle differences in time of onset may be of minor clinical import. A population-based study from the United Kingdom examined the time course of intercourse, from a man considering it, to agreeing with his partner, to beginning it, and found that on average it took 53 minutes from the initial thought to the start of intercourse, whether or not the patient had erectile dysfunction [8]. Therefore, all of the available PDE5is likely have appropriate onset of action.

Efficacy: short- and long-term

In short-term studies (12 weeks), sildenafil was found to lead to a 65% successful intercourse rate in general erectile dysfunction (ED) populations, compared with 20% with placebo. These trends are borne out when the ED population is stratified in terms of duration of ED, severity (mild/moderate versus severe), and origin (organic versus psychogenic versus mixed) [9]. Longer-term data are also available; in an open-label extension over 4 years, over 95% of patients continued to be satisfied with the effect of the medication on erections, with a cumulative drop-out rate of 6.3% for insufficient response and 1.2% for adverse events [10]. Vardenafil showed similar efficacy, with over 70% successful intercourse during a 12-week period [11] and over 85% at 2 years [12]. The same goes for tadalafil, with >70% successful intercourse when using 20 mg and over 60% using 10 mg [7].

Special populations

Sildenafil has been examined in a variety of more specific populations, showing increased efficacy when patients are stratified by age (>65), body mass index (>30), or ethnic group (Caucasians, African-Americans, Hispanics, and Asians) [9]. When specific etiologies are examined, sildenafil was found to work better than placebo in all groups (diabetes, ischemic heart disease, peripheral vascular disease, hypertension, postradical prostatectomy, antihypertensive medications, antidepressant medications, and depression), although overall efficacy was poorer in the postprostatectomy group [9] and for patients who had diabetes [13].

Side effects

Side effects of PDE5is are generally mild and well tolerated. For sildenafil, these include headache (16%), flushing (10%), dyspepsia (7%), and nasal congestion (4%), [14]. Vardenafil has a similar side-effect profile, with the FDA Web site listing headache (15%), flushing (11%), dyspepsia (9%), and rhinitis (4%) as side effects occurring appreciably more than in patients taking placebo. The FDA also reports that tadalafil induces somewhat less flushing (3%) than the other medications but may result in pain at different sites, most prominently the back (6%) and limbs (3%), and may result in general myalgia (3%).

Priapism, or a pathologic erection that lasts longer than 4 hours despite lack of sexual stimulation, is uncommon, with isolated case reports in the literature [15,16]. PDE5is, as endothelial regulators, may be helpful in the prevention of recurrent priapic episodes (eg, in patients who have sickle cell disease or trait) [17].

Absolute and relative contraindications

Due to the risk of profound and dangerous hypotension that may result from the use of PDE5is and nitrate-containing medication, regular or intermittent use of nitrates (eg, nitroglycerin, and isosorbide dinitrate) is an absolute contraindication to PDE5i use. Amyl nitrate inhalers ("poppers") are occasionally used as a drug of abuse, and the practitioner should ask about their use before prescribing a PDE5i. In isolation, sildenafil causes mild (<10 mm Hg) and transient effects on systolic and diastolic blood pressure [18].

Neither controlled nor postmarketing studies of the three available PDE5is has demonstrated any increase in rates of myocardial infarction or death; this was true in double-blind, placebo-controlled trials and in open-label studies (when compared with expected rates in the study populations) [19]. In patients who had known coronary artery disease or heart failure, the use of PDE-5 inhibitors did not lead to worse ischemia, coronary vasoconstriction, or worsening hemodynamics on exercise testing or cardiac catheterization. PDE-5 inhibitors have a minimal effect on QTc interval [20]. Vardenafil is not recommended in patients who take type-1A antiarrhythmics (eg, quinidine or procainamide) or type-3 antiarrhythmics (eg, sotalol or amiodarone) or in patients who have congenital prolonged QT syndrome.

Due to a lack of controlled clinical data, PDE5is should be used with caution, if at all, in patients who have recent serious cardiovascular events, uncontrolled hypertension, unstable angina, or retinitis pigmentosa. One proposed rule of thumb is that patients who have cardiovascular disease may be stratified into high, intermediate (which may be further stratified depending on subsequent testing), and low risk; low-risk patients may be treated with first-line agents, whereas high-risk patients (eg, patients who have unstable angina, uncontrolled hypertension, or a myocardial infarct or stroke within the last 2 weeks) should have their cardiovascular status stabilized before resuming sexual activity [21].

A lower starting dose (25 mg of sildenafil or 5 mg of vardenafil or tadalafil) should be used in patients who may attain and maintain higher plasma levels (eg, patients who are older than 65 years, have severe renal impairment, or take potent CYP450 3A4 inhibitors). Patients who take ritonavir should not take more than 25 mg of sildenafil in a 48-hour period [22]. To avoid symptomatic hypotension, PDE5is should not be taken within 4 hours of an α-blocker [23]. One study found a significant rate of hypotension (28% versus 6% with placebo) in patients taking concomitant doxazosin and tadalafil; however, the rate of hypotension matched that seen in placebo-treated patients and in patients taking tamsulosin and tadalafil [24], and some studies suggest that the interaction has less clinical relevance in patients who have undergone long-term α-blocker therapy [25]. The position of the American Urological Association is that all three PDE5is interact to some degree with α-blockers and that concurrent use of α-blockers and PDE5is may cause patients to develop orthostatic hypotension [26]. In hemodynamically stable patients treated with α-blockers, PDE5is should be used with caution and initiated at the lowest recommended starting dose. Similarly, patients using PDE5is and requiring α-blocker therapy should start at low doses and should be titrated gradually to effect. Other antihypertensive agents, such as calcium-channel blockers, are well tolerated by men concurrently taking any of the three PDE5 inhibitors. Concomitant administration of these drugs seems to cause no or only small additive drops in blood pressure.

Nonarteritic ischemic optic neuropathy (NAION) and PDE5i use has garnered a great deal of attention in scientific and lay publications. Spontaneous NAION is the most common acute optic neuropathy and ranks second only to glaucoma as a cause of acquired optic neuropathy for men aged 50 years and older [27]. The estimated annual incidence is 2.3 to 10.3 per 100,000. It is more common in Caucasians than African Americans, Asians, or Hispanics [28–30]. Most patients do not become legally blind, but the degree of visual acuity and visual field loss is usually significant [28]. Risk factors common to NAION and ED include hypertension, diabetes mellitus, hypercholesterolemia, age over 50 years, coronary artery disease, and smoking [27]. Given that an estimated 27 million men worldwide that have used sildenafil (up to 1 billion doses), not counting tadalafil or vardenafil users, the expected incidence of NAION in this group should be many-fold higher than the 43 cases reported to the FDA as of June 2005 [27,28,31]. If one bases calculations on the most conservative incidence of NAION in the general population (2.3 cases per 100,000) and the fact that there are at least 27 million users of PDE5is, one would expect at least 621 cases in this population.

This comparison therefore brings up the question of whether PDE5is exert a protective influence on the evolution of NAION. The FDA maintains that a causal relationship between NAION and PDE5is has not been established. Review of safety data from over 100 clinical studies of sildenafil (>13,000 men) did not identify any cases of NAION; with similar findings have been reported vardenafil and tadalafil [9,27,32]. Given current evidence, it is not possible to determine whether these events are directly related to the use of PDE5is or to other factors; however, men are instructed to stop taking these medications immediately and contact their physician should visual changes or loss occur [27]. Men who have a history of NAION should not use PDE5is.

PDE5i failures

Before moving to second-line treatments, several strategies may be pursued when a patient complains that their new medication is not having the desired effect. An important first step is re-education on the correct use of the medications. Many patients need to be reminded that these agents are reliant on central mechanisms and that they do not work well without erotic stimulation. Up to 55% of initial nonresponders to sildenafil experience improvement after education [33,34]. Dose titration may be necessary. Additionally, sildenafil may not work as well after a high-fat meal, although vardenafil and tadalafil seem to be less dependent on timing with regard to food [35,36]. Another step that can be taken is to check hormonal levels because these medications are at least partially androgen dependent [37]. There is also evidence in animal models that function may improve with chronic use [38,39].

Other oral agents

Yohimbine is a centrally acting α2-adrenergic receptor antagonist produced from the bark of the yohim tree and is discussed in great detail by Tamler and Mechanick elsewhere in this issue. Its effect on erectile function is at best marginal, and it is therefore not recommended in patients who have organic ED. A meta-analysis of several placebo-controlled studies of 419 men who had predominantly nonorganic ED has shown some benefit over placebo [40]. Frequent side effects include gastrointestinal intolerance, headache, palpitation, fine tremor, elevation of blood pressure, and anxiety.

Oral phentolamine (Vasomax, Schering-Plough, New Jersey) has been reported to improve erectile function compared with placebo [41,42]. Side effects include headache, facial flushing, and nasal congestion. Oral phentolamine has not been approved by the FDA, but it is available in several South American countries.

Apomorphine (Uprima, Abbott, Illinois), a dopaminergic agonist, is a sublingual medication that is available for use in Europe. Apomorphine is a potent emetic that acts on central dopaminergic (D1/D2) receptors. When injected subcutaneously, it induces erections in rats and humans, but the side effects, notably nausea, limit its clinical usefulness [43]. Sublingual apomorphine has not received FDA approval.

Bremelanotide is a melanocortin analog that acts centrally and has been investigated in subcutaneous [44] and intranasal [45] administration. These studies reported statistically significant improvements in erections compared with placebo in healthy men and in men who did not respond well to sildenafil. Common side effects include flushing and nausea. The medication has not been approved by the FDA because phase 3 trials are not complete.

Other second-line treatments

If oral agents cannot be used or have insufficient efficacy despite appropriate dosing and education, second-line treatments should be addressed. These include vacuum erection devices (VEDs), transurethral suppositories, and intra-avernous injection (ICI) therapy.

Vacuum erection devices

A variety of VEDs are available. Medical-grade VEDs work by applying negative pressure to the penile shaft and glans, which provokes ingress and storage of blood in the sinusoidal tissue. An elastic band is applied to the base of the penis, which prevents egress of the trapped blood. There are several advantages to VEDs. Despite an initial expense, they are overall the most economical therapy for ED. There are few contraindications and no systemic side effects, and they have an extremely high efficacy [46]. However, they are cumbersome and give an unnatural erection. They also require manual dexterity, and the patient may have to shave his pubic hair to facilitate the creation of a seal for the vacuum. Side effects include petechiae, pain, numbness or coldness, delayed ejaculation, and a sense of trapped ejaculate. Despite almost uniformly allowing erections, satisfaction rates are approximately 55% [47]. This type of therapy is preferred for older patients in stable relationships; younger and single patients are rarely willing to continue using VEDs.

Although VEDs are often touted as means of penile lengthening, this has not been shown to be an effective method, although patient satisfaction with VEDs for this purpose was found to be 30% [48].

Intracavernosal injections

There are several ICI medications available, the most popular of which are alprostadil, papaverine, and phentolamine. These may be used individually or in combination. In general, ICI has the advantage of provoking a rapid, predictable, and reliable erection once the patient has had proper instruction and training. Men (and preferably their partners) must receive appropriate training and education by medical personnel before beginning home injections. The goal is to achieve an erection that is adequate for sexual intercourse but does not last for more than 1 hour. In comparison to VEDs, ICI imitates the natural erectile physiology and uses less bulky equipment, leading to more subtle use. Erections resulting from ICI have normal sensation, and no interference with ejaculation volume, sensation, or fertility has been reported.

Alprostadil has the highest efficacy of any of the individual agents and results in erections in more than 70% of treated men [49]. The usual dose ranges from 5 to 20 μg. The most frequent side effect is painful erections, which occur in 17% to 34% of men [49,50]. This hyperalgesic effect is most prominent in men who have partial nerve injury, such as patients who have diabetic neuropathy or a history of radical pelvic surgery. Alprostadil has a relatively low incidence of priapism (0.35%–4%) and fibrosis (1%–23%) [50–52].

Papaverine is a nonspecific phosphodiesterase inhibitor that increases cyclic AMP and cGMP concentrations in penile erectile tissue [53]. Its usual dose ranges from 15 to 60 mg. It is more effective in psychogenic and neurogenic erectile dysfunction (up to 80% effective) compared with vasculogenic etiology (36%–50% effective). Its advantages include low cost and stability at room temperature. Major disadvantages are priapism (up to 35%), corporal fibrosis (up to 33%), and occasional increases in liver function tests.

Phentolamine is a competitive α-adrenergic receptor antagonist. It must be used in combination with papaverine to produce rigid erections (63%–87% success rates) [54,55]. Many urologists use a combination of 30 mg papaverine and 0.5 to 1 mg phentolamine (Bimix). The side effects of phentolamine include hypotension and reflex tachycardia.

Vasoactive intestinal polypeptide is a potent smooth muscle relaxant originally isolated from the small intestine. This treatment is only available in Europe. Injection of vasoactive intestinal polypeptide alone does not produce a rigid erection [56], but when combined with phentolamine, it produces erections sufficient for sexual intercourse in up to 67% of men [57]. Common side effects include transient facial flushing (53%), bruising (20%), pain at the injection site (11%), and truncal flushing (9%).

Although individual agents have a role, the most effective intracavernous therapy used in the United States is a three-drug mixture containing papaverine, phentolamine, and alprostadil (Trimix). The usual dose of Trimix solution ranges from 0.1 to 0.5 mL. The response rate to this solution is as high as 90% [58]. In spite of its widespread use in the United States, it is not approved by the FDA. Other combinations of medications, such as papaverine and alprostadil [59], ketanserin and alprostadil [60], and phentolamine and alprostadil [61], have been proven to be superior to single medications in efficacy of response.

Side effects

Two major side effects of injection are priapism and fibrosis (penile deviation, nodules, or plaque). In adults, intracavernous therapy with papaverine, phentolamine, alprostadil, or combinations of these agents is the most common cause of ischemic priapism [62]. Zorgniotti and Lefleur [42] first reported the use of a combination of 30 mg papaverine and 0.5 mg phentolamine for self-injection. Prolonged erection occurred in 1.6% of patients during titration and in one patient on home therapy. In a review of the literature, Linet and Neff [49] found that doses of 10 to 20 μg alprostadil led to prolonged erection/priapism in 1.3% of patients. The incidence was found to be about five times lower with alprostadil than with papaverine or papaverine/phentolamine (1.3% versus 10% versus 7%), a finding supported by an Australian study [63]. In the clinical trials conducted by the Alprostadil Study Group worldwide in 1996 [49], prolonged erection (4–6 hours) was noted in 5% of patients, and priapism (>6 hours) was noted in 1% [49]. In an Argentinean study, a much higher rate of priapism was reported, reaching 18% and 15% for papaverine plus phentolamine and prostaglandin E1, respectively [64]. These figures are substantially higher than those found in other studies, which is likely secondary to testing patients with neurologic or psychologic impotence who are often sensitive to the medication. Priapism is largely preventable through in-office instruction and at-home careful dose titration.

To prevent fibrosis, we routinely instruct men to compress the injection site for 3 to 5 minutes (up to 10 minutes in men taking anticoagulants). Intracavernous injection therapy is contraindicated in men who have sickle-cell anemia and in those taking medication for schizophrenia or other severe psychiatric disorder due to the risk of priapism. Additionally, injection therapy may be difficult to perform if patients are obese or have poor manual dexterity; teaching the partner to administer the injection may circumvent some of these barriers.

Although offering several advantages over VEDs, the drop-out rate is very high; in long-term studies, 38% to 80% of men dropped out [65,66]. To avoid the cumbersome nature of injection therapy, some men alternate injection therapy with sildenafil or MUSE (Medicated Urethral System for Erection), preferring injection in circumstances when an erection of longer duration is desired. Alternatively, in men for whom injection therapy alone fails or is insufficient, we recommend the use of injection therapy in combination with a vacuum constriction device.

Transurethral medication

Transurethral alprostadil (MUSE) has been extensively studied in Europe and in the United States and was found to be effective in 43% of men who have erectile dysfunction of various organic causes. The most common side effects were penile pain (32%) and urethral pain or burning (12%) [67,68].

Placing an adjustable constriction device (Actis, VIVUS, Mountain View, California) at the base of the penis after MUSE administration increased the rate of successful sexual intercourse to 69% of men [69]. Patients are initially started with a test dose of 500 µg in the office. Depending on the patient's response, this dose can be titrated from 250 to 1000 µg. It is important to administer the test dose in the office due to the risks of urethral bleeding, vasovagal reflex, hypotension, and priapism (occurring in <0.1%) [70].

Transdermal medications

No transdermal medication has been approved by the FDA for erectile dysfunction, and none is available for clinical use. Nitroglycerine cream or paste; alprostadil cream; and a cream containing aminophylline, isosorbide dinitrate, and codergocrine mesylate have been used in pilot studies in men who have ED with varying results [71].

Third-line/surgical treatments

Although some men who are unhappy with the results of oral medications or who cannot take them proceed directly to surgical intervention, most men try one or several second-line therapies before embarking on an operative course of management.

Penile prostheses

When there is lack of efficacy or when there is dissatisfaction with other modalities, penile prostheses are often the best alternative for ED. Unlike the other modalities, prosthesis surgery is irreversible in that the corporal tissue is permanently altered such that physiologic erections are no longer possible. If the prosthesis has to be removed, there will be complete ED, although devices are readily replaced should mechanical failure occur. Although a variety of exotic materials, flaps [72], and grafts have been used, most contemporary prostheses are hydraulic or semirigid/malleable. The malleable prostheses are made of silicone rubber with a central intertwined metallic core. Mechanical devices are also made of silicone rubber with interlocking rings in a column, which provide rigidity when the rings are lined up in a straight line and flaccidity when the penis is bent. The advantages of semirigid devices are that they are easy to implant, have few mechanical parts with minimal mechanical failure, and generally last longer than inflatable devices. The major disadvantage of the semirigid devices is that the penis is neither fully rigid nor fully flaccid. These devices may interfere with urination, are difficult to conceal, and have a higher likelihood of device erosion. About 15% of patients choose semirigid rod implants, and those with limited mental or manual dexterity are encouraged to use this type of device.

Inflatable prostheses come in two- or three-component setups. Two-piece inflatable prostheses consist of a pair of cylinders attached to a scrotal pump. The prosthesis can be deflated by bending the penis at midshaft. Three-piece inflatable prostheses consist of a pair of penile cylinders, a scrotal pump, and a suprapubic reservoir. They provide excellent rigidity when erect and a more natural appearance when flaccid. When fully erect, they are as rigid as the two-piece device. In the flaccid state, they surpass the flaccidity of two-piece prostheses. Of all the prosthesis types, hydraulic three-piece implants have been the most popular, accounting for 85% of the United States market. Most inflatable devices need replacement after 10 to 15 years. Repair or replacement rates of 5% to 20% in the first 5 years are realistic.

Of all the modalities for the management of ED, prostheses have the highest satisfaction rates [73], with two large studies demonstrating greater than 95% satisfaction [46,74]. This high satisfaction rate is likely due to multiple factors: Prostheses allow for spontaneous and repeated reliable erections without external medications or devices, and many men undergoing prostheses have tried, unsuccessfully or unsatisfactorily, many first- and second-line treatments before deciding on a prosthesis.

Infection remains the most devastating and feared complication. Modern prostheses allow for antibiotic impregnation and elution, and infection rates are approximately 3% for a first-time prosthesis. Although some studies [75] suggest that elevated HbA1c levels may predict a higher rate of infections in patients who have diabetes who are having penile prosthesis surgery, more recent studies refute this. A large study from Wilson and colleagues [10] demonstrated that neither diabetic status nor preoperative HgA1c were risk factors for prosthesis infection. A more recent study [76] finds that elevated HbA1c is not a risk factor for infection but notes that short-term sugar control is (as defined by morning fasting glucose levels > 200 ng/mL), although the data are hampered by low numbers of patients within that cohort. Penile shortening and eventual mechanical failure of the device are other common side effects.

Vascular surgery

Men often complain that the various modalities of treatment, although potentially effective, are not "natural" in that they require assistance from a pill, injection, or device and do not allow for the same level of spontaneity that men previously enjoyed. Rather than symptom management, men desire a cure. With the exception of reversible endocrinopathies, no other available treatments address this fundamental desire. Because erectile dysfunction often has a vascular component, it stands to reason that practitioners have tried to develop surgical methods to re-establish penile vascular integrity. In general, these methods have addressed inflow problems (ie, increasing the delivery of arterial flow to the corpora cavernosa) or outflow problems (ie, obstruction of pathologic leak of veins draining the corpora). Work-up of these problems generally requires invasive testing, such as angiography or dynamic infusion cavernosometry and cavernosography. Despite the theoretical appeal of improving the underlying pathology, results of vascular reconstructive surgery, venous and arterial, have been disappointing unless the patients are highly selected [77–80]. Optimal candidates for surgery are young men who have no vascular comorbidities and who have discrete, singular lesions. Very few men who have erectile dysfunction fall into this category, although young men may have congenital anomalous venous leakage or vascular lesions induced by perineal trauma.

Summary

A wide variety of medications, devices, and surgical interventions are available to patients who have ED. These range from first-line oral agents to second-line therapy with injections or vacuum devices to third-line options, such as penile prosthesis implantation. A few patients may be candidates for curative vascular reconstructive surgery. With this variety and the generally high efficacies of the treatments, men and their partners need not suffer from ED. In the future, tissue, cellular, or gene-based therapies, such as stem cell implantation or gene transfer [81–83], may allow curative therapies through the regeneration or growth of healthy vascular and neural tissue.

References

[1] Lue TF. Erectile dysfunction. N Engl J Med 2000;342(24):1802–13.
[2] Francis SH. Phosphodiesterase 11 (PDE11): is it a player in human testicular function? Int J Impot Res 2005;17(5):467–8.
[3] Boolell M, Allen MJ, Ballard SA, et al. Sildenafil: an orally active type 5 cyclic GMP-specific phosphodiesterase inhibitor for the treatment of penile erectile dysfunction. Int J Impot Res 1996;8(2):47–52.
[4] Padma-Nathan H, Stecher VJ, Sweeney M, et al. Minimal time to successful intercourse after sildenafil citrate: results of a randomized, double-blind, placebo-controlled trial. Urology 2003;62(3):400–3.
[5] Klotz T, Sachse R, Heidrich A, et al. Vardenafil increases penile rigidity and tumescence in erectile dysfunction patients: a RigiScan and pharmacokinetic study. World J Urol 2001; 19(1):32–9.
[6] Stark S, Sachse R, Liedl T, et al. Vardenafil increases penile rigidity and tumescence in men with erectile dysfunction after a single oral dose. Eur Urol 2001;40(2):181–8 [discussion 189–90].
[7] Brock GB, McMahon CG, Chen KK, et al. Efficacy and safety of tadalafil for the treatment of erectile dysfunction: results of integrated analyses. J Urol 2002;168(4 Pt 1):1332–6.
[8] Eardley I, Dean J, Barnes T, et al. The sexual habits of British men and women over 40 years old. BJU Int 2004;93(4):563–7.
[9] Carson CC, Burnett AL, Levine LA, et al. The efficacy of sildenafil citrate (Viagra) in clinical populations: an update. Urology 2002;60(2 Suppl 2):12–27.
[10] Wilson SK, Carson CC, Cleves MA, et al. Quantifying risk of penile prosthesis infection with elevated glycosylated hemoglobin. J Urol 1998;159(5):1537–9.

[11] Porst H, Rosen R, Padma-Nathan H, et al. The efficacy and tolerability of vardenafil, a new, oral, selective phosphodiesterase type 5 inhibitor, in patients with erectile dysfunction: the first at-home clinical trial. Int J Impot Res 2001;13(4):192–9.

[12] Stief C, Porst H, Saenz De Tejada I, et al. Sustained efficacy and tolerability with vardenafil over 2 years of treatment in men with erectile dysfunction. Int J Clin Pract 2004; 58(3):230–9.

[13] Park K, Ku JH, Kim SW, et al. Risk factors in predicting a poor response to sildenafil citrate in elderly men with erectile dysfunction. BJU Int 2005;95(3):366–70.

[14] Morales A, Gingell C, Collins M, et al. Clinical safety of oral sildenafil citrate (VIAGRA) in the treatment of erectile dysfunction. Int J Impot Res 1998;10(2):69–73 [discussion 73–4].

[15] Sur RL, Kane CJ. Sildenafil citrate-associated priapism. Urology 2000;55(6):950.

[16] King SH, Hallock M, Strote J, et al. Tadalafil-associated priapism. Urology 2005;66(2): 432.

[17] Burnett AL, Bivalacqua TJ, Champion HC, et al. Long-term oral phosphodiesterase 5 inhibitor therapy alleviates recurrent priapism. Urology 2006;67(5):1043–8.

[18] Zusman RM, Morales A, Glasser DB, et al. Overall cardiovascular profile of sildenafil citrate. Am J Cardiol 1999;83(5A):35C–44C.

[19] Kloner RA. Cardiovascular effects of the 3 phosphodiesterase-5 inhibitors approved for the treatment of erectile dysfunction. Circulation 2004;110(19):3149–55.

[20] Morganroth J, Ilson BE, Shaddinger BC, et al. Evaluation of vardenafil and sildenafil on cardiac repolarization. Am J Cardiol 2004;93(11):1378–83, A1376.

[21] DeBusk R, Drory Y, Goldstein I, et al. Management of sexual dysfunction in patients with cardiovascular disease: recommendations of The Princeton Consensus Panel. Am J Cardiol 2000;86(2):175–81.

[22] Physicians' desk reference. Montvale (NJ): Thomson PDR; 2005.

[23] Physicians' desk reference. 58th edition. Montvale (NJ): Thomson PDR; 2004.

[24] Kloner RA, Jackson G, Emmick JT, et al. Interaction between the phosphodiesterase 5 inhibitor, tadalafil and 2 alpha-blockers, doxazosin and tamsulosin in healthy normotensive men. J Urol 2004;172(5 Pt 1):1935–40.

[25] Kloner RA. Pharmacology and drug interaction effects of the phosphodiesterase 5 inhibitors: focus on alpha-blocker interactions. Am J Cardiol 2005;96(12B):42M–6M.

[26] Montague DK, Jarow JP, Broderick GA, et al. Chapter 1: the management of erectile dysfunction: an AUA update. J Urol 2005;174(1):230–9.

[27] Leung CM, Lee TS, Chan Ho MW, et al. A case of unrelenting pursuit of castration. Aust N Z J Psychiatry 1996;30(1):150–2.

[28] Tomsak R. PDE5 inhibitors and permanent visual loss. Int J Impot Res 2005;17(6): 547–9.

[29] Johnson CW, Bingham JB, Goluboff ET, et al. Transurethral resection of the ejaculatory ducts for treating ejaculatory symptoms. BJU Int 2005;95(1):117–9.

[30] Hattenhauer MG, Leavitt JA, Hodge DO, et al. Incidence of nonarteritic anterior ischemic optic neuropathy. Am J Ophthalmol 1997;123(1):103–7.

[31] Nagy V, Steiber Z, Takacs L, et al. Trombophilic screening for nonarteritic anterior ischemic optic neuropathy. Graefes Arch Clin Exp Ophthalmol 2006;244(1):3–8.

[32] van Ahlen H, Zumbe J, Stauch K, et al. The real-life safety and efficacy of vardenafil: an international post-marketing surveillance study–results from 29 358 German patients. J Int Med Res 2005;33(3):337–48.

[33] Levine LA. Diagnosis and treatment of erectile dysfunction. Am J Med 2000;109(Suppl 9A): 3S–12S [discussion 29S-30S].

[34] Hatzichristou D, Moysidis K, Apostolidis A, et al. Sildenafil failures may be due to inadequate patient instructions and follow-up: a study on 100 non-responders. Eur Urol 2005; 47(4):518–22 [discussion 522–3].

[35] Forgue ST, Patterson BE, Bedding AW, et al. Tadalafil pharmacokinetics in healthy subjects. Br J Clin Pharmacol 2006;61(3):280–8.

[36] Rajagopalan P, Mazzu A, Xia C, et al. Effect of high-fat breakfast and moderate-fat evening meal on the pharmacokinetics of vardenafil, an oral phosphodiesterase-5 inhibitor for the treatment of erectile dysfunction. J Clin Pharmacol 2003;43(3):260–7.

[37] Shabsigh R, Kaufman JM, Steidle C, et al. Randomized study of testosterone gel as adjunctive therapy to sildenafil in hypogonadal men with erectile dysfunction who do not respond to sildenafil alone. J Urol 2004;172(2):658–63.

[38] Musicki B, Champion HC, Becker RE, et al. Erection capability is potentiated by long-term sildenafil treatment: role of blood flow-induced endothelial nitric-oxide synthase phosphorylation. Mol Pharmacol 2005;68(1):226–32.

[39] Musicki B, Champion HC, Becker RE, et al. In vivo analysis of chronic phosphodiesterase-5 inhibition with sildenafil in penile erectile tissues: no tachyphylaxis effect. J Urol 2005; 174(4 Pt 1):1493–6.

[40] Ernst E, Pittler MH. Yohimbine for erectile dysfunction: a systematic review and meta-analysis of randomized clinical trials. J Urol 1998;159(2):433–6.

[41] Gwinup G. Oral phentolamine in nonspecific erectile insufficiency. Ann Intern Med 1988; 109(2):162–3.

[42] Zorgniotti AW. Experience with buccal phentolamine mesylate for impotence. Int J Impot Res 1994;6(1):37–41.

[43] Heaton JP, Morales A, Adams MA, et al. Recovery of erectile function by the oral administration of apomorphine. Urology 1995;45(2):200–6.

[44] Rosen RC, Diamond LE, Earle DC, et al. Evaluation of the safety, pharmacokinetics and pharmacodynamic effects of subcutaneously administered PT-141, a melanocortin receptor agonist, in healthy male subjects and in patients with an inadequate response to Viagra. Int J Impot Res 2004;16(2):135–42.

[45] Diamond LE, Earle DC, Rosen RC, et al. Double-blind, placebo-controlled evaluation of the safety, pharmacokinetic properties and pharmacodynamic effects of intranasal PT-141, a melanocortin receptor agonist, in healthy males and patients with mild-to-moderate erectile dysfunction. Int J Impot Res 2004;16(1):51–9.

[46] Levine LA, Dimitriou RJ. Vacuum constriction and external erection devices in erectile dysfunction. Urol Clin North Am 2001;28(2):335–41, ix–x.

[47] Jarow JP, Nana-Sinkam P, Sabbagh M, et al. Outcome analysis of goal directed therapy for impotence. J Urol 1996;155(5):1609–12.

[48] Aghamir MK, Hosseini R, Alizadeh F. A vacuum device for penile elongation: fact or fiction? BJU Int 2006;97(4):777–8.

[49] Linet OI, Neff LL. Intracavernous prostaglandin E1 in erectile dysfunction. Clin Investig 1994;72(2):139–49.

[50] Porst H. The rationale for prostaglandin E1 in erectile failure: a survey of worldwide experience. J Urol 1996;155(3):802–15.

[51] Chew KK, Stuckey BG. Clinical course of penile fibrosis in intracavernosal prostaglandin E1 injection therapy: a follow-up of 44 patients. Int J Impot Res 2003;15(2):94–8.

[52] Canale D, Giorgi PM, Lencioni R, et al. Long-term intracavernous self-injection with prostaglandin E1 for the treatment of erectile dysfunction. Int J Androl 1996;19(1): 28–32.

[53] Jeremy JY, Ballard SA, Naylor AM, et al. Effects of sildenafil, a type-5 cGMP phosphodiesterase inhibitor, and papaverine on cyclic GMP and cyclic AMP levels in the rabbit corpus cavernosum in vitro. Br J Urol 1997;79(6):958–63.

[54] Stief CG, Wetterauer U. Erectile responses to intracavernous papaverine and phentolamine: comparison of single and combined delivery. J Urol 1988;140(6):1415–6.

[55] Fallon B. Intracavernous injection therapy for male erectile dysfunction. Urol Clin North Am 1995;22(4):833–45.

[56] Kiely EA, Bloom SR, Williams G. Penile response to intracavernosal vasoactive intestinal polypeptide alone and in combination with other vasoactive agents. Br J Urol 1989;64(2): 191–4.

[57] Dinsmore WW, Alderdice DK. Vasoactive intestinal polypeptide and phentolamine mesylate administered by autoinjector in the treatment of patients with erectile dysfunction resistant to other intracavernosal agents. Br J Urol 1998;81(3):437–40.

[58] Bennett AH, Carpenter AJ, Barada JH. An improved vasoactive drug combination for a pharmacological erection program. J Urol 1991;146(6):1564–5.

[59] Zaher TF. Papaverine plus prostaglandin E1 versus prostaglandin E1 alone for intracorporeal injection therapy. Int Urol Nephrol 1998;30(2):193–6.

[60] Mirone V, Imbimbo C, Fabrizio F, et al. Ketanserin plus prostaglandin E1 (PGE-1) as intracavernosal therapy for patients with erectile dysfunction unresponsive to PGE-1 alone. Br J Urol 1996;77(5):736–9.

[61] Meinhardt W, de la Fuente RB, Lycklama a Nijeholt AA, et al. Prostaglandin E1 with phentolamine for the treatment of erectile dysfunction. Int J Impot Res 1996;8(1):5–7.

[62] El-Bahnasawy MS, Dawood A, Farouk A. Low-flow priapism: risk factors for erectile dysfunction. BJU Int 2002;89(3):285–90.

[63] Earle CM, Stuckey BG, Ching HL, et al. The incidence and management of priapism in Western Australia: a 16 year audit. Int J Impot Res 2003;15(4):272–6.

[64] Bechara A, Casabe A, Cheliz G, et al. Comparative study of papaverine plus phentolamine versus prostaglandin E1 in erectile dysfunction. J Urol 1997;157(6):2132–4.

[65] Weiss JN, Badlani GH, Ravalli R, et al. Reasons for high drop-out rate with self-injection therapy for impotence. Int J Impot Res 1994;6(3):171–4.

[66] Gupta R, Kirschen J, Barrow RC 2nd, et al. Predictors of success and risk factors for attrition in the use of intracavernous injection. J Urol 1997;157(5):1681–6.

[67] Padma-Nathan H, Hellstrom WJ, Kaiser FE, et al. Treatment of men with erectile dysfunction with transurethral alprostadil. Medicated Urethral System for Erection (MUSE) Study Group. N Engl J Med 1997;336(1):1–7.

[68] Williams G, Abbou CC, Amar ET, et al. Efficacy and safety of transurethral alprostadil therapy in men with erectile dysfunction. MUSE Study Group. Br J Urol 1998;81(6): 889–94.

[69] Lewis RW. Transurethral alprostadil with MUSE (medicated urethral system for erection) vs intracavernous alprostadil: a comparative study in 103 patients with erectile dysfunction. Int J Impot Res 1998;10(1):61–2.

[70] Ekman P, Sjogren L, Englund G, et al. Optimizing the therapeutic approach of transurethral alprostadil. BJU Int 2000;86(1):68–74.

[71] Gomaa A, Shalaby M, Osman M, et al. Topical treatment of erectile dysfunction: randomised double blind placebo controlled trial of cream containing aminophylline, isosorbide dinitrate, and co-dergocrine mesylate. BMJ 1996;312(7045):1512–5.

[72] Akoz T, Kargi E, Kapucu MR, et al. The use of iliac bone flap as a penile stiffener in a diabetic patient with erectile dysfunction. Plast Reconstr Surg 1999;103(7):1975–8.

[73] Mulcahy JJ, Austoni E, Barada JH, et al. The penile implant for erectile dysfunction. J Sex Med 2004;1(1):98–109.

[74] Montorsi F, Rigatti P, Carmignani G, et al. AMS three-piece inflatable implants for erectile dysfunction: a long-term multi-institutional study in 200 consecutive patients. Eur Urol 2000;37(1):50–5.

[75] Bishop JR, Moul JW, Sihelnik SA, et al. Use of glycosylated hemoglobin to identify diabetics at high risk for penile periprosthetic infections. J Urol 1992;147(2):386–8.

[76] Cakan M, Demirel F, Karabacak O, et al. Risk factors for penile prosthetic infection. Int Urol Nephrol 2003;35(2):209–13.

[77] Berardinucci D, Morales A, Heaton JP, et al. Surgical treatment of penile veno-occlusive dysfunction: is it justified? Urology 1996;47(1):88–92.

[78] Sarramon JP, Bertrand N, Malavaud B, et al. Microrevascularisation of the penis in vascular impotence. Int J Impot Res 1997;9(3):127–33.

[79] Manning M, Junemann KP, Scheepe JR, et al. Long-term followup and selection criteria for penile revascularization in erectile failure. J Urol 1998;160(5):1680–4.

[80] Schultheiss D, Truss MC, Becker AJ, et al. Long-term results following dorsal penile vein ligation in 126 patients with veno-occlusive dysfunction. Int J Impot Res 1997;9(4):205–9.

[81] Melman A. Gene transfer for the therapy of erectile dysfunction: progress in the 21st century. Int J Impot Res 2006;18(1):19–25.

[82] Melman A, Bar-Chama N, McCullough A, et al. The first human trial for gene transfer therapy for the treatment of erectile dysfunction: preliminary results. Eur Urol 2005;48(2):314–8.

[83] Schiff JD, Melman A. Ion channel gene therapy for smooth muscle disorders: relaxing smooth muscles to treat erectile dysfunction. Assay Drug Dev Technol 2006;4(1):89–95.

ELSEVIER
SAUNDERS

Endocrinol Metab Clin N Am
36 (2007) 481–495

ENDOCRINOLOGY
AND METABOLISM
CLINICS
OF NORTH AMERICA

Performance-Enhancing Drugs in Sport

Paul C. Carpenter, MD, FACE

Divisions of Endocrinology-Metabolism and Bioinformatics Research, Mayo Clinic College of Medicine, Mayo Clinic, 200 First Street, S.W., Rochester, MN 55905, USA

The emphasis on winning in sports, and the lucrative incentives professional athletics hold, has amplified the means an athlete might use to gain an edge over competitors. The popular sport press has alleged use of performance-enhancing agents by many of sport's recognized star performers. It is easily understandable why an athlete might experiment with substances or methods above those of basic good coaching, equipment, and training in an attempt to improve athletic performance above normal physiological levels. The motivation to use such methods or substances may come from fellow athletes, coaches, trainers, business managers, the economic rewards of superior performance, and unfortunately, from physicians treating the competitor. Many times the incentive is also driven by peer-social pressures and the push of societal body image [1–4].

This discussion will review the concept and history of ergogenic aides, the penetration of use in society, some benefit/risk information, drug sources in our society, detection and regulation of these agents, and will provide a look to the future. It will also examine the role of the clinician/endocrinologist for these patients and use some cases as examples of drug use among adolescents/teens.

Ergogenic aids

The methods or substances used to enhance athletic performance are termed "ergogenic" aids. Some are "legal" in a regulatory sense, while many are either banned by various competition-governing bodies or carry considerable personal medical hazard in their use. These aids are classified into five broad categories: physiological, physical, psychological, nutritional, and chemical (or pharmacological). The chemical or pharmacological aids are the focus of this discussion.

E-mail address: pccarp@mayo.edu

0889-8529/07/$ - see front matter © 2007 Elsevier Inc. All rights reserved.
doi:10.1016/j.ecl.2007.03.006

History—winning through doping

The use of various physical and chemical aids in performance enhancement is not a novel problem but has been a feature of athletic competition since the beginning of recorded history. Athletes have sought foods and potions to transform their bodies into powerful, well-tuned machines. Greek wrestlers ate huge quantities of meat and sesame seeds to build muscle. Hallucinogenic mushrooms containing bufotenin were used by the legendary Berserkers in Norwegian mythology. The Andean Indians and the Australian aborigines chewed coca leaves and pituri plant for their stimulating and anti-fatiguing effects.

Enter anabolic steroids

Testosterone was first synthesized in the 1930s and introduced into the sporting arena in the 1940s and 1950s. When the Russian weightlifting team, thanks in part to synthetic androgens, walked off with a pile of medals at the 1952 Olympics, an American physician determined that US competitors should have the same advantage. By 1958 a US pharmaceutical firm had developed the first anabolic steroids. Although medicine soon realized the drugs had unwanted side effects, it was too late to halt its spread into the sports world. The first ergogenic use of anabolic steroids was reported to have occurred in the 1950s among weightlifters and bodybuilders. Since that time their use has permeated a myriad of sports. Use of anabolic steroids was a known, significant problem at the 1964 Olympic Games. By 1972, one third of a sample of elite track and field athletes in Sweden surveyed admitted to systematic anabolic steroid use. Of a sample of athletes interviewed at the 1976 Olympic Games from seven countries, who were competing in such diverse activities as throwing, jumping, vaulting, sprinting, and distance running, 68% admitted to having used anabolic steroids. Use has also been noted for norbolethone, and a number of other anabolic steroids that have never been through US Food and Drug Administration (FDA) approval or marketed. Several agents are normally used in the veterinary or animal husbandry arena.

In 1988, Congress passed the Anti-Drug Abuse Act, making the distribution or possession of anabolic steroids for nonmedical reasons a federal offense. Distribution to minors carried a prison sentence. In 1990, Congress toughened the laws, passing legislation that classifies anabolic steroids as a controlled substance. The law also increased penalties for steroid abuse and trafficking. Thirty-two states have passed laws and regulations to control steroid abuse, and many others are considering similar legislation.

Shock waves went through the sports world when Canadian track superstar Ben Johnson was denied his gold medal at the 1988 Olympics after tests showed he had taken anabolic steroids (stanozolol). The US Powerlifting Federation's National Championship in 1990 found 55% of survey respondents admitted previous anabolic steroid use.

Ergogenics and adolescents

In the past decade, it has become obvious that the use of performance-enhancing drugs has reached adolescents below college age. This includes both boys and girls. Use in this young age group has a number of physiologic and psychological consequences not felt to be major problems in their older peer drug users. Although it was suggested as early as 1973, it is now evident that the use of anabolic steroids is not limited to elite amateur and professional athletes. It has trickled down from the professional and college levels to even teens and pre-adolescents [5–11]. The prevalence of nonmedical anabolic steroid use and societal-public health implications prompted several scientific meetings. These include technical review at the National Institute on Drug Abuse, the American Medical Association (AMA), American Academy of Pediatrics, and a number of federal and state investigations. Efforts to reclassify anabolic steroids as controlled substances, despite initial nonconcurrence from the AMA, eventually led to a sequence of regulatory actions.

Today, it is not only the college football player or the professional weightlifter who may use anabolic steroids, it may be an 18-year-old who loathes his skinny body or a 15-year-old in a hurry to reach maturity. A series of surveys from 1988 to 2001 found that 3% to 8% of male and 0.5% to 3% of female adolescents in the United States have used or are currently using anabolic steroids [12–18]. It also appears that use in middle school students may be approaching that of high school teens. Steroids are used by nearly as many students as crack cocaine and by more pupils than the hallucinogenic drug PCP.

College athletic surveys in 1985 through 2003 found anabolic steroids were used in all men's sports, many women's sports, and that football (19%) had the greatest admitted use [19]. The overall anabolic agent use in all collegiate sports nationally rates at 8%. The largest proportional increase in the past 2 decades is certainly among women athletes. Others also note that the increase is not just among athletes but others just trying to improve their female body image. It should be noted that the quoted data are based on random surveys among the target population and has the usual possible errors using this method, including both under- and overreporting drug use. Many athletes would admit to use of cocaine before admitting steroid use. There have not been any randomized studies using drug detection methods for obvious reasons of confidentiality, human rights, and the reality of costs.

Other trends seen include:

(1) Even more (18%–25%) of 12- to 21-year-olds report use of over-the-counter (OTC) drugs (androstenedione, DHEA, creatine, ephedrine, and so forth).
(2) In general, use of OTCs and illicitly acquired drugs is higher in North American than in European or Asian adolescents and teens.

(3) In college sports the use is higher in Division I versus Division III schools.

(4) College athletes receive their anabolic steroid 32% of the time from a physician other than the team physician.

(5) Where one might get performance-enhancing drugs is broad knowledge to 12% of preteens, 29% of adolescents, and 38% of college students.

(6) Use of performance-enhancing drugs is also increasing in nonathletes to improve their performance outside of sports.

(7) Two thirds of those reporting performance-enhancing drug use are involved in organized sport. The observation that one third are may point to societal issues that would prompt a juvenile user to start.

The Monitoring the Future (MTF) study, a National Institute on Drug Abuse assessment of adolescents in 8th, 10th, and 12th grades that is administered by the University of Michigan, showed that during 2002, lifetime prevalence of anabolic steroid use was at an all-time high (4%) among 12th-graders, which represented a significant increase from 1999 [20]. While other drug use either remained unchanged or decreased among 12th-graders, anabolic steroids were the only drug class for which use increased significantly for lifetime, annual, and 30-day prevalence from 2000 to 2002. Although lifetime use of anabolic steroids among 10th-graders remained steady during 2002, its lifetime prevalence more than doubled since 1993 and remains at the highest level since steroid use data were first assessed by the MTF study. There may be a trend toward decreased use among 8th-graders since 2000, but the numbers are still worse than 1998, and many suspect the diversity of drugs used may be diluting the focused abuse reporting [21,22].

Many team physicians and sports medicine practitioners are unfamiliar with the benefits and risks of these products and thus are unable to educate young athletes on this topic. In spite of numerous reports on the health risks of anabolic steroid use, 1 to 3 million Americans have used them. Human growth hormone has been tried by 1% to 5% of 10th graders, although no scientific study has shown that it is an effective performance-enhancing drug.

The food-nutritional supplement industry, led by supplements such as creatine, ephedra, and androstenedione, remains near unregulated by the FDA and has serious issues with quality and side effects. Regulatory efforts have been blocked by economic interests. Ephedra was finally regulated after a recognized professional athlete suffered serious consequences from use of the agent.

Because of the increasingly younger target population, pediatricians have directed focus to this topic. Use in boys or girls as young as 8 years has been reported. Those caring for our young recognize the negative implications for growth and maturation. Programs for treatment and prevention in this group have demonstrated utility [7,21–29].

The broader approach to regulation of drug use has come from various sources including the following:

- Legislative/Administrative
- High school drug testing (determined to be constitutional)
- NCAA education and drug testing
- Collective bargaining in professional sport
- Turning over governance and testing to independent agencies (World Anti-Doping Agency [WADA], US Anti-Doping Agency [USADA])

Are anabolic steroids addictive?

Evidence that mega-doses of anabolic steroids affect the brain and produce mental changes in users prompts questions about possible addiction to the drugs. Long-term steroid users do experience many of the characteristics of classic addiction: cravings, difficulty in ceasing steroid use, and withdrawal symptoms. Formal psychiatric DSM-III (Diagnostic and Statistical Manual of Mental Disorders) classification was first proposed in 1996.

Individuals using anabolic steroids appear to believe that higher doses and continued use result in greater gains. When individuals discontinue using anabolic steroids, their size and strength diminish, often very dramatically. This outcome, as well as psychological effects of use that serve to create a new body image, improved self-esteem, heightened libido, and general euphoria, are thought to motivate continued use of anabolic steroids.

Twenty-five percent of adolescent anabolic users report behaviors, perceptions, and opinions consistent with psychological dependence [30–32]. High school users are significantly different from nonusers in several areas including self-perceptions of health and strength. The majority perceive their relative strength to be greater than average and their health as very good. Heavy users are more likely to use injectable anabolic steroids, express intentions to continue to use anabolic steroids regardless of health consequences, and take more than one anabolic drug at a time.

Adolescent users exhibit a prime trait of addicts: denial. They tend to overlook or simply ignore the physical dangers and moral implications of taking illegal substances [31]. Certain delusional behavior that is characteristic of addiction can occur. Some athletes who "bulk up" on anabolic steroids are unaware of body changes that are obvious to others, experiencing what is sometimes called reverse anorexia.

The range of DSM-IV symptoms covering abuse of and dependence on anabolics are reported in at least 78% of the users, and 25% qualify for a diagnosis of steroid dependence or drug abuse using DSM-IV criteria. There are no gender differences in anabolic abuse or dependence diagnoses. Twelve percent develop major depression while withdrawing from anabolic steroids. Weight and fluid loss may portend or be the cause of the impending depression. An interesting observation that illustrates the difficulties facing drug abuse researchers and educators was made in a study of the effects of testosterone enanthate on body image and behavior in young males with Klinefelter's syndrome. Results included not only a significant change from a feminine to a masculine body image, increased assertiveness, increased goal-directed behavior, and heightened sexual drive, but the majority of subjects expressed "…a desire to become further masculinized."

Steroid use is more common in males, non-white (especially some subsets of the Asian-American population), and in middle school students (as compared with high school). In males, steroid use is associated with poorer self-esteem, higher rates of depressed mood, attempted suicide, poorer knowledge and attitudes about health, greater participation in sports that emphasize weight and shape, greater parental concern about weight, and higher rates of disordered eating and substance use. Among females, steroid use was less consistent in its associations with other variables, although overall, a similar pattern is seen.

In 1993 the Canadian Center for Drug-free Sport estimated that 83,000 individuals between the ages of 11 and 18 had used anabolic steroids in the previous 12 months. Recent evidence suggests anabolic steroids are now the third most common starter drug for children in the United Kingdom, behind cannabis and amphetamines.

Finally, weight training per se may be addictive, perhaps by augmentation of certain neurochemicals, in the sense of promoting compulsive, stereotypic, and repetitive behavior to include not only the strength training but dieting, drug use, and a host of other lifestyle variables as well.

Anabolic steroid use in adolescence is associated with poor health-related attitudes and behaviors and exposure to socioenvironmental influences encouraging weight preoccupation. Attention needs to be directed toward youths who may be at increased risk for steroid use within clinical and community-based settings.

Do anabolic steroids work?

This question is difficult because there have been rare controlled, blinded, crossover studies of steroid effects on performance, particularly using the supraphysiologic dosing that the majority of athlete users receive. These doses would not likely be permitted by regulatory bodies overseeing human studies. There also have been rare checks on other drug use, medication blood levels, and so forth. Most studies have used admitted anabolic steroid users, leaving little control over truthfulness, drug types, or their doses. The athletes are confident they work (as is this author). There is no question they offer major performance enhancements in women. Examples were seen when the East German data were released after the "wall came down" and Germany's unification [33–41].

The hazards of anabolic steroid use

As endocrinologists, we have a good understanding of the potential consequences of overreplacement with androgenic medications. These include for men: testis atrophy, oligospermia, baldness, prostatic hypertrophy, and gynecomastia. Women may experience hirsutism, amenorrhea-infertility, clitoral hypertrophy, voice changes, and breast atrophy.

Both sexes may complain of acne, jaundice, tremor, edema, reduced HDL-cholesterol, hypertension, concentric cardiomyopathy, peliosis hepatitis, hepatic adenomatosis, polycythemia, thrombosis, and growth retardation in the young.

In addition, there are a number of other health hazards that include behavioral-psychological changes ("roid rage") and biomechanical (eg, tendon ruptures), and impairment of the exercise-induced growth of the cardiac capillary bed.

The insurance industry has become interested in studies suggesting serious health consequences and apparent major reduction in life expectancy that prolonged use of anabolic steroids carries [42–50].

Other drugs used by athletes (and others)

In the past 15 to 20 years there has been a major broadening of the categories of drugs that athletes and others are using in the quest for a more attractive body or for the sake of performance gains. The explosion has been so rapid that the athletic governing bodies (International Olympic Committee [IOC], Unites States Olympic Committee [USOC], National College Athletic Association [NCAA], Amateur Athletic Committee [AAU], and so forth) have not had the means or time to review the potential pharmacologics being used, assess whether they should be banned, and prepare for suitable testing of competitive athletes [39,51–57].

This pharmaceutical warehouse now consists of numerous central nervous system (CNS) stimulants, human growth hormone, neurotransmitters (gammahydroxybutyrate, gamma aminobutyric acid), human growth hormone, insulin, tamoxifen, clomiphene citrate, cocaine, erythropoietin (EPO), and a variety of agents taken to mask or alter drug-detection methods. When one interviews a person using insulin for anabolic enhancement use it is often obvious what sophisticated knowledge they have of the metabolic properties of insulin and now the rapid-acting synthetics. Evidence for use of EPO in sport dates back to just a short time after the bioengineered product was on the market. In parallel there were a burst of deaths among world elite cyclists starting in the mid-1980s.

The 1994 Dietary Supplement and Health Education Act made possible the sale of a variety of nonprescription products. The most discussed are androstenedione and DHEA, both of which are discussed by Tamler and Mechanick elsewhere in this issue.

These "weak" androgens may have very legitimate medical uses but the majority of use is among those seeking performance or physical enhancements...now also including many members of our aging community.

Supply and demand: the black market

Most users maintain their anabolic steroid habit acquired through a highly organized black market handling up to $950 million worth of the drugs per year in the United States. The market is $46 billion worldwide with some 30,000 products. Until the mid-1980s most underground steroids were legitimately manufactured pharmaceuticals that were diverted to the black market through theft and fraudulent prescriptions. Some came from the veterinary medicine arena. More effective law enforcement and greater demand forced black marketers to seek new sources. Now black market anabolic steroids and other drugs are either produced offshore and smuggled into the United States or are produced in clandestine laboratories in this country. These counterfeit drugs present greater health risks because they are manufactured without controls and thus may be impure, mislabeled, or simply bogus. Several studies have analyzed street-sold performance drugs and note a high incidence of mislabeling, additional toxic substances, or complete absence of any significant pharmacological agents [58].

Sales are made in gyms, health clubs, on campuses, through the mail, and now through numerous Internet sites. Users report that suppliers may be drug dealers, trainers, physicians, pharmacists, friends...or the unknown at the other end of an Internet URL. When last checked the author could identify over 60 Web sites selling ergogenic drugs. Many ergogenic aide Web sites also have detailed schedule information about initiation, use cycles, taper/discontinuation schedules, and details about avoiding drug detection. It is remarkably easy for users to buy the drugs and learn how to use them.

Ergogenic agents—the future

The year 2004 marked the discovery of "designer" steroids. Tetrahydrogestrinone (THG) was found in a submitted sample from a syringe, and structure was determined by high-pressure liquid chromatography (HPLC) and tandem mass spectrometry (MS-MS). Never marketed, the steroid had been obviously designed to not withstand the conditions of usual detection methods, disintegrating to avoid discovery. As a potent androgen and progestin with unspecified properties, its distribution for use at high doses without any prior biological or toxicological evaluation poses significant health risks [59,60]. This also raises the suspicion that many similar designs are on the market [61]. Designer androgens also offer the possibility of tissue-specific effects, enhancing the beneficial effects of androgens while mitigating the undesirable ones. Once this drug had been identified, the WADA and the IOC rapidly put detection methods in place for the 2004 Olympics in Athens. This event also marked the first time that illicit growth hormone use could be detected.

The specter of human bioengineering or "gene doping" has also now been raised. WADA has already initiated discussions about what sort of testing methods might be used to detect an athlete who has had alteration in their genome or other tissue alterations to promote expression of chemical agents, eg, in muscle, that could promote muscle development or strength. Viral-mediated expression of IGF-1 in mouse muscle has been demonstrated, resulting in "ripped" or "Schwarzenegger" mice with increased muscle mass and diminished usual muscle aging deterioration. A virus carrying an IGF-1 structural and control gene is inserted into muscle cells. The gene is established in the nucleus and the muscle produces IGF-1 and increases in mass and strength (up to 27% in elderly mice, when losing one third of muscle mass is the norm) [62]. Modulators of muscle metabolism have also come into focus. An example is the use of investigative drug GW501516, a peroxisome proliferator-activated receptor-delta (PPARδ) agonist, to significantly enhance (50%) the endurance of mice on treadmill exercise. The agent promises resistance to weight gain, increased "slow-twitch" muscle fibers, and dramatically increased endurance, hence leading to "marathon mice" [63,64].

Drug use regulation in sport

WADA, created in 1999, is a shared initiative of sport *and* governments promoting and coordinating the fight against doping internationally and nationally through education, advocacy, research, and leadership. The USADA was created as a result of the recommendations of the USOC's Select Task Force on Externalization. USADA's responsibility is to develop a comprehensive national antidoping program for the Olympic Movement in the United States. USADA has full authority for testing, education, research, and adjudication for US Olympic and Pan Am Games and Paralympic athletes. Specific information about the banned substances, testing, and education is available on the IOC and WADA Web sites: www.olympic.org, www.wada-ama.org.

Drug detection has become quite sophisticated. Natively synthesized testosterone is produced with a fixed molar ratio of epitestosterone, an isomer of the biologically active product. Established acceptable maximum ratios are the basis to detect use of synthesized testosterone. With the advent of HPLC-MS-MS methods for steroid detection the analysts have tools for detection of a huge spectrum of steroid and other small molecules. "Reverse engineering" of molecular fragments to determine structure of parent steroids is also possible. Detection of growth hormone or EPO was a challenge as the bioengineered peptides have short half-lives requiring sampling within 24 hours of last use. The focus is now on examination of downstream products reflecting their use (IGF-1, IGFBP, etc.) [65–70].

The role of the physician-endocrinologist

As physicians we have some opportunities to see patients who are using these ergogenic drugs, eg, the adolescent with more than average or recurrent gynecomastia, the high school football player with raging acne resistant to usual therapies, the athletic woman with secondary amenorrhea, the teen athlete with unusual tendon injuries, new type-2 diabetes in a trim teen, a history of sexual aggression, aberrant rage behaviors, and so forth. Through their physical and psychosocial assessment of young people, health care professionals can play a role in identifying, counseling, and appropriate referrals for adolescents at risk. Remaining alert to the possibility of this hidden medication use is important. Health care providers, particularly endocrinologists, are the logical specialists to be approached when advice about these agents is sought. Maintaining knowledge of what is being used and abused is important in our practices.

We as health care providers should care about the regrettable messages that are being sent to our youth and aspiring athletes who seek nothing more than fair and ethical competition on a level playing field. Five to seven percent of Major League Baseball players have tested positive for anabolic steroids, and an apparently never-ending stream of athletes is caught and suspended for doping. Maybe we should care that 4.5% of boy and 2.4% of girl 12th graders and 2.0% of 8th graders have used anabolic steroids in their lifetime—a 50% increase since 1995. What we are witnessing is a violation of the public trust and a corrosion of the public health.

Case examples

Case #1

A 17-year-old male is referred for evaluation of gynecomastia. His parents recall some breast enlargement when 13 years old that resolved, but now has returned dramatically over the past 1 year along with severe acne. He works out daily in a gym. He is involved in high school football in the fall and field track in the spring season. The patient denies use of any medications.

Examination
    Ht = 185 cm, Wt = 98 kg. Muscular upper body.
    Acne lesions jaw line and abundant across upper back.
    Pale striae over pectorals, deltoids.

Significant bilateral gynecomastia, no breast masses, no secretions. Testes 12–14 mL each (nl 18–22 mL).

Discussion

The clues that suggest possible anabolic steroid use are the recurrent gynecomastia and worsening acne. Although the patient denied drug use, labs find the following: Total testosterone = 86 ng/mL (nl 250–950), bio-available T = 6 ng/mL (nl 50–190), LH = 0.4 IU, estradiol = 4.1, Urine high pressure liquid chromatography/mass spectrometry = oxandrolone, boldenone (no FDA approval). IGF-1 = 150 (nl 90–360). He later admits to polysteroid injection and hGH. Urine drug screen also finds trace levels of tamoxifen.

Case #2

A 16-year-old male is incarcerated for physical and sexual aggression. Several previous aggression incidences were reported. The current event was brought on by a female refusing his sexual advances resulting in severe physical injuries and sexual assault. Parents have noted an increasing isolation, poor school performance, and rage or abusive language outbursts during the past year. On high school disciplinary detention several times. Involved in no organized sport. Since 7th grade he has gained 13 cm in height and remarkable 34 kg muscular weight. Now at Ht = 180 cm, Wt = 99 kg. Law enforcement with search warrant finds a wide variety of drug paraphernalia hidden in his room and school locker. Drugs recovered include vials of testosterone enanthate, stanozolol [Winstrol], marijuana, and crack cocaine.

Increasing physical/sexual aggressiveness in teen males, particularly when there is no history of same in them or family may be a clue to anabolic steroid use. The majority of teen male steroid users, particularly those not involved in sport, also abuse other drugs.

Case #3

An 18-year-old female is seen by a sports medicine physician because of increasing number of tendon-ligament injuries coming from her workout in the weight room.

She is a nationally recognized competitive swimmer, involved in organized competition since age 7. Many NCAA Division I scholarship offers and Olympic trials competition. Spurred on by her swim club coaches she has been weight training for the past 5 years. In the past year her performances have been outstanding and in nearly all swim meets she has improved on her personal best times and won many events. Exam: superior upper and lower body development. More than average skin oiliness. No menses for 4 months. Pelvic exam by GYN finds some degree of clitoral hypertrophy. Lab: Hgb: 17.7 Hct: 50% LH 2.0.

The multiple tendon injuries can be a clue to anabolic steroid use. The cause is thought to be related to an accelerated muscle mass development without the supporting attachment tissues developing in parallel. This young woman is involved seriously in competitive sport.

She was using Nandrolone, Winstrol, and Procrit (EPO).

Further readings

Evans NA. Current concepts in anabolic-androgenic steroids. Am J Sports Med 2004;32(2): 534–42.

Fraser AD. Doping control from a global and national perspective. Ther Drug Monit 2004;26(2): 171–4.

Kutscher EC, Lund BC, Perry PJ. Anabolic steroids: a review for the clinician. Sports Med 2002; 32:285–96.

Yesalis CE, Bahrke MS. Anabolic-androgenic steroids and related substances. Curr Sports Med Rep 2002;1(4):246–52.

References

[1] Labre MP. Adolescent boys and the muscular male body ideal. J Adolesc Health 2002;30: 233–42.

[2] Kanayama G, Barry S, Hudson JI, et al. Body image and attitudes toward male roles in anabolic-androgenic steroid users. Am J Psychiatry 2006;163(4):697–703.

[3] Faigenbaum AD, Zaichkowsky LD, Gardner DE, et al. Anabolic steroids used by male and female middle school students. Pediatrics 1998;101:916–7.

[4] Field AE, Austin SB, Camargo CA Jr, et al. Exposure to the mass media, body shape concerns, and use of supplements to improve weight and shape among male and female adolescents. Pediatrics 2005;116(2):e214–20.

[5] Radakovich J, Broderick P, Pickell G. Rate of anabolic-androgenic steroid use among students in junior high school. J Am Board Fam Pract 1993;6(4):341–5.

[6] Tanner SM, Miller DW, Alongi C. Anabolic steroid use by adolescents: prevalence, motives, and knowledge of risks. Clin J Sport Med 1995;5(2):108–15.

[7] Anonymous. Adolescents and anabolic steroids: a subject review. Am Acad Pediatrics. Committee on Sports Medicine and Fitness. Pediatrics 1997;99(6):904–8.

[8] Metzl JD. Performance-enhancing drug use in the young athlete. Pediatr Ann 2002;31(1): 27–32.

[9] Irving LM, Wall M, Neumark-Sztainer D, et al. Steroid use among adolescents: findings from Project EAT. J Adolesc Health 2002;30:243–52.

[10] Gomez JE. Performance-enhancing substances in adolescent athletes. Tex Med 2002;98:41–6.

[11] Laure P, Lecerf T, Friser A, et al. Drugs, recreational drug use and attitudes towards doping of high school athletes. Int J Sports Med 2004;25(2):133–8.

[12] Metzl JD. Anabolic steroids and the pediatric community. Pediatrics 2005;116(6):1542.

[13] Naylor AH, Gardner D, Zaichkowsky L. Drug use patterns among high school athletes and nonathletes. Adolescence 2001;36(144):627–39.

[14] Metzl JD. Sports medicine in pediatric practice: keeping pace with the changing times. Pediatr Ann 2000;29:146–8.

[15] Stilger VG, Yesalis CE. Anabolic-androgenic steroid use among high school football players. J Community Health 1999;24(2):131–45.

[16] Whitehead R, Chillag S, Elliott D. Anabolic steroid use among adolescents in a rural state. J Fam Pract 1992;35(4):401–5.

[17] Scott DM, Wagner JC, Barlow TW. Anabolic steroid use among adolescents in Nebraska schools. Am J Health Syst Pharm 1996;53(17):2068–72.

[18] National Household Survey on Drug Abuse. United States Department of health and human services. Available at: http://www.samhsa.gov/oas/nhsda.htm#NHSDAinfo.

[19] Green GA, Uryasz FD, Petr TA, et al. NCAA study of substance use and abuse habits of college student-athletes. Clin J Sport Med 2001;11(1):51–6.

[20] Johnston LD, O'Malley PM, Bachman JG. Demographic subgroup trends for various licit and illicit drugs, 1975–2001. Monitoring the future—occasional paper No. 57. Ann Arbor (MI): Institute for Social Research; 2002.

[21] Calfee R, Fadale P. Popular ergogenic drugs and supplements in young athletes. Pediatrics 2006;117(3):e577–89.

[22] Moore MJ, Werch CE. Sport and physical activity participation and substance use among adolescents. J Adolesc Health 2005;36(6):486–93.

[23] Golberg L, Elliot D, MacKinnon D, et al. Drug testing athletes to prevent substance abuse: background and pilot study results of the SATURN (Student Athlete Testing Using Random Notification) study. J Adolesc Health 2003;32:16–25.

[24] Elliot DL, Goldberg L, Moe EL, et al. Preventing substance use and disordered eating: initial outcomes of the ATHENA (athletes targeting healthy exercise and nutrition alternatives) program. Arch Pediatr Adolesc Med 2004;158(11):1043–9.

[25] Elliot D, Goldberg L. Intervention and prevention of steroid use in adolescents. Am J Sports Med 1996;24(6 Suppl):S46–7.

[26] Goldberg L, MacKinnon DP, Elliot DL, et al. The adolescents training and learning to avoid steroids program: preventing drug use and promoting health behaviors. Arch Pediatr Adolesc Med 2000;154(4):332–8.

[27] Fritz MS, MacKinnon DP, Williams J, et al. Analysis of baseline by treatment interactions in a drug prevention and health promotion program for high school male athletes. Addict Behav 2005;30(5):1001–5.

[28] Gomez JE. American Academy of Pediatrics Committee on Sports Medicine and Fitness. Use of performance-enhancing substances. Pediatrics 2005;115(4):1103–6.

[29] Estrin I, Sher L. The constitutionality of random drug and alcohol testing in secondary schools. Int J Adolesc Med Health 2006;18(1):21–5.

[30] Pope HG, Kanayama G, Ionescu-Pioggia M, et al. Anabolic steroid users' attitudes towards physicians. Addiction 2004;99(9):1189–94.

[31] Anshel MH, Russell KG. Examining athletes' attitudes toward using anabolic steroids and their knowledge of the possible effects. J Drug Educ 1997;27(2):121–45.

[32] Porcerelli JH, Sandler BA. Narcissism and empathy in steroid users. Am J Psychiatry 1995; 152(11):1672–4.

[33] Tokish JM, Kocher MS, Hawkins RJ. Ergogenic aids: a review of basic science, performance, side effects, and status in sports. Am J Sports Med 2004;32:1543–53.

[34] Blue JG, Lombardo JA. Steroids and steroid-like compounds. Clin Sports Med 1999;18(3): 667–89.

[35] Bemben MG, Lamont HS. Creatine supplementation and exercise performance: recent findings. Sports Med 2005;35(2):107–25.

[36] Kouri EM, Pope HG Jr, Katz DL, et al. Fat-free mass index in users and nonusers of anabolic-androgenic steroids. Clin J Sport Med 1995;5(4):223–8.

[37] Ninot G, Connes P, Caillaud C. Effects of recombinant human erythropoietin injections on physical self in endurance athletes. J Sports Sci 2006;24(4):383–91.

[38] Pope HG Jr, Katz DL. Psychiatric and medical effects of anabolic-androgenic steroid use. A controlled study of 160 athletes. Arch Gen Psychiatry 1994;51(5): 375–82.

[39] Healy ML, Gibney J, Russell-Jones DL, et al. High dose growth hormone exerts an anabolic effect at rest and during exercise in endurance-trained athletes. J Clin Endocrinol Metab 2003;88(11):5221–6.

[40] Seehusen DA, Glorioso JE. Tamoxifen as an ergogenic agent in women body builders. Clin J Sport Med 2002;12(5):313–4.

[41] Stacy JJ, Terrell TR, Armsey TD. Ergogenic aids: human growth hormone. Curr Sports Med Rep 2004;3(4):229–33.

[42] Bryden AA, Rothwell PJ, O'Reilly PH. Anabolic steroid abuse and renal-cell carcinoma. Lancet 1995;346(8985):1306–7.

[43] Kanayama G, Pope HG, Cohane G, et al. Risk factors for anabolic-androgenic steroid use among weightlifters: a case-control study. Drug Alcohol Depend 2003;71(1):77–86.

[44] Parssinen M, Kujala U, Vartiainen E, et al. Increased premature mortality of competitive powerlifters suspected to have used anabolic agents. Int J Sports Med 2000;21(3):225–7.

[45] Cooper CJ, Noakes TD, Dunne T, et al. A high prevalence of abnormal personality traits in chronic users of anabolic-androgenic steroids. Br J Sports Med 1996;30(3):246–50.

[46] Midgley SJ, Heather N, Davies JB. Levels of aggression among a group of anabolic-androgenic steroid users. Med Sci Law 2001;41(4):309–14.

[47] Dickerman RD, McConathy WJ, Zachariah NY. Testosterone, sex hormone-binding globulin, lipoproteins, and vascular disease risk. J Cardiovasc Risk 1997;4(5–6):363–6.

[48] Bahrke MS, Yesalis CE, Kopstein AN, et al. Risk factors associated with anabolic steroids use among adolescents. Sports Med 2000;29:397–406.

[49] Kennedy MC, Lawrence C. Anabolic steroid abuse and cardiac death. Med J Aust 1993; 158(5):346–8.

[50] Bizzarini E, De Angelis L. Is the use of oral creatine supplementation safe? J Sports Med Phys Fitness 2004;44(4):411–6.

[51] Karila T, Hovatta O, Seppala T. Concomitant abuse of anabolic androgenic steroids and human chorionic gonadotrophin impairs spermatogenesis in power athletes. Int J Sports Med 2004;25(4):257–63.

[52] Evans PJ, Lynch RM. Insulin as a drug of abuse in body building. Br J Sports Med 2003; 37(4):356–7.

[53] Okudan N, Gokbel H. The effects of creatine supplementation on performance during the repeated bouts of supramaximal exercise. J Sports Med Phys Fitness 2005;45(4):507–11.

[54] Karila T, Koistinen H, Seppala M, et al. Growth hormone induced increase in serum IGFBP-3 level is reversed by anabolic steroids in substance abusing power athletes. Clin Endocrinol (Oxf) 1998;49(4):459–63.

[55] Konrad C, Schupfer G, Wietlisbach M, et al. Insulin as an anabolic: hypoglycemia in the bodybuilding world. Anasthesiol Intensivmed Notfallmed Schmerzther 1998;33(7):461–3 [in German].

[56] Healy ML, Russell-Jones D. Growth hormone and sport: abuse, potential benefits, and difficulties in detection. Br J Sports Med 1997;31(4):267–8.

[57] Handelsman DJ. Clinical review: the rationale for banning human chorionic gonadotropin and estrogen blockers in sport. J Clin Endocrinol Metab 2006;91(5):1646–53.

[58] Pearce PZ. Sports supplements: a modern case of caveat emptor. Curr Sports Med Rep 2005; 4(3):171–8.

[59] Orchard JW, Fricker PA, White SL, et al. The use and misuse of performance-enhancing substances in sport. Med J Aust 2006;184(3):132–6.

[60] Sekera MH, Ahrens BD, Chang YC, et al. Another designer steroid: discovery. Synthesis and detection of 'madol' in urine. Rapid Commun Mass Spectrom 2005;19(6):781–4.

[61] Handelsman DJ. Designer androgens in sport: when too much is never enough. Sci STKE 2004;27:e41.

[62] Barton-Davis ER, Shoturma DI, Musaro A, et al. Viral mediated expression of IGF-I blocks the aging-related loss of skeletal muscle function. Proc Natl Acad Sci U S A 1998;95:15603–7.

[63] Wang XY, Zhang C-L, Yu RT, et al. Regulation of muscle fiber type and running endurance by PPARδ. PLoS Biol 2004;2(10):e294.

[64] Dressel U, Allen TL, Pippal JB, et al. The peroxisome proliferator-activated receptor ß/δ agonist, GW501516, regulates the expression of genes involved in lipid catabolism and energy uncoupling in skeletal muscle cells. Mol Endocrinol 2004;17(12):2477–93.

[65] Rigamonti AE, Cella SG, Marazzi N, et al. Growth hormone abuse: methods of detection. Trends Endocrinol Metab 2005;16(4):160–6.

[66] Thevis M, Thomas A, Delahaut P, et al. Doping control analysis of intact rapid-acting insulin analogues in human urine by liquid chromatography-tandem mass spectrometry. Anal Chem 2006;78(6):1897–903.

[67] Maughan RJ. Contamination of dietary supplements and positive drug tests in sport. J Sports Sci 2005;23(9):883–9.

[68] Thevis M, Geyer H, Mareck U, et al. Screening for unknown synthetic steroids in human urine by liquid chromatography-tandem mass spectrometry. J Mass Spectrom 2005;40(7): 955–62.

[69] Goebel C, Alma C, Howe C, et al. Methodologies for detection of hemoglobin-based oxygen carriers. J Chromatogr Sci 2005;43(1):39–46.

[70] Healy ML, Dall R, Gibney J, et al. Toward the development of a test for growth hormone (GH) abuse: a study of extreme physiological ranges of GH-dependent markers in 813 elite athletes in the post-competition setting. J Clin Endocrinol Metab 2005;90(2):641–9.

ELSEVIER
SAUNDERS

Endocrinol Metab Clin N Am
36 (2007) 497–519

ENDOCRINOLOGY
AND METABOLISM
CLINICS
OF NORTH AMERICA

Gynecomastia

Harmeet Singh Narula, MD, Harold E. Carlson, MD*

*Division of Endocrinology, Diabetes, and Metabolism, Health Sciences Center, T15-060,
Stony Brook University, Stony Brook, NY 11794–8154, USA*

Gynecomastia refers to benign enlargement of the male breast attributable to proliferation of the ductular elements and not merely excessive breast adipose tissue, a condition termed *lipomastia* or *pseudogynecomastia*. The two can generally be differentiated by careful palpation, in which subareolar tissue is compared with adjacent subcutaneous fat. Gynecomastia can be unilateral or bilateral and may be asymmetric (ie, one breast larger than the other). Although it is a common finding on routine physical examination, it can be a source of psychologic or, less often, physical discomfort; can raise fears of breast cancer; and can occasionally be a sign of serious endocrine or systemic disease. In this article, the authors review recent advances in the understanding of the pathogenesis, evaluation, and management of gynecomastia.

Prevalence

Gynecomastia is common: 50% to 70% of all boys develop breast enlargement during puberty [1], and 30% to 65% of men have palpable breast tissue [2–4]. In hospitalized men, the proportion with gynecomastia is even higher (70%) [5]. In autopsy studies, histologic evidence of gynecomastia is found in 40% to 55% of all men [6].

Histology

Histologically, gynecomastia is characterized by the proliferation of the mammary ductules in a fibroconnective tissue stroma [4,7]. True terminal acini, as seen in the adult female breast, are rarely seen in men with gynecomastia, because such acini require the presence of estrogen and progesterone.

---

* Corresponding author.
E-mail address: harold.carlson@stonybrook.edu (H.E. Carlson).

0889-8529/07/$ - see front matter © 2007 Elsevier Inc. All rights reserved.
doi:10.1016/j.ecl.2007.03.013   *endo.theclinics.com*

In the early or florid stage of gynecomastia, ductal hyperplasia and proliferation are extensive and the stroma is loose and edematous. Over time, the glandular elements become less prominent and stromal fibrosis is the predominant histologic finding (quiescent or fibrous stage) [7]. Medical therapy is likely to be most effective in the early stage; in late stages, when the breast tissue consists mostly of dense fibrotic stroma, medical therapy may be ineffective and patients may require surgery for cure. There is no relation between the cause of the gynecomastia and its histologic appearance [7].

Pathogenesis

Male breast tissue has estrogen receptors and androgen receptors (ARs). Estrogens stimulate and androgens inhibit breast tissue proliferation; gynecomastia is usually caused by an imbalance between these two influences, which may be attributable to excessive estrogen action, deficient androgen action, or a combination of these effects on the breast tissue (Box 1) [8–11].

In addition to circulating hormones, local tissue factors in the breast may be important. Increased local production of estrogens attributable to enhanced aromatase activity in the breast, decreased local estrogen inactivation, decreased local production of testosterone from androstenedione, and changes in ARs or estrogen receptors could all contribute to the genesis of gynecomastia. Absent or defective ARs lead to deficient androgen action at breast tissue and may result in gynecomastia. In addition, expanded CAG trinucleotide repeats in exon 1 of the AR gene can lead to partial androgen insensitivity and gynecomastia, as in Kennedy disease (Online Mendelian Inheritance in Man [OMIM] 313200), a rare X-linked motor neuron disorder [12]. This may be related to modulation of AR activity by CAG repeats: the longer the sequence of repeats, the lower is the transcriptional activation by the AR. In the general population, it is possible that variation in the number of CAG repeats may lead to increased or decreased sensitivity of the AR to circulating androgens and may explain why some men develop gynecomastia, even with normal circulating androgen levels.

In normal men, serum estrogens are primarily derived from peripheral aromatization of androgens [13,14]. Adipose tissue is a major site of aromatization; with increasing age, there is often increasing adiposity. In addition, there is evidence that there may be increased aromatase activity in adipose cells with aging [15]. Inflammatory cytokines may also play a role in increasing aromatase expression with aging and with certain medical illnesses [16–18]. Thus, increased peripheral aromatase activity may partly explain the gynecomastia seen with aging and some diseases.

Although prolactin receptors have been demonstrated in breast tissue, including gynecomastia [19], hyperprolactinemia probably plays an indirect role in gynecomastia by causing central hypogonadism. Most men with gynecomastia do not have elevated serum prolactin levels, and not all men with hyperprolactinemia develop gynecomastia. Nevertheless, it has been shown in cultured breast cancer cells that prolactin and sex steroid receptors (especially the progesterone receptor [PgR]) may be coexpressed and may cross-regulate each other's expression [20,21]; acute prolactin treatment produced an increase in PgR and a decrease in AR content. If this were to occur in the breast tissue of hyperprolactinemic men, the resulting increase in PgR expression and decrease in AR expression could promote breast tissue growth and result in gynecomastia. Similar cross-talk may exist among other hormones and may play an important role in the genesis of gynecomastia. For example, growth hormone (GH) probably plays an important permissive role in breast development in normal girls during puberty; GH receptor or insulin-like growth factor (IGF)-I receptor knockout mice fail to have normal mammary duct elongation, similar to estrogen receptor knockout mice [22,23]. Estrogens increase the expression of the IGF-I receptor in cultured breast cancer cells [24] and may thereby enhance the action of IGF-I in pubertal breast development, including a possible role in gynecomastia.

Progesterone plays an important role in lobuloalveolar differentiation in normal female breast tissue, but PgR knockout mice have normal breast development at puberty; however, they fail to lactate, similar to prolactin receptor knockout mice [25]. The role of progesterone in male breast enlargement is less clear; PgRs have been demonstrated in male breast tissue [8], and elevated serum progesterone concentrations have been reported in men with cirrhosis and hyperthyroidism [26,27]. Progesterone may synergize with local IGF-I and stimulate breast ductular morphogenesis [28].

Luteinizing hormone (LH)/human chorionic gonadotropin (hCG) receptors have also been demonstrated in the male breast [29]. Although the role of this receptor in the male breast remains to be further elucidated, binding of LH or hCG to this receptor may modulate androgen action on breast tissue. LH and hCG decrease levels of AR and type 2 5α-reductase proteins in samples of women's skin in vitro [30]; a similar effect in the breast could decrease the inhibitory effect of androgens on breast ductular proliferation.

Breast tissue can produce, and respond to, numerous growth factors, including epidermal growth factor (EGF), platelet-derived growth factor (PDGF), IGF-I, IGF-II, transforming growth factor (TGF)-α, and TGFβ [22,23,31,32]. The role of these local growth factors (acting in a paracrine or autocrine fashion in the breast) in the genesis of gynecomastia remains to be further investigated.

Causes of gynecomastia

Absolute estrogen excess

An absolute excess of circulating estrogens (ie, elevated serum concentrations of estrogens) directly stimulates growth of the male breast. It can also suppress LH secretion and further alter the balance of estrogens and androgens. The absolute increase in serum estrogens may be attributable

Box 1. Pathogenesis of gynecomastia

I. Absolute excess of estrogens
   A. Administration of exogenous estrogens
      1. Intentional therapeutic use: estrogens in prostate cancer
      2. Unintentional exposure to estrogens
         a. Occupational
         b. Dietary exposure (phytoestrogens): soy, alcoholic beverages
         c. Percutaneous absorption: antibalding creams, from partner's estrogen cream
   B. Increased endogenous estrogen production
      1. Increased secretion of estrogens
         a. From testis
            (1) Leydig cell tumors
            (2) Stimulation of normal Leydig cells by human chorionic gonadotropin (hCG)
         b. From adrenals
            Feminizing adrenocortical tumors
      2. Increased aromatization of androgens to estrogens
         a. Aromatase excess syndrome
         b. Drugs (eg, androgens, ethanol)
         c. Alcoholic cirrhosis of liver
         d. Aging
         e. Obesity
         f. Hyperthyroidism
         g. hCG-secreting tumors
II. Absolute deficiency of androgens
   A. Hypogonadism
      1. Primary hypogonadism
         a. Klinefelter syndrome
         b. Testicular trauma
         c. Cancer chemotherapeutic agents
         d. Testicular radiation
         e. Infections (eg, mumps orchitis, leprosy)
         f. Disordered enzymes of testosterone biosynthesis
            (1) Drugs (eg, ketoconazole, spironolactone, metronidazole)
            (2) Inherited defects in androgen biosynthesis
      2. Secondary hypogonadism (pituitary/hypothalamic disease/surgery/radiation)

III. Altered serum androgen/estrogen ratio
  A. Puberty
  B. Aging
  C. Refeeding gynecomastia
  D. Renal failure and dialysis
  E. Hepatic cirrhosis
  F. Hyperthyroidism
  G. Drugs
IV. Decreased androgen action
  A. Drugs (eg, spironolactone, cimetidine)
  B. AR defects
    1. Absent or defective ARs (complete and partial androgen insensitivity syndromes)
    2. Expansion of CAG repeats in AR gene (Kennedy disease)

to endogenous overproduction of estrogens or to exogenous estrogen administration.

Endogenous estrogen overproduction
Excess testicular secretion of estrogens
  Leydig cell tumors. Leydig cell tumors of the testis are rare, and most are benign (85%–90%). These are generally seen in young and middle-aged men, although they can occur at any age. The tumor often tends to be small and may not be palpable. Testicular ultrasound examination is helpful in localization. Surgery is the treatment of choice [33].
  Leydig cell tumors directly secrete estradiol, which raises serum estrogen levels and suppresses LH release from the pituitary, leading to a reduction in the testicular production of testosterone [34]. Estrogens also stimulate the production and glycosylation of sex hormone–binding globulin (SHBG), raising serum SHBG levels. Because testosterone is more tightly bound to SHBG than estradiol, a rise in the SHBG level leads to a decrease in the free testosterone concentration, further increasing the ratio of free estrogen to free androgen.
  Sertoli cell tumors. Sertoli cell tumors of the testis are rare; most are benign, occur in boys and young men, and do not have any endocrine effects. Sertoli cell tumors in the Peutz-Jeghers syndrome (PJS) often present with rapid growth, gynecomastia, and advancing bone age, however. These tumors overexpress aromatase, leading to significant production of estrogens and markedly elevated serum estrogen levels [35]. PJS seems to be caused by a mutation in the serine-threonine kinase gene STK11 on chromosome 19p; it is unclear how this mutation leads to Sertoli cell tumors with the characteristic increase in aromatase activity [36]. Sertoli cell

tumors with increased aromatase activity may also be seen in the Carney complex [37].

Human chorionic gonadotropin–secreting tumors. The placental hormone hCG is similar to LH in its structure and its action on the testis. Many malignant germ cell tumors of the testis (especially those with chorionic elements) secrete hCG, and tumors arising from other organs can secrete hCG ectopically. Like LH, hCG stimulates normal Leydig cells of the testes to secrete estradiol preferentially [38]. In addition, many hCG-secreting tumors can take up steroid precursors (eg, dehydroepiandrosterone [DHEA]-sulfate) from the circulation and aromatize them into active estrogens [39], leading to a relative or absolute systemic excess of estrogens. Serum β-hCG is useful as a tumor marker in these patients. Although LH/hCG receptors have been described in the male breast [29], a direct role for hCG in the genesis of gynecomastia has yet to be demonstrated.

Excess adrenal production of estrogens

Feminizing adrenocortical tumors. Unlike Leydig cell tumors of the testis, which are mostly benign, feminizing adrenal tumors are generally malignant poorly differentiated tumors that are often large at presentation (half have a palpable abdominal mass). The peak incidence is in young and middle-aged men [40]. These cancers may secrete estrogens directly [41], along with steroid precursors (eg, DHEA, androstenedione) that may be aromatized into estrogens in peripheral tissues [40]. As with Leydig cell tumors, the elevated serum estrogens may suppress LH-mediated testosterone production, further increasing the estrogen-to-androgen ratio.

Abdominal CT can localize most of these tumors; biochemically, two thirds of the patients have elevations in urinary 17-ketosteroids, and many have elevated serum levels of DHEA-sulfate or androstenedione. The prognosis is poor because of extensive local invasion and distant metastases; surgery is the initial treatment of choice, and palliation may be attempted with mitotane and other chemotherapeutic agents.

Increased peripheral aromatization to estrogens: familial aromatase excess syndrome. The enzyme aromatase (P450 arom, or CYP19A1), or estrogen synthetase, catalyzes the conversion of C19 steroid precursors to C18 estrogens. It is present in adipose tissue, the major site of peripheral aromatization of androgens to estrogens as well as in the testis, bone, brain, muscle, and hair follicles [13,14]. The CYP19A1 gene resides on chromosome 15 and is flanked by the tropomodulin (TMOD3) and FLJ genes, which are constitutively expressed. Shozu and colleagues [42] described two patients (a father and a son) who had an inversion in 15q21.2-q21.3, which brought the promoter of the TMOD3 gene (or FLJ gene in another patient) immediately upstream of the coding region of the CYP19A1 gene, leading to its overexpression, with marked increases in aromatization of adrenal androgens to estrogens. Affected male patients presented with precocious puberty and gynecomastia occurring at the time of adrenarche (OMIM 139300 and 107910), although gonadotropins may be suppressed because of elevated estrogens; even though testosterone concentrations and testicular volume may be decreased, fertility and libido are usually normal in affected men. Affected female patients may have precocious puberty, premature thelarche, and macromastia [43]. Aromatase inhibitors lead to a decrease in estrogen levels and reversal of estrogen excess–induced hypogonadotropic hypogonadism, with recovery of normal testicular function [42,43].

Exogenous estrogen administration

Therapeutic administration of estrogens. Estrogens are used therapeutically in the treatment of men with prostate cancer and often lead to breast pain, tenderness, and enlargement (gynecomastia in men with prostate cancer is reviewed later in detail). Estrogens are also used to stimulate breast development in male-to-female transsexuals.

Unintentional exposure to estrogens. Unintentional exposure to estrogens may occur percutaneously from estrogen in skin creams and antibalding lotions used by men or by absorption during sexual intercourse from vaginal estrogen cream applied by the partner [44]. Unintentional exposure to estrogens may also be related to one's occupation (a barber who massaged an estrogen-containing ointment into the scalps of his clients [45]; a mortician who applied an estrogen-containing embalming cream to corpses [46]; factory workers involved in manufacturing estrogens [47]; and even children of such a factory worker, who absorbed the drug from their father's clothes [48]). Boys and young men are especially susceptible to estrogens and may develop gynecomastia with small exposures [49]. Unintentional estrogen exposure may also occur by means of food, including ingestion of milk or meat from estrogen-treated cows, endogenous estrogens in foods (plant and animal sources), and certain beers and wines [50,51]. Dietary estrogen intake is not likely to be a significant contributing factor in most men with gynecomastia, however, unless large amounts of these foods are consumed.

Absolute deficiency in serum androgens

Primary hypogonadism

Primary hypogonadism of any cause can result in gynecomastia. A deficiency of testosterone itself contributes to a relative estrogen excess. The elevation in serum LH also leads to increased estradiol synthesis in the remaining Leydig cells in the testis. Peripheral conversion of adrenal androgens (eg, DHEA, androstenedione) to estrogens additionally contributes to the relative or absolute excess of estrogens. Estrogen excess leads to increased SHBG levels; because testosterone is more tightly bound to SHBG than estradiol, free testosterone levels fall more substantially than free estradiol, again perturbing the ratio of androgens to estrogens. Testosterone replacement therapy in men with primary hypogonadism often leads to a reduction in the gynecomastia.

Klinefelter syndrome (KS) is the most common chromosomal disorder associated with hypogonadism and infertility in men, and it often leads to gynecomastia, which is seen in approximately 50% to 70% of cases [52,53]. KS is the only cause of gynecomastia in which there is a clearly established increase in the risk of developing breast cancer; compared with normal men, men with KS have a 20-fold elevated risk of developing breast cancer [54]. Classically, men with KS have a 47,XXY karyotype (90%), although approximately 10% are mosaic (46,XY/47,XXY karyotype). The role of the additional X chromosome in the development of the gynecomastia and the increased risk of breast cancer is unclear. Men with KS must be counseled regarding their increased risk of breast cancer and should be encouraged to perform periodic breast self-examinations to look for any suspicious breast masses. The role of screening mammograms in patients with KS is unclear.

Defects in genes coding for critical enzymes in the testosterone biosynthetic pathway can lead to decreased testosterone production. These include defects in the CYP17A1 (encoding 17 α-hydroxylase and 17/20 lyase; OMIM 609300) and HSDB3 (encoding 3β-hydroxysteroid dehydrogenase; OMIM 201810) genes. Several drugs, including ketoconazole and spironolactone, can inhibit various enzymes in the testosterone biosynthetic pathway and lead to decreased testosterone production and gynecomastia.

Secondary hypogonadism

As in men with primary hypogonadism, a decreased serum testosterone level but continued estrogen production from peripheral aromatization of adrenal precursors alters the androgen-to-estrogen ratio in secondary hypogonadism of any cause, leading to gynecomastia.

Deficient androgen action at tissues (androgen receptor defects)

In partial and complete androgen insensitivity syndromes, defective ARs result in decreased androgen action in spite of elevated serum testosterone and lead to gynecomastia. The elevated gonadotropins (because of lack of inhibitory androgen feedback on the pituitary) lead to increased estradiol synthesis in the testis, which also promotes gynecomastia.

Relative estrogen excess: altered androgen-to-estrogen ratio

Pubertal gynecomastia

Fifty percent to 70% of healthy boys develop gynecomastia during puberty, with a peak incidence in early to midpuberty. The breast enlargement may be asymmetric and tender. It resolves spontaneously within 1 to 2 years in most boys, and only 20% of men still have gynecomastia by the age of 20 years [1,3].

In boys who develop pubertal gynecomastia, there may be a relative imbalance in the androgen-to-estrogen ratio; serum estrogen levels may rise sooner than testosterone early in puberty, leading to transient gynecomastia. Later in puberty, as the normal androgen-to-estrogen balance is restored, gynecomastia often resolves [55,56]. The rise in serum IGF-I levels at puberty may also play a role in the pathogenesis of pubertal gynecomastia [22,57].

In recent years, increasing numbers of boys are using anabolic steroids for body building; some anabolic steroids are aromatized to estrogens and may lead to gynecomastia. Because of the underreporting of steroid abuse, the clinician should raise the issue with the adolescent and discuss the risks associated with anabolic steroid abuse (this is reviewed in detail by Carpenter in a separate article in this issue).

A boy with age-appropriate physical and sexual development who has palpable gynecomastia and no worrisome findings on a comprehensive history and physical examination may need no further workup and may simply be observed, because there is a high rate of spontaneous regression. If the boy has bothersome breast pain or tenderness or the gynecomastia is the cause of anxiety and social stress, however, one could attempt medical therapy with antiestrogens [58], aromatase inhibitors [59], or androgens (danazol [60]). The best experience so far is with tamoxifen and raloxifene, selective estrogen receptor modulators (SERMs) that act as estrogen receptor antagonists at breast tissue. Various studies have used tamoxifen at a dose of 10 to 20 mg/d or raloxifene at a dose of 60 mg/d for 3 to 9 months and have reported clinical improvement in up to 90% of cases [58].

Gynecomastia of aging

Aging is associated with an increase in the prevalence of hypogonadism; in the Baltimore Longitudinal Study of Aging, 20% of men older than 60 years of age and 50% of men older than 80 years of age were hypogonadal using total testosterone criteria; an even greater percentage were hypogonadal using free testosterone criteria [61]. The hypothalamic-pituitary-testis axis is variable in the age-related decline in testosterone; in some men, serum gonadotropins are elevated, whereas they are normal in most [62]. Aging is often accompanied by increased adiposity, leading to increased aromatization of androgens to estrogens. Also, serum SHBG levels rise with increasing age, further decreasing the free and bioavailable testosterone. Additionally, older men often have multiple medical problems and require multiple medications, some of which may contribute to gynecomastia.

Refeeding gynecomastia

Refeeding gynecomastia was first recognized after World War II when some men liberated from prison camps developed tender gynecomastia after resuming a normal diet [63,64]. It is usually transient and remits spontaneously in most patients in 1 or 2 years. Starvation and substantial weight loss are associated with hypogonadotropic hypogonadism, and when these men return to eating a healthy diet and regain weight, the hypothalamic-pituitary-testicular axis returns to normal, leading to a "second puberty," with a transient imbalance of estrogens to androgens and self-limited gynecomastia. A similar phenomenon has been seen in refugee populations, in impoverished groups, and after therapeutic dieting [63,65–67]. Refeeding gynecomastia may partly explain the gynecomastia seen in several medical illnesses, including dialysis-associated gynecomastia. It may also explain the gynecomastia associated with drugs like isoniazid and digoxin, which lead to significant improvement in the clinical status of chronically ill malnourished patients.

Renal failure and hemodialysis

Many men with chronic renal failure (CRF) develop gynecomastia on initiation of dialysis. Dialysis-associated gynecomastia may be similar in pathogenesis to refeeding gynecomastia; before dialysis, these men are often nauseated and anorectic, are on protein-restricted diets, and often lose weight. After initiation of dialysis, their nutritional status improves. Dialysis-associated gynecomastia often resolves spontaneously after 1 or 2 years [68].

CRF is accompanied by many changes in the gonadal axis. Men with renal failure are often hypogonadal with defects in testicular steroidogenesis and spermatogenesis. This defect is usually not corrected by hemodialysis, although renal transplantation does improve testicular function. Men with CRF usually have low total and free serum testosterone as well as normal or elevated LH; follicle-stimulating hormone (FSH) may be normal but is often elevated in men with azoospermia [69]. Decreased production and increased metabolism of testosterone probably lead to low testosterone levels. Serum prolactin levels are often elevated because of decreased renal clearance and increased production, which is likely related to a functional disturbance in the hypothalamic regulation of prolactin secretion. Several medications (eg, metoclopramide) used in patients with CRF can also elevate prolactin.

Cirrhosis of the liver

It has long been believed that men with liver disease, especially cirrhosis, have an increased prevalence of gynecomastia. In 1990, however, Cavanaugh and colleagues [70] reported that the prevalence of gynecomastia in cirrhotics is no different from that of hospitalized age-matched controls. Nonetheless, there are several hormonal changes in chronic liver disease that theoretically increase the risk of developing gynecomastia. Cirrhotics have decreased clearance of androstenedione; more substrate is therefore available for aromatization to estrone in the peripheral tissues, leading to increased serum estrogens. SHBG levels are also increased, decreasing free testosterone levels [71]. Alcohol also has direct toxic effects on gonadal function; cirrhotics often have testicular atrophy and are frequently hypogonadal [72]. In addition, it has been reported that serum progesterone levels may be elevated in men with cirrhosis [26]; insofar as progesterone may possibly play some role in breast development and ductular proliferation, this observation may be relevant to the occurrence of gynecomastia.

Hyperthyroidism

Ten percent to 40% of men with thyrotoxicosis may develop gynecomastia that resolves with correction of the hyperthyroid state. This is likely attributable to increased peripheral conversion of androgens to estrogens and increased serum SHBG levels in hyperthyroidism, leading to decreased serum free testosterone [73,74]. Elevated serum levels of progesterone have also been reported in hyperthyroid men [27], although the biologic significance of this observation and its relation to gynecomastia remain to be further evaluated.

Gynecomastia in men with prostate cancer

Gynecomastia is frequently seen in men with prostate cancer. Because prostate cancer is an androgen-dependent neoplasm, hormonal therapy using androgen deprivation or androgen blockade is often used and is frequently associated with new-onset breast pain, tenderness, and enlargement. Estrogen agonists have also been used for hormonal therapy of prostate cancer and commonly lead to gynecomastia. Dobs and Darkes [75] found that the prevalence of gynecomastia in men with prostate cancer is highest in those treated with systemic estrogens (71%), less with luteinizing hormone releasing–hormone (LHRH) analogues (1%–25%) or nonsteroidal antiandrogens (eg, flutamide, bicalutamide; generally 16%–49%), and least with bilateral orchiectomy (approximately 10%) (this topic is reviewed in further detail by Hall in a separate article in this issue).

Prophylactic radiation therapy of the breast tissue has been reported to be effective in decreasing the risk of developing gynecomastia in these men [76–78], although the long-term increased risk of breast cancer is a theoretic concern. Tamoxifen seems to be even more effective than radiation in decreasing the risk of gynecomastia in men with prostate cancer who are about to start antiandrogen or estrogen agonist therapy [78]. The aromatase inhibitor anastrazole was found to be significantly less effective than tamoxifen in preventing gynecomastia in bicalutamide-treated men with advanced prostate cancer. In a double-blind placebo-controlled trial, 73% of patients on bicalutamide and placebo developed gynecomastia; only 10% of the men treated with bicalutamide and tamoxifen developed gynecomastia compared with 53% receiving bicalutamide plus anastrazole [79].

Gynecomastia in HIV-positive men

Gynecomastia has increasingly been recognized in men with HIV disease, although breast enlargement in these men could also be attributable to lipomastia (because of generalized adiposity or HIV-related lipodystrophy), Kaposi sarcoma, Paget disease of the breast, lymphoma, and breast infections [80]. Gynecomastia in HIV-positive men is often multifactorial in cause, and it may be difficult to ascertain the exact mechanism because of the multiple comorbidities and concomitant confounding factors present in these men. First, many medications used to treat HIV as part of highly active antiretroviral therapy (HAART) have been associated with gynecomastia, including protease inhibitors (PIs) and nucleoside reverse transcriptase inhibitors (NRTIs) [81,82]. Second, the use of illicit drugs, such as marijuana and heroin, that may be associated with gynecomastia may be increased [80]. Third, many HIV-infected men have concomitant liver disease (hepatitis B or C or alcoholic liver disease). Fourth, some patients with HIV infection and some men on HAART therapy have hypogonadotropic hypogonadism, although the exact mechanism for this is unclear [83]. Finally, a refeeding mechanism could also contribute in some patients. Gynecomastia may develop within a few months or as late as a few years after starting HAART therapy. It may resolve spontaneously over several months, even when medications are continued, or may be persistent.

Benveniste and colleagues [84], reported the use of topical dihydrotestosterone (DHT) gel applied to the breast in four men with HIV and gynecomastia; DHT gel resulted in significant and rapid (within 10–30 days) improvement in gynecomastia in all four men and was well tolerated without any serious side effects. Although no well-designed clinical trials have been reported to date with tamoxifen in HIV-associated gynecomastia, it seems reasonable to try it for 3 months; because of the multiple medications these men often take, it would be advisable to monitor liver function studies closely. If gynecomastia persists in spite of a trial of medical therapy and is bothersome to the patient, surgery may be helpful.

Diabetic mastopathy

Although diabetic mastopathy was originally described in women with long-standing type 1 diabetes, it is now known that men may also develop this breast disease, which may be unilateral or bilateral [85,86]. Patients may present with a painless or painful breast lump or with diffuse enlargement of one or both breasts. Physical examination may reveal a discrete breast mass or diffuse nodularity, especially in the subareolar region. Histologically, the lesion is characterized by lymphocytic (B-cell) infiltration of the mammary ducts and lobules, with varying degrees of fibrosis and vasculitis [85,87]. Although the exact mechanism is still unclear, autoimmunity may play a role in the pathogenesis of this inflammatory lesion, because it has also been described in nondiabetics with Hashimoto thyroiditis or systemic lupus erythematosus. In men, the breast lesion may be indistin-guishable clinically and radiologically from gynecomastia [86]. It may re-gress spontaneously [88] but often persists and may recur after excision. Diabetic mastopathy does not seem to increase the risk for subsequent de-velopment of breast cancer or lymphoma.

Drug-induced gynecomastia

Many medications and recreational drugs have been associated with gy-necomastia. Although a causal relation is well established with some drugs, the mechanism is unclear for most drugs; there are often only anecdotal re-ports, and the association may be merely coincidental (Box 2). Drugs may be responsible for one in four cases of new-onset gynecomastia in adults [2].

Male breast cancer

Fortunately, breast cancer is rare in men; approximately 1400 men are di-agnosed with invasive breast cancer in the United States each year—1 percent of the risk of developing breast cancer in women. Men with a family history of breast cancer in female relatives have a 2.5 times increased risk of developing breast cancer, however, and those with an inherited germline BRCA2 mutation are at a 100-fold greater risk of developing a breast malig-nancy. With the exception of KS, gynecomastia does not increase the risk of future development of breast carcinoma [89]. Men with breast cancer seem to have a prognosis similar to women with the same stage of cancer at the time of diagnosis [89].

Clinical features worrisome for breast malignancy include a hard eccentri-cally located asymmetric mass, often with fixation to the skin or underlying structures, ulceration, axillary lymphadenopathy, or a bloody nipple dis-charge. Any breast mass suspicious for malignancy should be biopsied; the biopsy provides the definitive diagnosis (or excludes) malignancy. It is important to remember that gynecomastia is far more common than male breast cancer; hence, it is unnecessary and impractical to perform a breast bi-opsy on all men with gynecomastia (Box 3; Fig. 1). As in women with breast cancer, treatment includes surgery, chemotherapy, or radiation therapy, depending on the stage of the disease.

Evaluation of a patient with gynecomastia

As reviewed previously, gynecomastia is common, even among healthy men, and is often incidentally noted on routine physical examination. In an asymptomatic healthy man with long-standing stable gynecomastia and a benign history and detailed physical examination, no further hor-monal evaluation is necessary. Men with new-onset breast pain, tenderness,

Box 2. Mechanisms of drug-induced gynecomastia

I. Increased serum estrogens or estrogen-like activity
    A. Exogenous estrogens (intentional or unintentional exposure)
    B. Increased aromatization of androgens to estrogens
        1. Androgens
        2. Ethanol abuse
    C. Estrogen agonist activity (digitoxin)
II. Decreased serum testosterone
    A. Hypogonadotropic hypogonadism
        1. LHRH agonists/antagonists
        2. Possibly HAART therapy for HIV
    B. Hypergonadotropic hypogonadism
        1. Destruction or inhibition of Leydig cells: chemotherapeutic/cytotoxic agents (eg, alkylating agents, vincristine, methotrexate, nitrosoureas, cisplatin, imatinib)
        2. Decreased testosterone or DHT biosynthesis
            a. Ketoconazole
            b. Metronidazole
            c. Spironolactone (high doses)
            d. Finasteride and dutasteride
III. AR blockade
    A. Flutamide, bicalutamide
    B. Cimetidine
    C. Marijuana
    D. Spironolactone
IV. Increased serum prolactin
    A. Antipsychotic agents
    B. Metoclopramide
    C. Possibly calcium channel blockers
V. Possible refeeding gynecomastia
    A. Isoniazid
    B. Digoxin
    C. Effective HAART therapy for HIV disease
VI. Unknown
    A. HAART
    B. Human GH
    C. Amiodarone
    D. Calcium channel blockers (eg, nifedipine, verapamil, diltiazem)
    E. Amphetamines
    F. Diazepam
    G. Antidepressants (tricyclics and selective serotonin reuptake inhibitors)

or enlargement should be evaluated to rule out serious underlying systemic or endocrine disease, however.

Clinical evaluation of a man with gynecomastia is focused on differentiating true gynecomastia from fatty breasts (pseudogynecomastia), excluding breast malignancy, and determining the probable cause of the gynecomastia. True enlargement of breast tissue may be differentiated from fatty breasts on careful clinical examination by comparing subareolar tissue with the adjacent subcutaneous fat. The presence of an unusually firm asymmetric breast mass in an eccentric location with fixation to the skin or to the underlying structures, ulceration, nipple retraction or discharge, or axillary lymphadenopathy is worrisome for malignancy and should be biopsied. A mammogram or breast sonogram may also be useful in evaluating suspicious masses before biopsy. It is important to remember, however, that gynecomastia may be unilateral or more pronounced on one side.

To determine the possible cause of the gynecomastia, it is important to obtain a detailed history of the onset and duration of gynecomastia; associated breast pain or tenderness; systemic disease (eg, chronic liver or kidney disease, hyperthyroidism, hypogonadism, prostate or testicular

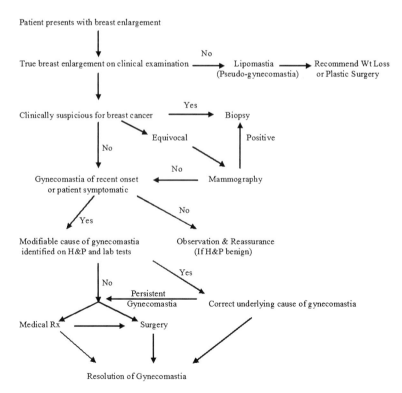

Fig. 1. Suggested algorithm for the management of gynecomastia. H&P, history and physical examination; Rx, therapy; Wt, weight.

Box 3. Diagnostic evaluation of gynecomastia

I. History
    A. Related to breast enlargement:
        1. Duration of breast enlargement
        2. Presence of breast pain or tenderness
        3. Worrisome symptoms of breast cancer
    B. Systemic illness
        1. Recent abnormal weight loss or weight gain
        2. Liver disease
        3. CRF or dialysis
        4. Symptoms of hyperthyroidism
    C. Changes in libido, sexual functioning, or other symptoms of hypogonadism
    D. Medication use
    E. Recreational drug use (eg, marijuana, heroin)
    F. Occupational/dietary/accidental exposure to estrogen
II. Physical examination
    A. Degree of virilization: voice, facial and body hair, muscular development
    B. Breast examination
        1. True gynecomastia versus pseudogynecomastia
        2. Signs suspicious for breast cancer
        3. Breast tenderness
    C. Examination of genitalia
        1. Testicular size
        2. Testicular masses
        3. Phallus size and development
        4. Pubic hair development
    D. Stigmata of chronic liver or kidney disease
    E. Examination of thyroid and signs of hyperthyroidism
III. Laboratory evaluation
    A. Kidney function (blood urea nitrogen/creatinine)
    B. Liver function tests
    C. Thyroid function (thyroid-stimulating hormone with or without free thyroxine)
    D. Serum testosterone (total and bioavailable or free), LH, FSH, prolactin
    E. Serum estrogens (serum estradiol)
    F. Tumor markers for germ cell neoplasms (β-hCG, α-fetoprotein)
    G. Adrenal androgens (serum DHEA-sulfate or urinary 17-ketosteroids)

IV. Radiologic examination[a]
    A. Mammogram[a]
    B. Breast ultrasound[a]

---

[a] Radiologic examination is not recommended for routine evaluation of gynecomastia (see text for detailed discussion).

malignancy); recent weight gain or loss; use of medications (including over-the-counter supplements); and possible unintentional exposure to estrogens through occupation, diet, or cosmetics.

On physical examination, in addition to a detailed breast examination, careful examination of the genitalia should be done for documenting testicular size and detecting testicular masses. On general physical examination, attention should be paid to signs of chronic liver or kidney disease, hyperthyroidism, abdominal masses (for possible adrenal tumor), the degree of virilization, and secondary sexual development.

Routine biochemical testing should include evaluation of kidney, liver, and thyroid function and measurement of serum testosterone (total or, preferably, bioavailable), LH, FSH, and prolactin. Serum tumor markers, such as hCG or α-fetoprotein (AFP), should be measured in the appropriate clinical setting. If a testicular tumor is suspected, an ultrasound examination may be helpful in locating the neoplasm. Similarly, a CT scan of the adrenals may be helpful if an adrenal neoplasm is suspected on clinical grounds or biochemical testing. Given the low prevalence of male breast cancer, mammograms or breast ultrasound examinations are not indicated in the routine evaluation of gynecomastia unless breast malignancy is suspected clinically [90,91].

Management of gynecomastia

For asymptomatic men with long-standing stable gynecomastia, no specific treatment is necessary. Men with new-onset breast pain, tenderness, or enlargement should be evaluated as detailed previously (see Fig. 1).

In men with a possible medication, recreational drug, or nutritional exposure, the inciting agent should be withdrawn if possible; the gynecomastia should improve over the next few weeks. If there is no improvement over several months or if the medication cannot be stopped, medical therapy may be attempted.

Because gynecomastia is often the result of a relative excess of estrogens, medical therapy of gynecomastia aims to block estrogen effects in the breast tissue (with antiestrogens [eg, tamoxifen, raloxifene, clomiphene]), decrease estrogen production (using aromatase inhibitors [eg, testolactone, anastrazole]), or give androgens to counteract the effects of estrogens. Unfortunately, there are few well-designed prospective studies assessing the effect of medical therapy on gynecomastia.

Tamoxifen blocks estrogen effects on breast tissue and is commonly used as an effective breast cancer chemotherapeutic agent. In men with gynecomastia attributable to a variety of causes, tamoxifen has been used in doses of 10 to 20 mg/d for 3 to 9 months; resolution of gynecomastia has been noted in up to 90% of men [92,93]. If the gynecomastia recurs on stopping the medication, a second course of therapy may be attempted. Tamoxifen is usually well tolerated. Raloxifene is another SERM related to tamoxifen; in a retrospective chart review, Lawrence and colleagues [58] found raloxifene to be more effective than tamoxifen in reducing breast size in boys with persistent pubertal gynecomastia. Clomiphene has also been used in the management of gynecomastia, although the results have been less promising than with tamoxifen [94].

Testolactone, an older aromatase inhibitor, has been reported in small studies to be beneficial in treating gynecomastia, although the treatment was less effective than tamoxifen [95]. Anastrazole, a potent new aromatase inhibitor frequently used as breast cancer chemotherapy, was found to be no better than placebo in a randomized controlled trial in 80 boys with pubertal gynecomastia, however [59]. Similarly, in men with prostate cancer with bicalutamide-related gynecomastia, tamoxifen was significantly more effective than anastrazole in decreasing breast pain, tenderness, and gynecomastia [79]. Danazol, a weak androgen, has also been used to suppress gonadotropins, and hence decrease testicular estradiol production, with some reduction in gynecomastia reported [60].

Testosterone replacement leads to the resolution of gynecomastia in many hypogonadal men. Because it can be aromatized to estradiol, testosterone therapy may also lead to new-onset gynecomastia in some men. For this reason, nonaromatizable androgens like DHT have been tried, systemically and topically, for the treatment of gynecomastia. Topical application of DHT gel to the breast was found to be effective in HIV-associated gynecomastia [84]. DHT gel is not yet available in the United States, however.

Radiation therapy directed at the breast has been used in men with prostate cancer to prevent new-onset breast pain, tenderness, and gynecomastia associated with antiandrogen therapy [75–78]. It has also been tried in the past to treat pubertal boys with gynecomastia; in young men, the long-term risk of breast cancer after radiation exposure is a significant concern.

In men with long-standing symptomatic gynecomastia, medical therapy is less likely to be effective, because the stroma is mostly fibrotic. Surgery may be the preferred treatment in these men and also in men who fail, do not tolerate, or decline medical therapy as well as in the patient who prefers surgical removal for cosmetic reasons. Surgery usually involves excision of the glandular tissue by means of a periareolar incision and may include suction lipectomy [96].

Summary

Although gynecomastia is a common asymptomatic physical finding, it may also be a sign of underlying disease or an undesirable drug side effect. Proper evaluation may identify the cause and serve to guide treatment. Administration of tamoxifen is emerging as an effective therapy in many instances of symptomatic gynecomastia.

References

[1] Nydick M, Bustos J, Dale JH Jr, et al. Gynecomastia in adolescent boys. JAMA 1961;178: 449–54.

[2] Carlson HE. Gynecomastia. N Engl J Med 1980;303:795–9.

[3] Nutall FQ. Gynecomastia as a physical finding in normal men. J Clin Endocrinol Metab 1979;48:338–40.

[4] Bannayan GA, Hajdu SI. Gynecomastia: clinicopathologic study of 351 cases. Am J Clin Pathol 1972;57:431–7.

[5] Niewoehner CB, Nuttall FQ. Gynecomastia in a hospitalized male population. Am J Med 1984;77:633–8.

[6] Williams MJ. Gynecomastia: its incidence, recognition and host characterization in 447 autopsy cases. Am J Med 1963;34:103–12.

[7] Nicolis GL, Modlinger RS, Gabrilove JL. A study of the histopathology of human gynecomastia. J Clin Endocrinol Metab 1971;32:173–8.

[8] Sasano H, Kimura M, Shizawa S, et al. Aromatase and steroid receptors in gynecomastia and male breast carcinoma: an immunohistochemical study. J Clin Endocrinol Metab 1996;81:3063–7.

[9] Dimitrikakis C, Zhou J, Bondy CA. Androgens and mammary growth and neoplasia. Fertil Steril 2002;77(Suppl 4):S26–33.

[10] Kanhai RCJ, Hage JJ, VanDiest PJ, et al. Short-term and long-term histologic effects of castration and estrogen treatment on breast tissue of 14 male-to-female transsexuals in comparison with two chemically castrated men. Am J Surg Pathol 2000;24: 74–80.

[11] Burgess HE, Shousha S. An immunohistochemical study of the long-term effects of androgen administration on female-to-male transsexual breast: a comparison with normal female breast and male breast showing gynecomastia. J Pathol 1993;170:37–43.

[12] Dejager S, Bry-Gauillard H, Bruckert E, et al. A comprehensive endocrine description of Kennedy's disease revealing androgen insensitivity linked to CAG repeat length. J Clin Endocrinol Metab 2002;87(8):3893–901.

[13] Bulun SE, Fang Z, Gurates B, et al. Aromatase in health and disease. Endocrinologist 2003; 13(3):269–76.

[14] Braunstein GD. Aromatase and gynecomastia. Endocr-Relat Cancer 1999;6:315–24.

[15] Cleland WH, Mendelson CE, Simpson ER. Effects of aging and obesity on aromatase activity of human adipose cells. J Clin Endocrinol Metab 1985;60:174–7.

[16] Reed MJ, Purohit A. Breast cancer and the role of cytokines in regulating estrogen synthesis: an emerging hypothesis. Endocr Rev 1997;18(5):701–15.

[17] Ryde CM, Nicholls JE, Dowsett M. Steroid and growth factor modulation of aromatase activity in MCF7 and T47D breast carcinoma cell lines. Cancer Res 1992;52:1411–5.

[18] Christeff N, Benassayag C, Carli-Vielle C, et al. Elevated oestrogen and reduced testosterone levels in the serum of male septic shock patients. J Steroid Biochem 1988;29(4): 435–40.

[19] Gill S, Peston D, Vonderhaar BK, et al. Expression of prolactin receptors in normal, benign, and malignant breast tissue: an immunohistological study. J Clin Pathol 2001;54:956–60.

[20] Ormandy CJ, Hall RE, Manning DL, et al. Coexpression and cross-regulation of the prolactin and sex steroid hormone receptors in breast cancer. J Clin Endocrinol Metab 1997;82(11): 3692–9.

[21] Gutzman JH, Miller KK, Schuler LA. Endogenous human prolactin and not exogenous human prolactin induces estrogen receptor α and prolactin receptor expression and increases estrogen responsiveness in breast cancer cells. J Steroid Biochem Mol Biol 2004;88:69–77.

[22] Kleinberg DL. Role of IGF-I in normal mammary development. Breast Cancer Res Treat 1998;47(3):201–8.

[23] Ruan W, Kleinberg DL. Insulin-like growth factor I is essential for terminal end bud formation and ductal morphogenesis during mammary development. Endocrinology 1999;
140(11):5075–81.

[24] Stewart AJ, Johnson MD, May FEB, et al. Role of insulin-like growth factors and the type I
insulin-like growth factor receptor in the estrogen-stimulated proliferation of human breast
cancer cells. J Biolumin Chemilumin 1990;265:21172–8.

[25] Humphreys RC, Lydon JP, O'Malley BW, et al. Use of PRKO mice to study the role of progesterone in mammary gland development. J Mammary Gland Biol Neoplasia 1997;2:
343–54.

[26] Farthing MJG, Green JRB, Edwards CRW, et al. Progesterone, prolactin, and gynecomastia in men with liver disease. Gut 1982;23:276–9.

[27] Nomura K, Suzuki H, Saji M, et al. High serum progesterone in hyperthyroid men with
Graves' disease. J Clin Endocrinol Metab 1988;66(1):230–2.

[28] Ruan W, Monaco ME, Kleinberg DL. Progesterone stimulates mammary gland ductal morphogenesis by synergizing with and enhancing insulin-like growth factor-1 action. Endocrinology 2005;146:1170–8.

[29] Carlson HE, Kane P, Lei ZM, et al. Presence of luteinizing hormone/human chorionic
gonadotropin receptors in male breast tissues. J Clin Endocrinol Metab 2004;89:4119–23.

[30] Bird J, Li X, Lei ZM, et al. Luteinizing hormone and human chorionic gonadotropin
decrease type 25α-reductase and androgen receptor protein levels in women's skin. J Clin
Endocrinol Metab 1998;83:1776–82.

[31] Nahta R, Hortobagyi GN, Esteva FJ. Growth factor receptors in breast cancer: potential for
therapeutic intervention. Oncologist 2003;8(1):5–17.

[32] Peres R, Betsholtz C, Westermark B, et al. Frequent expression of growth factors for mes-
enchymal cells in human mammary carcinoma cell lines. Cancer Res 1987;47:3425–9.

[33] Gabrilove JL, Nicolis GL, Mitty HA, et al. Feminizing interstitial cell tumor of the testis:
personal observations and a review of the literature. Cancer 1975;35:1184–202.

[34] Bercovici JP, Nahoul K, Tater D, et al. Hormonal profile of Leydig cell tumors with gynecomastia. J Clin Endocrinol Metab 1984;59:625–30.

[35] Young S, Gooneratne S, Straus FH, et al. Feminizing Sertoli cell tumors in boys with Peutz-
Jeghers syndrome. Am J Surg Pathol 1995;19:50–8.

[36] Amos CI, Keitheri-Cheteri MB, Sabripour M, et al. Genotype-phenotype correlations in
Peutz-Jeghers syndrome. J Med Genet 2004;41:327–33.

[37] Stratakis CA, Kirschner LS, Carney JA. Clinical and molecular features of the Carney complex: diagnostic criteria and recommendations for patient evaluation. J Clin Endocrinol
Metab 2001;86:4041–6.

[38] Forest MG, Lecoq A, Saez JM. Kinetics of human chorionic gonadotropin-induced ste-
roidogenic response of the human testis. II. Plasma 17 alpha-hydroxy-progesterone,
delta⁴-androstenedione, estrone, and 17 beta-estradiol: evidence for the action of human
chorionic gonadotropin on intermediate enzymes implicated in steroid biosynthesis. J Clin
Endocrinol Metab 1979;49:284–91.

[39] Kirschner MA, Lippman A, Berkowitz R, et al. Estrogen production as a tumor marker in
patients with gonadotropin-producing neoplasms. Cancer Res 1981;41:1447–50.

[40] Gabrilove JL, Sharma DC, Wotiz HH, et al. Feminizing adrenal cortical tumors in the male:
a review of 52 cases including a case report. Medicine 1965;44:37–79.

[41] Young J, Bulun SE, Agarwal V, et al. Aromatase expression in a feminizing adrenocortical
tumor. J Clin Endocrinol Metab 1996;81:3173–6.

[42] Shozu M, Sebastian S, Takayama K, et al. Estrogen excess associated with novel
gain-of-function mutations affecting the aromatase gene. N Engl J Med 2003;348:1855–65.

[43] Binder G, Iliev DI, Dufke A, et al. Dominant transmission of prepubertal gynecomastia due
to serum estrone excess: hormonal, biochemical, and genetic analysis in a large kindred.
J Clin Endocrinol Metab 2005;90:484–92.

[44] Di Raimondo CV, Roach AC, Meador CK. Gynecomastia from exposure to vaginal estrogen cream. N Engl J Med 1980;302:1089–90.

[45] Cimorra GA, Gonzalez-Peirona E, Ferrandez A. Percutaneous oestrogen-induced gynaecomastia: a case report. Br J Plast Surg 1982;35(2):209–10.

[46] Finkelstein J, McCully W, MacLaughlin D, et al. The mortician's mystery: gynecomastia and reversible hypogonadotropic hypogonadism in an embalmer. N Engl J Med 1988;319:961–5.

[47] Harrington JM, Stein GF, Rivera RO, et al. The occupational hazards of formulating oral contraceptives—a survey of plant employees. Arch Environ Health 1978;33(1):12–5.

[48] Pacynski A, Budzynska A, Przylecki S, et al. Hyperestrogenism in pharmaceutical factory workers and their children as an occupational disease. Endokrynol Pol 1971;22(2):149–54.

[49] Aksglaede L, Juul A, Leffers H, et al. The sensitivity of the child to sex steroids: possible impact of exogenous estrogens. Hum Reprod Update 2006;12(4):341–9.

[50] Daxenberger A, Ibarreta D, Meyer HH. Possible health impact of animal oestrogens in food. Hum Reprod Update 2001;7(3):340–55.

[51] Gavaler JS, Rosenblum ER, Deal SR, et al. The phytoestrogen congeners of alcoholic beverages: current status. Proc Soc Exp Biol Med 1995;208(1):98–102.

[52] Smyth CM, Bremner WJ. Klinefelter syndrome. Arch Intern Med 1998;158(12):1309–14.

[53] Lanfranco F, Kamischke A, Zitzmann M, et al. Klinefelter's syndrome. Lancet 2004;364:273–83.

[54] Swerdlow AJ, Schoemaker MJ, Higgins CD, et al. Cancer incidence and mortality in men with Klinefelter syndrome: a cohort study. J Natl Cancer Inst 2005;97(16):1204–10.

[55] Large DM, Anderson DC. Twenty four hour profiles of circulating androgens and oestrogens in male puberty with or without gynecomastia. Clin Endocrinol (Oxf) 1979;11:505–21.

[56] Moore DC, Schlaepfer LV, Paunier L, et al. Hormonal changes during puberty. V. Transient pubertal gynecomastia: abnormal androgen-estrogen ratios. J Clin Endocrinol Metab 1984;58:492–9.

[57] Juul A, Bang P, Hertel NT, et al. Serum insulin-like growth factor-1 in 1030 healthy children, adolescents, and adults: relation to age, sex, stage of puberty, testicular size, and body mass index. J Clin Endocrinol Metab 1994;78:744–52.

[58] Lawrence SE, Faught KA, Vethamuthu J, et al. Beneficial effects of raloxifene and tamoxifen in the treatment of pubertal gynecomastia. J Pediatr 2004;145(1):71–6.

[59] Plourde PV, Reiter EO, Jou HC, et al. Safety and efficacy of anastrozole for the treatment of pubertal gynecomastia: a randomized, double-blind, placebo-controlled trial. J Clin Endocrinol Metab 2004;89(9):4428–33.

[60] Buckle R. Danazol in the treatment of gynaecomastia. Drugs 1980;19:356–61.

[61] Harman SM, Metter EJ, Tobin JD, et al. Longitudinal effects of aging on serum total and free testosterone levels in healthy men. Baltimore Longitudinal Study of Aging. J Clin Endocrinol Metab 2001;86:724–31.

[62] Allan CA, McLachlan RI. Age-related changes in testosterone and the role of replacement therapy in older men. Clin Endocrinol (Oxf) 2004;60(6):653–70.

[63] Platt SS, Schulz RZ, Kunstadter RH. Hypertrophy of the male breast associated with recovery from starvation. Bulletin of U.S. Army Medical Department 1947;7:403–5.

[64] Jacobs EC. Effect of starvation on sex hormones in the male. J Clin Endocrinol Metab 1948;8:227–32.

[65] Sattin RW, Roisin A, Kafrissen ME, et al. Epidemic of gynecomastia among illegal Haitian entrants. Public Health Rep 1984;99(5):504–10.

[66] Linn S, Almagor G, Lamm S. Gynecomastia among Ethiopian Jews. Public Health Rep 1986;101(3):237.

[67] Smith SR, Chhetri MK, Johanson AJ, et al. The pituitary-gonadal axis in men with protein-calorie malnutrition. J Clin Endocrinol Metab 1975;41:60–9.

[68] Schmitt GW, Shehadeh I, Sawin CT. Transient gynecomastia in chronic renal failure during chronic intermittent hemodialysis. Ann Intern Med 1968;69:73–9.

[69] Karagiannis A, Harsoulis F. Gonadal dysfunction in systemic disease. Eur J Endocrinol 2005;152:501–13.

[70] Cavanaugh J, Niewoehner CB, Nuttall FQ. Gynecomastia and cirrhosis of the liver. Arch Intern Med 1990;150(3):563–5.

[71] Kley HK, Niederau C, Stremmel W, et al. Conversion of androgens to estrogens in idiopathic hemochromatosis: comparison with alcoholic liver cirrhosis. J Clin Endocrinol Metab 1985;61(1):1–6.

[72] Van Thiel DH. Ethanol: its adverse effects upon the hypothalamic-pituitary-gonadal axis. J Lab Clin Med 1983;101:21–33.

[73] Ford HC, Cooke RR, Keightley EA, et al. Serum levels of free and bound testosterone in hyperthyroidism. Clin Endocrinol 1992;36:187–92.

[74] Ridgway EC, Maloof F, Longcope C. Androgen and estrogen dynamics in hyperthyroidism. J Endocrinol 1982;95:105–15.

[75] Dobs A, Darkes M. Incidence and management of gynecomastia in men treated for prostate cancer. J Urol 2005;174:1737–42.

[76] McLeod DG, Iversen P. Gynecomastia in patients with prostate cancer: a review of treatment options. Urology 2000;56:713–20.

[77] Van Poppel H, Tyrrell CJ, Haustermans K, et al. Efficacy and tolerability of radiotherapy as treatment for bicalutamide-induced gynaecomastia and breast pain in prostate cancer. Eur Urol 2005;47:587–92.

[78] Perdona S, Autorino R, De Placido S, et al. Efficacy of tamoxifen and radiotherapy for prevention and treatment of gynaecomastia and breast pain caused by bicalutamide in prostate cancer: a randomised controlled trial. Lancet Oncol 2005;6(5): 295–300.

[79] Boccardo F, Rubagotti A, Battaglia M, et al. Evaluation of tamoxifen and anastrozole in the prevention of gynecomastia and breast pain induced by bicalutamide monotherapy of prostate cancer. J Clin Oncol 2005;23(4):808–15.

[80] Evans DL, Pantanowitz L, Dezube BJ, et al. Breast enlargement in 13 men who were seropositive for human immunodeficiency virus. Clin Infect Dis 2002;35:1113–9.

[81] Piroth L, Grappin M, Petit JM, et al. Incidence of gynecomastia in men infected with HIV and treated with highly active antiretroviral therapy. Scand J Infect Dis 2001;33:559–60.

[82] Manfredi R, Calza L, Chiodo F. Gynecomastia, lipodystrophy syndrome, and dyslipidemia occurring or worsening during antiretroviral regimens other than protease inhibitor-based ones. J Acquir Immune Defic Syndr 2004;35:99–102.

[83] Biglia A, Blanco JL, Martinez E, et al. Gynecomastia among HIV-infected patients is associated with hypogonadism: a case-control study. Clin Infect Dis 2004;39:1514–9.

[84] Benveniste O, Simon A, Herson S. Successful percutaneous dihydrotestosterone treatment of gynecomastia occurring during highly active antiretroviral therapy: four cases and a review of the literature. Clin Infect Dis 2001;33:891–3.

[85] Ely KA, Tse G, Simpson JF, et al. Diabetic mastopathy. A clinicopathologic review. Am J Clin Pathol 2000;113:541–5.

[86] Weinstein SP, Conant EF, Orel SG, et al. Diabetic mastopathy in men: imaging findings in two patients. Radiology 2001;219:797–9.

[87] Valdez R, Thorson J, Winn WJ, et al. Lymphocytic mastitis and diabetic mastopathy: a molecular, immunophenotypic and clinicopathologic evaluation of 11 cases. Mod Pathol 2003; 16(3):223–8.

[88] Bayer U, Horn L-C, Schulz H-G. Bilateral, tumorlike diabetic mastopathy: progression and regression of the disease during 5-year follow up. Eur J Radiol 1998;26:248–53.

[89] Fentiman IS, Fourquet A, Hortobagyi GN. Male breast cancer. Lancet 2006;367:595–604.

[90] Hanavadi S, Monypenny IJ, Mansel RE. Is mammography overused in male patients? Breast 2006;15(1):123–6.

[91] Chen L, Chantra PK, Larsen LH, et al. Imaging characteristics of malignant lesions of the male breast. Radiographics 2006;26:993–1006.

[92] Ting ACW, Chow LWC, Leung YF. Comparison of tamoxifen with danazol in the management of idiopathic gynecomastia. Am Surg 2000;66:38–40.

[93] Khan HN, Rampaul R, Blamey RW. Management of physiological gynecomastia with tamoxifen. Breast 2004;13:615.

[94] Plourde PV, Kulin HE, Santner SJ. Clomiphene in the treatment of adolescent gynecomastia. Clinical and endocrine studies. Am J Dis Child 1983;137(11):1080–2.

[95] Zachmann M, Eiholzer R, Muritano M, et al. Treatment of pubertal gynaecomastia with testolactone. Acta Endocrinol 1986;113(Suppl 279):218–26.

[96] Fruhstorfer BH, Malata CM. A systematic approach to the surgical management of gynaecomastia. Br J Plast Surg 2003;237–46.

ELSEVIER
SAUNDERS

Endocrinol Metab Clin N Am
36 (2007) 521–531

ENDOCRINOLOGY
AND METABOLISM
CLINICS
OF NORTH AMERICA

Psychosocial Aspects
of Andrologic Disease

Nigel Hunt, PhD[a],*, Sue McHale, PhD[b]

[a]Institute of Work, Health, and Organisations, University of Nottingham,
University Boulevard, Nottingham, NG7 2RQ, United Kingdom
[b]Psychology Group, Sheffield Hallam University, Collegiate Crescent Campus,
Collegiate Crescent, Sheffield, S10 2BP, United Kingdom

Although clinicians and researchers used to focus on medical treatments of andrologic diseases with limited consideration of the psychologic sequelae, psychosocial aspects have recently received more attention. This article reviews the evidence available regarding the psychosocial impact of andrologic diseases on men and women and on their relationships. We briefly outline the key principles in health psychology regarding stress and coping as it is relevant for andrologic disease. We focus on infertility, hypospadias, and erectile dysfunction (ED) because research in these areas highlights the general problems faced by men who have andrologic diseases and because ED is strongly linked to psychosocial circumstances (eg, stress or relationship issues). We conclude with an outline of therapies and areas demanding further research in the future.

Many years ago, there was a call for research to recognize men as a whole and integrated organism [1]; this should be reflected not only in medical aspects of health and illness, but also in psychosocial factors.

Stress and coping

Much psychologic research has been performed on stress and coping. The impact of stress on the human organism is now well understood, as are the responses people have to stressors in terms of styles and strategies of coping, coping capacity, and individual differences; however, many controversial aspects of stress remain [2,3].

---

* Corresponding author.
E-mail address: nigel.hunt@nottingham.ac.uk (N. Hunt).

0889-8529/07/$ - see front matter © 2007 Elsevier Inc. All rights reserved.
doi:10.1016/j.ecl.2007.03.001

There are well-established sex differences in health status and mortality among men and women. Ivancevich and Matteson [4] note that men are four times more likely to die of coronary heart disease and five times more likely to die of alcohol-related diseases and have a life expectancy that is 8 years less than women. On the other hand, women seem to report more stress-related symptoms and are more likely to visit the doctor or physician than men. Several studies found that women were twice as likely to report symptoms of depression [5–7]. The discrepancies may relate to cultural differences rather than the physiologic response to stress. Women are more likely to report symptoms than men in many cultures. Given current understanding, it is not possible to determine whether these reported differences occur because of biologic sex differences or because of complex cultural and environmental factors [2].

Extensive research links stress and illness, with stress as a cause and consequence of illness [8]. Regarding androgenic diseases, coping styles such as denial and repression have associations with poorer health outcomes [9,10]. Research consistently shows that non-expression of emotion is harmful for health, and because men are less likely to express emotion, they are more likely to experience stress-related disorders. This has implications for psychosocial factors in androgenic diseases.

A thorough review of the measures available for the assessment of psychologic stress, coping, and related psychosocial issues in relation to medical interventions is not possible here, but there are some key issues to consider. Many widely available measures are too generic and may not be suitable for people who have particular disorders. Newly devised, more specific measures, may not have adequate reliability, comparability, or validity because they may have been used on a single occasion. This fact limits attempts at meta-analysis or comparison across studies. Conflicting evidence may be explained by aforementioned differences in measures.

Cousineau and colleagues [11] developed and validated a valuable measure of perceived self-efficacy for people coping with infertility treatment. The scale was validated using extant measures of fertility problem distress, perceived stress, and coping style. The authors produced a reliable and valid scale that presents a useful measure of cognitive/affect regulation in infertile men and women and that may benefit practitioners who treat such patients.

Infertility

The most extensive psychosocial research relating to andrologic diseases has taken place with respect to infertility. Most studies have looked at male and female infertility and combined the results. Men and women, at least in the Western world, are treated differently for infertility. This in itself is likely to have psychosocial consequences. Although women usually receive extensive and invasive testing and treatment in relation to infertility, there has, over the last 25 years, been an increase and then a decline in the use of intensive andrology testing in men, particularly in the United States. Improved assisted reproductive technologies have made it easier for clinicians to implement the techniques quickly; some physicians may therefore forgo full diagnostic male testing [12]. This is a potential health risk because infertility can be a marker of serious medical problems.

Infertility and relationships

The literature relating to infertility and its impact on relationships is ambiguous. For many men and women, infertility places a serious strain on their relationship [13]. Earlier qualitative research has shown that infertility treatment can be a threat or a challenge to the relationship or that it can strengthen the relationship [14]. The experience of infertility forced partners to discuss its emotional aspects and the more general existential aspects of life. Individual difference factors play an important role, but they have never been clearly defined.

Peterson and colleagues [15] found no gender differences in marital benefit in a group of men and women who had infertility problems. Another study on a cohort of 2250 married couples beginning infertility treatment in Denmark found that 26% of women and 21% of men reported high marital benefit from the experiences of infertility; around two thirds reported at least some marital benefit [16].

In one study of infertile men, men and women perceived the men as less masculine [17]. Men and women displayed moderate problems, with men being more neurotic than in the general population and women displaying more anxiety and social desirability. The authors found that there were few serious marital problems and that there was less conflict than in normal marriages. What is not clear from the research is whether there are differences when it is the man who is infertile.

The wider social context

The secrecy and shame that often surround infertility and infertility treatment can lead to problems. This is illustrated by the case of an artificial donor insemination couple who experienced the sudden infant death of their child [18]. The couple was assessed at 6 months and 6 years after the incident. Bereavement was mixed with feelings of anger and shame associated with male infertility, which made it impossible for the couple to communicate their feelings to each other or to friends and relations. At 6 years, the couple planned to divorce. Men who do not communicate their infertility problem to others beyond the marital relationship have a lower level of well-being compared with those who do talk about it [19].

Coping and infertility

Approach-oriented (problem-focused) coping can predict decreased distress among couples receiving insemination treatment [20]. Other studies have found differences between the coping styles of men and women [21]. Men who coped well tended to use a range of coping styles, including active-confronting (eg, showing feelings, asking others for advice), passive-avoidance (eg, hoping for a miracle, believing that the only thing to do is wait), and meaning-based coping (eg, thinking about infertility in a positive light, believing there is a meaning). Women used an active-confronting coping style and a secrecy communication strategy that involves discussing the problem with others but not telling their partner. Less effective coping was observed in men and women using an active-avoidance coping strategy (eg, avoiding being with pregnant women and children).

An analysis of the association between coping with infertility and occupational social class found that women from lower social classes and men from the middle social classes used more active-confronting coping [16]. Women from lower social classes also used significantly more meaning-based coping. Men and women from lower social classes used more passive-avoidant coping and less active avoidant coping. The results suggest that elements of coping may be learned from one's social network and reference group.

Couples adjust more effectively when they use appraisal-oriented coping as opposed to avoidant coping [20,22]. To complicate this further, there is evidence that coping styles are cyclical and that individuals and couples sometimes prefer an active cognitive processing style where problems are discussed and addressed and at other times prefer a more avoidant or suppressed style where the problems are not talked about [23]. This approach can be beneficial for couples when their coping cycles match, but it may create problems if they do not. Infertile couples who reflect on their experiences (ie, use cognitive processing) are more likely to experience a positive psychosocial outcome [24] and experience emotional support [25].

Kowalcek and colleagues [26] found sex differences in emotional demand during the course of an assisted reproductive treatment cycle for male subfertility. They measured emotional demand using a questionnaire and found that it was at its highest during follicular puncture and after pregnancy testing. Keeping a diary helped the patients begin to cope with the diagnosis of infertility, providing the scope to admit emotional demands, hurt self-esteem, feelings of mourning and depression, and aggression.

Stress as cause of infertility

Mental stress can affect semen quality and should be taken into account when assessing men for infertility [27]. Spermatozoa concentrations, motility index, and percentage of progressive motility decrease under examination stress [28]. Other studies have found an association between high stress levels and subfertility in a sample of men [29]. Mental stress may cause oxidative stress in semen, which can result in male subfertility [28,30,31] and in a decrease in the proportion of sperm that are progressively or rapidly motile. Animal data support the theory that environmental causes of stress may induce changes in male fertility [32]. Another possible effect of stress is highlighted by a significant change in the sex ratio observed in Slovenia 9 months after the brief war of 1991 [33]. The same researchers also found that stress factors should be taken into account in the management of infertile couples, particularly in relation to depression and the reaction to stress [34].

There has been limited research examining the role of occupational stress and infertility. Although the evidence for women is weak [35], there is evidence that for men infertility is associated with industry and construction jobs and with job burnout [36]. Male reproductive function is sensitive to environmental factors such as weight loss, diet, exercise, disease, and psychologic stress [37]. Although the exact mechanisms of action of many factors are poorly understood, some interesting connections are discussed in the article by Dobs elsewhere in this issue.

Psychologic treatment can contribute to the reduction of stress in couples who are attempting in vitro fertilization treatment, but this rarely increases the probability of pregnancy [38]. Stress may not be a key factor for many infertile couples, although it might be for a subpopulation. The problems relating to infertility do not only concern stress and coping. Several studies have found higher levels of alexithymia and somatization in infertile men [39].

Hypospadias

Hypospadias is a disease found in boys who, at birth, have an ectopic opening of the urethral meatus on the penis or scrotum, an abnormal distribution of the penile skin, and occasionally abnormal curvature of the penis. Unlike infertility, this entity is included in this article as an example of a visible disorder and is part of a growing body of psychologic literature on the impact of disfigurement [40]. The prevalence of hypospadias in the United States doubled between 1970 and 1990 [41], suggesting a possible environmental cause. A recent review outlined a range of psychosocial issues relating to the disorder but did not provide concrete conclusions or recommendations for practice [42]. A study of boys who had hypospadias showed that they had more behavioral problems and weaker social skills than boys without this problem [43]. This study was replicated with a larger sample (175 children, aged 6–10 years). Boys who had hypospadias had problems with social competency and were less likely to externalize their problems. Poor cosmetic appearance of the genitals was related to worse school performance [44].

Another study found that boys who have hypospadias were more inhibited than control subjects in initiating sexual contacts, and fear of sexual contact increased with age [45]. The same team found that boys who had hypospadias were more inhibited concerning nudity than normal control subjects [46]. These problems persist into adulthood. Adult men operated on for hypospadias were shyer and more socially isolated and had lower self-esteem, a decreased capacity for relationships, and poorer occupations [47]. They were more inhibited in seeking sexual contacts and had a more negative appraisal of their genitals, and a lower proportion reported full sexual intercourse than control subjects [48].

Practical difficulties with sex may compound psychosocial problems. In one study, 24% of patients who had hypospadias experienced erection problems, compared with 7% of circumcised patients. Furthermore, 13% of the patients who had hypospadias had ejaculatory problems [49]. Patients also report other sexual relationship difficulties relating to dissatisfaction or pain [47,49].

The research available on men operated on as adults provides little information about psychosocial issues, apart from one observation that 40% of patients did not have sexual relations before surgery [50]. It is feasible to assume that shyness and social embarrassment were the cause. Operations had been delayed for a number of reasons, including cultural, religious, and sociodemographic reasons.

Men who have hypospadias, even after treatment that has medical and cosmetic benefits, may still experience problems with developing relationships. This fear of being seen as different, which is common among adolescents, can seriously interfere with their lives and demonstrates the importance of early treatment that is effective and cosmetically acceptable. Psychologic work into disfigurement suggests that personal perceptions of disfigurement predict a range of psychosocial problems. It is the perception that matters rather than the disfigurement per se [40].

The only observation of untreated men with hypospadias showed that they had greater difficulty in initiating sexual contact than those who had been operated on, although the conclusions are tentative and hampered by the small study size [48].

Erectile dysfunction

ED is a cause and a consequence of psychologic distress. Much of the research focusing on the risk factors for ED does not adequately consider the psychosocial variables that can contribute to the disorder, although there is evidence that stress and anxiety are associated with ED [51–53]. There are exceptions. One study that focused on risk factors such as age and specific urologic and nonurologic somatic conditions recognized that knowing about patient-reported psychologic or relationship stress was useful in determining the risk of ED [54,55]. There is also limited research on the role of psychologic and interpersonal factors with regard to the treatment of ED [56]. For ED, there is a clear association between the social (relationship), the psychologic (stress and anxiety), and the biologic factors that can interact to negatively affect sexual functioning [54]. Furthermore, impotence is a common symptom of most major diseases, and male physiology is sensitive to general physical health and to environmental and psychologic stressors [57].

As men age, they are increasingly likely to experience ED [58] and concomitant psychosexual problems. Up to 50% of men over 40 years of age experience at least some level of ED, and the incidence increases to 65% or more for men over 70 years of age [58]. Antidepressants can cause ED; if the physician prescribes them for the psychosocial problems arising from ED, the problem can be exacerbated [59,60].

The treatment for ED changed fundamentally with the introduction of sildenafil, which means that men often no longer have to resort to more invasive or less effective regimens [61]. When sildenafil works, it improves well-being. Men who are not successfully treated may experience an exacerbation of the psychosocial problems and a confirmation of a lack of self-worth [61]. For this reason, it is important that a person prescribed sildenafil be informed of the potential risk for the drug not being successful, and patient should be followed to determine whether there have been detrimental psychologic effects.

Psychologic treatment and counseling

There has been limited work regarding the efficacy of psychosocial interventions for men who have andrologic disorders. One study investigated the effectiveness of support counseling by the embryologist acting as counselor during assisted reproduction procedures to determine whether people receiving such support would have more effective coping mechanisms [62]. Patients in the counseling group experienced a significant reduction in anxiety levels after the counseling intervention, along with increased use of problem-focused coping. The study did not use blinded procedures, and the counseling was not performed by a trained counselor.

Discussion

Studies examining the psychosocial impact of andrologic diseases are relatively rare, and the results are contradictory. Difficulties in obtaining and retaining suitable sample sizes and response rates to questionnaires and the frequently found lack of a control group mean that conclusions must be tentative. One of the reasons for the low response rates may be that of embarrassment on the part of patients, a psychosocial problem in itself.

This article has highlighted some of the key psychosocial factors that affect andrologic diseases. Our focus illustrates problems associated with physical appearance (hypospadias, ED) and perceptions (infertility, hypospadia, and ED). It is likely that these problems occur across the full range of andrologic diseases. For instance, serious forms of alopecia are associated with serious psychosocial problems and can seriously damage or destroy relationships [63]. Problems may not stem from the medical disorder itself but from the effect it has on self-perception and the perceptions of their spouses, family, and friends.

The psychosocial consequences of andrologic disease should be incorporated into a single model accounting for all disorders, taking into account the key areas of stress (as etiologic factor and consequence), coping (individual differences), and psychosocial disorders such as anxiety and depression. Such a model must focus on the sexes individually. It must include the importance of the development of relationships (for disorders present at birth or as a child) and the sustainability of relationships (for disorders that may emerge once a relationship has started). For visible and invisible disorders, men are likely to experience consequences relating to the construction of self and identity [64], particularly with regard to the notion of masculinity and the damage to conceptions of masculinity that are perceived by men and women.

Many infertile couples cope well with infertility, and particular coping styles, active cognitive processing, and discussion are effective at reducing the distress caused by infertility. Psychologic therapy should encourage such coping styles. The majority of people rarely use positive styles [23], and there are difficulties encouraging such an approach for many couples. This may affect the suitability of people receiving infertility treatment. Linking the treatment to effective psychosocial coping may be one way forward. It may assist in cases where man male is subfertile and where problems may be associated with environmental stress. Using cognitive processing techniques may reduce such stress and enhance the chances of pregnancy. Further research may highlight particular subgroups for whom such an approach may be beneficial. Cyclical coping in couples dealing with infertility also deserves a closer look. If one partner is using active styles and the other is using passive styles, the result may be difficulties in adjusting as a couple to the situation.

The area of individual differences is rarely explored. Most research considers groups. Little is understood about the individual factors that determine whether someone experiences a negative reaction to an andrologic disease, and there are implications for treatment. We know that men who have more confident and outgoing coping styles deal more effectively with disease in general and with regard to androgenic diseases. Personality factors relate to coping styles, but personality is difficult to change. Eysenck [65] and Cloninger [66] have provided detailed theories of the biologic basis of personality. The positive coping literature regarding infertility may relate more to a biased sample than objective truth because it is likely that only men who have confidence and a positive coping style enter infertility treatment. This is also likely to be associated with wealth and with social class, so the samples used may not reflect what many infertile couples are experiencing.

Clinicians should take into account the psychosocial impact of the disease and the treatment. The physician should account for the perspective of the person who may undergo a course of treatment and the longer-term consequences for the individual and for any relevant partner. Whatever the disease, if a person is aware that treatment is likely to be ineffective or will take a long time, be expensive, or be painful, there are likely to be psychologic consequences. Psychosocial treatment should take account of these factors and should be coordinated with medical treatment where appropriate. There should be no separation of medical and psychosocial interventions for the treatment of andrologic disease.

References

[1] Alexander NJ. Andrology in the year 2000. Schaumberg (IL): the American Society of Andrology, Inc.; 1980.

[2] Jones F, Bright J, Clow A. Stress: myth, theory and research. Upper Saddle River (NJ): Prentice Hall; 2001.

[3] Lazarus RS. Coping theory and research: past, present, and future. Psychosom Med 1993; 55(3):234–47.

[4] Ivancevich JM, Matteson MT. Stress and work: a managerial perspective. Glenview (IL): Scott, Foresman; 1980.

[5] Holmes DS. Abnormal psychology. New York: Longman; 1997.

[6] Lucas RE, Gohm CL. Age and sex differences in subjective well-being across cultures. In: Diener E, Suh EM, editors. Culture and subjective well-being. Cambridge (MA): Bradford; 2000. p. 291–318.

[7] Fuhrer R, Stansfeld SA, Chemali J, et al. Gender, social relations and mental health: prospective findings from an occupational cohort (Whitehall II study). Soc Sci Med 1999; 48(1):77–87.

[8] Ogden J. Health psychology: a textbook. Buckingham (UK): Open University Press; 1996.

[9] Gross JJ, Levenson RW. Hiding feelings: the acute effects of inhibiting negative and positive emotion. J Abnorm Psychol 1997;106(1):95–103.

[10] Myers LB. Identifying repressors: a methodological issue for health psychology. Psychology and Health 2000;15:205–14.

[11] Cousineau TM, Green TC, Corsini EA, et al. Development and validation of the infertility self-efficacy scale. Fertil Steril 2006;85(6):1684–96.

[12] Prins GS, Bremner W. The 25th volume: President's message: andrology in the 20th century: a commentary on our progress during the past 25 years. J Androl 2004;25(4):435–40.

[13] Greil AL. Infertility and psychological distress: a critical review of the literature. Soc Sci Med 1997;45(11):1679–704.

[14] Greil AL, Leitko TA, Porter KL. Infertility: his and hers. Gend Soc 1988;2(2):172–99.

[15] Peterson BD. Examining the congruence between couples' perceived infertility-related stress and its relationship to depression and marital adjustment in infertile men and women. Blacksburg (VA): Virginia Polytechnic Institute and State University; 2000.

[16] Schmidt L, Holstein B, Christensen U, et al. Does infertility cause marital benefit? An epidemiological study of 2250 women and men in fertility treatment. Patient Educ Couns 2005; 59(3):244–51.

[17] Weiss P, Mateju L, Urbanek V. Personality and characteristics of couples in infertile marriage. Ceska Gynekol 2004;69(1):42–7.

[18] Conrad R, Schilling G, Liedtke R. Parental coping with sudden infant death after donor insemination: case report. Hum Reprod 2005;20(4):1053–6.

[19] van Balen F, Trimbos-Kemper TC. Factors influencing the well-being of long-term infertile couples. J Psychosom Obstet Gynaecol 1994;15(3):157–64.

[20] Berghuis JP, Stanton AL. Adjustment to a dyadic stressor: a longitudinal study of coping and depressive symptoms in infertile couples over an insemination attempt. J Consult Clin Psychol 2002;70(2):433–8.

[21] Schmidt L, Christensen U, Holstein BE. The social epidemiology of coping with infertility. Hum Reprod 2005;20(4):1044–52.

[22] Litt MD, Tennen H, Affleck G, et al. Coping and cognitive factors in adaptation to in vitro fertilization failure. J Behav Med 1992;15(2):171–87.

[23] Horowitz MJ. Stress response syndromes. 2nd editon. Northvale (NJ): J. Aronson; 1986.

[24] Cudmore L. Becoming parents in the context of loss. Sexual and Relationship Therapy 2005; 20(3):299–308.

[25] Abbey A, Andrews FM, Halman LJ. Provision and receipt of social support and disregard: what is their impact on the marital life quality of infertile and fertile couples? J Pers Soc Psychol 1995;68(3):455–69.

[26] Kowalcek IWJ, Lauter MB, Diedrich K. Strain and gender-specific coping with a fertility treatment cycle for male subfertility. Gynakol Prax 2003;27(1):55–65.

[27] Schneid-Kofman N, Sheiner E. Does stress effect male infertility?–a debate. Med Sci Monit 2005;11(8):SR11–3.

[28] Eskiocak S, Gozen AS, Kilic AS, et al. Association between mental stress & some antioxidant enzymes of seminal plasma. Indian J Med Res 2005;122(6):491–6.

[29] Harth W, Linse R. Male fertility: endocrine stress parameters and coping. Dermatology and Psychosomatics/Dermatologie und Psychosomatik 2004;5(1):22–9.

[30] Eskiocak S, Gozen AS, Taskiran A, et al. Effect of psychological stress on the L-arginine-nitric oxide pathway and semen quality. Braz J Med Biol Res 2006;39:581–8.

[31] Eskiocak S, Gozen AS, Yapar SB, et al. Glutathione and free sulphydryl content of seminal plasma in healthy medical students during and after exam stress. Hum Reprod 2005;20(9): 2595–600.

[32] Mor I, Grisaru D, Titelbaum L, et al. Modified testicular expression of stress-associated "read-through" acetylcholinesterase predicts male infertility. FASEB Journal 2001;15(11):2039–41.

[33] Zorn B, Sucur V, Stare J, et al. Decline in sex ratio at birth after 10-day war in Slovenia. Hum Reprod 2002;17(12):3173–7.

[34] Zorn B, Virant-Klun I, Kolbezen M, et al. Facteurs de stress psychologique et qualité du sperme dans une population de 450 hommes infertiles slovènes. Andrologie 2001;11:76–85.

[35] Sheiner E, Sheiner EK, Potashnik G, et al. The relationship between occupational stress and female fertility. Occupational Medicine (London) 2003;53:265–9.

[36] Sheiner EK, Sheiner E, Carel R, et al. potential association between male infertility and occupational psychological stress. J Occup Environ Med 2002;44(12):1093–9.

[37] Campbell BC, Leslie PW. Reproductive ecology of human males. Yearb Phys Anthropol 1995;21:1–26.

[38] Wischmann T. [Psychosocial aspects of fertility disorders]. Urologe A 2005;44(2):185–94 [quiz: 195] [in German].

[39] Conrad R, Schilling G, Hagemann T, et al. Somatization and alexithymia in male infertility: a replication study. Hautarzt 2003;54(6):530–5.

[40] Rumsey N, Harcourt D. The psychology of appearance. Maidenhead: Open University Press; 2005.

[41] Paulozzi LJ. International trends in rates of hypospadias and cryptorchidism. Environ Health Perspect 1999;107(4):297–302.

[42] Mieusset R, Soulie M. Hypospadias: psychosocial, sexual, and reproductive consequences in adult life. © Copyright 2005 by the American Society of Andrology, Inc.; 2005.

[43] Sandberg DE, Meyer-Bahlburg HF, Aranoff GS, et al. Boys with hypospadias: a survey of behavioral difficulties. J Pediatr Psychol 1989;14:491–514.

[44] Sandberg DE, Meyer-Bahlburg HFL, Hensle TW, et al. Psychosocial adaptation of middle childhood boys with hypospadias after genital surgery. J Pediatr Psychol 2001;26(8): 465–75.

[45] Mureau MA, Slijper FM, Slob AK, et al. Psychosocial functioning of children, adolescents, and adults following hypospadias surgery: a comparative study. J Pediatr Psychol 1997; 22(3):371–87.

[46] Mureau MAM, Slijper FME, Slob AK, et al. Satisfaction with penile appearance after hypospadias surgery: the patient and surgeon view. J Urol 1996;155(2):703–6.

[47] Berg R, Berg G, Edman G, et al. Androgens and personality in normal men and men operated for hypospadias in childhood. Acta Psychiatr Scand 1983;68(3):167–77.

[48] Mondaini N, Ponchietti R, Bonaf M, et al. Hypospadias: incidence and effects on psychosexual development as evaluated with the minnesota multiphasic personality inventory test in a sample of 11,649 young Italian men. Urol Int 2002;68(2):81–5.

[49] Aho MO, Tammela OK, Somppi EM, et al. Sexual and social life of men operated in childhood for hypospadias and phimosis: a comparative study. Eur Urol 2000;37(1):95–100 [discussion: 101].

[50] Moudouni S, Tazi K, Nouri M, et al. [Hypospadias in adults]. Prog Urol 2001;11(4):667–9.

[51] Corona G, Mannucci E, Petrone L, et al. Psycho-biological correlates of hypoactive sexual desire in patients with erectile dysfunction. Int J Impot Res 2004;16:275–81.

[52] Štulhofer A, Bajic Ž. Prevalence of erectile and ejaculatory difficulties among men in Croatia. Croat Med J 2006;47:114–24.

[53] Gheiler J, Sharpe I. Improving the quality of life of erectile dysfunction (ED) patients through penile implants. Ethn Dis 2005;15(3 Suppl 4):41–2.

[54] Rowland DL, Thornton JA, Burnett AL. Recognizing the risk of erectile dysfunction in a urology clinic practice. BJU Int 2005;95(7):1034–8.

[55] Ponholzer A, Temml C, Mock K, et al. Prevalence and risk factors for erectile dysfunction in 2869 men using a validated questionnaire. Eur Urol 2005;47(1):80–5.

[56] Rosen R, Janssen E, Wiegel M, et al. Psychological and interpersonal correlates in men with erectile dysfunction and their partners: a pilot study of treatment outcome with sildenafil. J Sex Marital Ther 2006;32(3):215–34.

[57] Cellerino A, Jannini EA. Why humans need type 5 phosphodiesterase inhibitors. Int J Androl 2005;28:14–7.

[58] Johannes CB, Araujo AB, Feldman HA, et al. Incidence of erectile dysfunction in men 40 to 69 years old: longitudinal results from the Massachusetts Male Aging Study. J Urol 2000; 163(2):460–3.

[59] Rosen RC, Lane RM, Menza M. Effects of SSRIs on sexual function: a critical review. J Clin Psychopharmacol 1999;19(1):67–85.

[60] Mrcpsych MJT, Mrcpsych LR, Frcpsych K, et al. Strategies for managing antidepressant-induced sexual dysfunction: systematic review of randomised controlled trials. J Affect Disord 2005;88:241–54.

[61] Tomlinson J, Wright D. Impact of erectile dysfunction and its subsequent treatment with sildenafil: qualitative study. Br Med J 2004;328(7447):1037–9.

[62] van Zyl C, van Dyk AC, Niemandt C. The embryologist as counsellor during assisted reproduction procedures. Reprod BioMed Online 2005;11(5):545–51.

[63] Hunt N, McHale S. The psychological impact of alopecia. BMJ 2005;331(7522):951–3.

[64] Leary MR, Tangney JP. The self as an organizing construct in the behavioral and social sciences. Handbook of self and identity. London: Guilford Press; 2005. p. 3–14.

[65] Eysenck HJ. The structure of human personality. Methuen; 1970.

[66] Cloninger CR. The genetics and psychobiology of the seven-factor model of personality. In: Silk KR, editor. Biology of personality disorders. Washington DC: American Psychiatric Press; 1998. p. 63–92.

ELSEVIER
SAUNDERS

Endocrinol Metab Clin N Am
36 (2007) 533–552

ENDOCRINOLOGY
AND METABOLISM
CLINICS
OF NORTH AMERICA

Dietary Supplements and Nutraceuticals in the Management of Andrologic Disorders

Ronald Tamler, MD, PhD, MBA, CNSP*,
Jeffrey I. Mechanick, MD, FACP, FACE, FACN

*Division of Endocrinology, Diabetes and Bone Disease, Mount Sinai School of Medicine,
1 Gustave L. Levy Place, Box 1055, New York, NY 10029, USA*

Men have relied on dietary aides to alleviate andrologic ailments for centuries and across cultures: starfish were sold as aphrodisiacs on the streets of ancient Rome, potable gold was heralded as the path to eternal youth and sexual prowess in medieval times, and even the biblical King David may have sought remedies for impotence [1].

In spite of the availability of more evidence-based therapeutics, approximately $21 billion were spent in 1997 out of pocket in the United States for alternative care [2]. Sales of dietary supplements and nutraceuticals (DS/N) in particular have increased from $9 billion in 1994 to $ 16 billion in 2000. This increase may be connected to the Dietary Supplement Health and Education Act (DSHEA), which was passed by the US Congress in 1994 [3,4]. It defined dietary supplements and resulted in freely traded preparations not limited to their commonly perceived nutritional benefits. Nutraceuticals have been defined as "dietary supplements that contain a concentrated form of a presumed bioactive substance originally derived from a food, but now present in a non-food matrix, and used to enhance health in dosages exceeding those obtainable from normal foods" [5].

A survey of more than 60,000 Americans between 50 and 76 years showed that approximately 30% of all men were using at least one dietary supplement (as opposed to 40% of all women surveyed). Whereas the most popular agents, glucosamine and chondroitin, relate to joint problems, andrologic remedies like saw palmetto, ginkgo, ginseng, and DHEA follow closely [6]. Another survey of over 12,000 men in a prostate cancer screening

* Corresponding author.
E-mail address: ronald.tamler@mssm.edu (R. Tamler).

0889-8529/07/$ - see front matter © 2007 Published by Elsevier Inc.
doi:10.1016/j.ecl.2007.03.005

clinic revealed that 21% of participants were using herbal supplements, but only 10% were using prescription medications for lower urinary tract symptoms (LUTS) [7]. The impact on endocrinologists' practices has become so significant that the American Association of Clinical Endocrinologists (AACE) established guidelines for the use of dietary supplements and nutraceuticals [8].

This review will focus on the use of DS/N and associated problems in the following andrologic areas: erectile dysfunction (ED), decreased libido, and prostate health. The aim is to present the evidence in humans for the most popular and best-studied agents.

Common problems

Three problems can occur when dealing with dietary supplements and nutraceuticals.

First, the ingredients on the label may not be present in the indicated dosage, or may even be completely absent. This was the case in a US Food and Drug Administration (FDA) study that found little or no yohimbine in most of the 18 supplements tested [9]. DHEA concentrations in supplements were determined at 0% to 150% of the amount indicated on the package [10]. Of 13 tested isoflavone preparations, 9 contained less than 90% of the advertised amount [11], and wide fluctuations were found in the concentration of ginseng products [12], saw palmetto, lycopene, selenium, and vitamin E [13].

Second, the supplement can be laced with impurities, such as undisclosed active pharmacologic agents requiring a prescription or toxic contaminants [14]. For instance, of seven tested dietary supplements for ED, two contained significant amounts of the phosphodiesterase (PDE)-5 inhibitors sildenafil and tadalafil [15]. The FDA issued a statement in July of 2006 in which it warned of seven dietary supplements illegally containing PDE-inhibitors [16]. While aflatoxin, yeast, and mold have been found in ginseng preparations [17–19], other DS/N were found to contain lead, methomyl, and steroids [19–22]. In fact, one large study investigating 103 supplements found high amounts of an anabolic steroid in 4 preparations, and compounds not disclosed by the manufacturer in 14 prohormone products [23].

Finally, many manufacturers of DS/N make inappropriate claims not permitted under DSHEA. In a large Internet survey, more than 50% of Web sites selling DS/N illegally made specific health claims or omitted the federal disclaimer [24]. In spite of quality initiatives, these issues continue to complicate the safe prescribing of DS/N [25].

ED and decreased libido

From 10 to 30 million American men suffer from ED [26,27], and with a population that is aging and increasingly suffering from risk factors such as hypertension, diabetes, and obesity, the prevalence is bound to increase [28]. Although ED and decreased libido are different entities that do not necessarily overlap, many DS/N claim to improve both conditions. Unfortunately, the quality of many studies is hampered by small sample sizes, inappropriate or poorly controlled study designs, and a significant placebo effect [29,30]. One should keep in mind that 25% to 41% of men experience improved erections with placebo in trials of PDE-5 inhibitors [31,32]. This fact puts claims of success for many agents studied in an uncontrolled setting into perspective.

Several agents discussed here not only have purported benefits on erectile function, but also on the cardiovascular system in general. This mirrors recent findings that erectile function and cardiovascular health are not only affected by the same risk factors, but that impotence is frequently a precursor of cardiovascular disease [33].

DHEA

Dehydroepiandrosterone (DHEA) is a mildly androgenic prohormone stemming from the adrenal gland that can be converted to estrogens at the target tissue level [34]. Low levels of DHEA have been associated with Alzheimer disease, depression, diabetes mellitus, and normal aging [35]. It is often marketed as an "anti-aging hormone" [36]. Levels of DHEA and its sulfate metabolite correlate strongly with erectile function [37–39].

Encouraged by a successful controlled study of DHEA, 50 mg orally daily, versus placebo over 6 months in 40 Austrian men with low DHEA levels and erectile dysfunction [40], a larger uncontrolled trial by the same group yielded significant improvements in patients with ED due to hypertension or nonorganic reasons, but not in patients with diabetes or neurologic disease [41].

In another uncontrolled trial of DHEA given to aging men with partial androgen deficiency, there was subjective improvement in mood, fatigue, and joint pain [42].

However, DHEA should be used with caution in men undergoing androgen deprivation therapy, as it may significantly elevate levels of testosterone or IGF-1 in this group of patients [43,44]. It should also be noted that protodioscin, which is extracted from *Tribulus terrestris* and is frequently advertised as plant-derived DHEA, in fact does not increase DHEA levels unless chemically altered [45], and that the plant's protodioscin contents depend on the soil it grows in [46].

Androstenedione is another preandrogen that can be converted to testosterone and is produced in the testicles and the adrenals [47]. Plant-derived androstenedione was advertised to promote muscle growth, improve muscular strength, reduce fat, improve libido and erectile function, and slow aging [48–50], but some studies did not show any effect on muscle strength [51] or testosterone levels. Instead, an increase in estrogen levels was seen [49].

Whereas 100 mg daily had no effect, oral doses of 300 mg daily were shown to increase testosterone levels in one study and to more than double estradiol levels [52,53] in young men. Only the estradiol effect has been demonstrated in middle-aged men [54]. Other herbal ingredients do not prevent the significant metabolization to estradiol [55]. Although the FDA took androstenedione off the market in 2004 [56], it continues to be popular with athletes [57,58]. Androstenedione probably has no benefit for prostate health, libido, or erectile function.

L-arginine

Nitric oxide plays a central role in mediating an erection through vasorelaxation, by way of increased levels of cyclic guanosine monophosphate and decreased calcium levels in vascular smooth muscle cells [59]. The amino acid L-arginine acts as an NO donor for neuronal and endothelial NO synthase [60] and has been shown to increase NO production when consumed in supraphysiologic doses of more than 3 g per day. Although a small uncontrolled trial over 2 weeks showed improved erectile function in 40% of participants [61], 31% of men in a controlled study over 6 weeks felt an improvement [62]. However, a small controlled crossover trial with just 1.5 g L-arginine per day did not show any benefits over placebo [63]. To boost NO levels, L-arginine is often combined with the NO synthase stimulant pygnogenol, a pine bark derivative [64]. Only one study investigated this combined approach in humans; it showed improved erectile function in 92% of the subjects [65].

Yohimbine

Yohimbine is an extract from the bark of the Yohim tree. As a pharmacological agent, this centrally active alpha-2 antagonist has been prescribed for over 70 years and was a popular choice for ED before the advent of PDE-5 inhibitors [66]. A meta-analysis of seven randomized controlled trials found that, while yohimbine was in general effective and inexpensive when treating ED, it was particularly successful in patients with nonorganic ED [67,68]. Two of the largest trials found doses of 5.4 mg three times a day to 10.8 mg four times a day to improve ED in 34% to 42% of the patients [69]. One more recent trial in 18 men that appeared after the meta-analysis found that yohimbine was effective in men with nonsevere ED [70]. No new trials with yohimbine alone have been published in the past 5 years, but combinations with L-arginine have yielded favorable results [71,72]. It should be noted that yohimbine can have a multitude of side effects, such as palpitations, anxiety, fine tremor, hypertension, and arterial vasoconstriction [73] and that yohimbine was placed on the "unsafe herb" list by the FDA in 1997. Because of the aforementioned variability of the ingredient in over-the-counter (OTC) preparations, the prescription version should be used.

Ginkgo biloba

Although ginkgo has been used frequently to improve cerebrovascular perfusion in patients with dementia, its central effects have also been postulated to ameliorate antidepressant-induced ED. A single study claiming significant improvements in men experiencing ED with selective serotonin reuptake inhibitors (SSRIs) [74] was not only uncontrolled, but also yielded multiple discrepancies on closer analysis [75]. Two other studies in patients taking SSRIs did not demonstrate any significant improvement over placebo [76,77]. In addition to the discouraging data on gingko, its many interactions with prescription drugs, potentially leading to seizures and increased bleeding time, need to be taken into account [78–81].

Ginseng

Of the different ginseng varieties (Brazilian, Indian, Siberian, Asian, North American) that are frequently found in dietary supplements in the United States and are taken regularly by up to 4.5% of the US population, it is Korean Red Ginseng (also called Panax ginseng) that has been most extensively studied in relation to ED. Animal models suggest that the saponin glycosides in Panax ginseng induce penile vasorelaxation through NO synthase induction [82], cavernosal NO release, and intracellular calcium decrease [83,84], but it has also been described as a scavenger of free radicals [85] and, surprisingly, nitric oxide itself [86]. One three-way trial of Panax ginseng versus trazodone and placebo demonstrated improved erectile function in 60% of all subjects in the ginseng group, as opposed to 30% in the two other groups [87]. A small crossover study over 8 weeks demonstrated encouraging results in 60% of participants [88] as measured by International Index for Erectile Function and penile blood flow. Patients with a history of prostatectomy, neurological damage, or possible drug-induced ED were excluded. Remarkably, these two studies alone (combined n = 135) managed to prompt a recommendation to treat ED with ginseng from the *Journal of Family Practice,* citing its safety and low cost (6 cents per 500-mg pill) [89].

Propionyl-L-carnitine and acetyl-L-carnitine

The purported mechanism of action of propionyl-L-carnitine (PLC) and acetyl-L-carnitine (ALC) is prostaglandin-induced vasorelaxation of arterioles [90]. In a three-way trial, a combination of these agents proved to raise mood and libido as well as oral testosterone undecanoate and fared significantly better than placebo [91]. Seventy percent of diabetic patients with ED receiving a combination of sildenafil and PLC experienced significant improvements in erectile function as opposed to 34% with sildenafil alone [92]. A three-way trial of placebo, sildenafil alone, and a combination of ALC and PLC with sildenafil in patients after radical prostatectomy showed improved erections by questionnaire in more than 85% of patients in the combined group. This result was corroborated by a positive intracavernous injection test after the combined therapy [93].

Prostate health

A Canadian survey among over 1000 men newly diagnosed with prostate cancer found that 39% of responders were using alternative therapies, particularly DS/N [94]. A similar study in the United States showed that of over 2500 men with prostate cancer surveyed, about one third were using complementary or alternative medicine [95]. A smaller survey of men whose brothers had been diagnosed with prostate cancer revealed that 55% of responders were using complementary medicine [7]. The most popular agents in these surveys were saw palmetto and vitamin E.

Saw palmetto

The popularity of saw palmetto in the management of benign prostate hyperplasia (BPH) has made it the most extensively investigated dietary supplement in the urologic literature. Saw palmetto is the extract of the American dwarf palm tree; a standardized lipid extract is marketed as permixon. Its active ingredient and mechanism of action on the prostate remain unknown. According to the more than 30,000 responders to the National Health Interview Survey (NHIS), saw palmetto was used among 1.1% of the adult male population, which can be extrapolated to over 2 million men in the United States alone [96].

This practice was supported by a large number of studies showing some improvement with saw palmetto extract in patients with BPH. A French study of more than 1000 patients over 6 months showed that both permixon and finasteride reduced LUTS-related symptoms in two thirds of the subjects. In contrast to finasteride, phytotherapy fared well with regard to sexual side effects but did not reduce prostate size or prostate-specific antigen (PSA) values [97]. A meta-analysis of 14 randomized controlled trial (RCT)s brought to light the immense variability in sample size and study quality, but still postulated beneficial effects of permixon on nocturia and peak flow [98]. In one of the better studies, Gerber and colleagues [99] showed symptomatic improvement, but no change in flow rate when compared with placebo. Summarizing the common perception, a recent review highlighted the safety and efficacy of saw palmetto for BPH [100].

However, saw palmetto has garnered less enthusiasm after a rigorous and well-published RCT in 225 men with BPH found no difference in symptoms or objective measures when compared with placebo [101] over 1 year.

Antioxidants

Epidemiologic studies have linked decreased rates of prostate cancer in some regions of the world to the ingestion of fruit and vegetables rich in antioxidants (reviewed by Chan and colleagues [102]). The concept is that oxidative stress can facilitate mutations leading to cancer, and that antioxidants help prevent that development by restoring the balance with pro-oxidant compounds [103,104].

Lycopene, a carotenoid typically found in tomatoes, is known as one of the most effective antioxidants in our diet [105] and has relatively high concentrations in prostate tissue [106]. Lycopene ingestion, which in the United States mainly occurs through tomato sauce, and high plasma lycopene levels have been connected in multiple studies to significant reductions on the order of 25% to 80% in the incidence of prostate cancer [107–113]. A meta-analysis of 21 studies also suggested decreased incidence of prostate cancer in subjects eating more tomatoes, and even showed this effect to be more pronounced with cooked tomatoes [114]. Negative studies [115–118] have been criticized as being underpowered or containing insufficient lycopene in the subjects' diet [108]. In response, a recently published multicentric observational study of almost 30,000 men found no association between lycopene intake and prostate cancer risk [119].

The evidence for other carotenoids is not nearly as convincing. Vitamin A was shown to reduce the incidence of prostate cancer in men with low plasma levels of beta-carotene [120,121], but had the opposite effect in men with high plasma levels [122]. Overall, no solid correlation between beta-carotene intake and prostate cancer risk could be established.

Vitamin E (Tocopherol) also has significant antioxidant properties. Low levels of vitamin E have been found to correlate with increased incidence of prostate cancer [123–126]. The Alpha-Tocopherol Beta-Carotene (ATBC) cancer prevention trial, which had demonstrated no significant effect with beta-carotene in almost 30,000 smokers, showed 40% decreased incidence of prostate cancer with vitamin E supplementation [122]. This result was confirmed by observational studies around the globe [127–129] as well as data from smokers participating in the Health Professionals Follow-up Study (HPFS) [130]. However, the data in smaller studies that did not target smokers is mostly negative [131–134] and showed no effect on PSA or IGF-1 levels [135]. Lately, gamma-tocopherol, as opposed to the more common alpha-tocopherol, has been touted as effective in reducing the incidence of prostate cancer [136,137].

Selenium (Se) and Se-containing compounds such as the amino acid selenomethionine are also antioxidants commonly used in dietary supplements aiming to reduce the risk of prostate cancer by inducing apoptosis and preventing damage from free radicals [138–140]. Se has also been shown to be involved in the regulation of androgen and estrogen effects [141–143]. Low Se levels have been tied to higher rates of prostate cancer [144–148], although other studies could not confirm this observation [149–152]. The Nutritional Prevention of Cancer Trial, originally aimed at investigating melanoma, showed significant reductions in the incidence of prostate cancer with Se supplementation in patients with low baseline Se or PSA levels

Table 1
Select dietary supplements and nutraceuticals in andrologic diseases

Name, synonyms	Purported effects	Evidence
Damiana, damiane, oreganillo, the bourrique, Mexican damiana, Mexican holly, damiana de Guerrero	Increases libido, relieves depression	No studies in the modern literature
Quibracho bark, also called aspidosperma quebracho, aspidospermine, aspidospermatine, aspidosamine, quebrachine, hypoquebrachine	Vasodilation, smooth muscle relaxation	In vitro data show effects are related to yohimbe content [195]
Radix morindae	Improves erectile function	Animal data [196]
L-Methionine	Improves erectile function, free radical scavenger	2 studies in patients with AIDS-associated myelopathy [197,198]
Catuaba bark, trichilia catigua, meliaceae	Improves erectile function	No studies in the modern literature
Licorice	Aphrodisiac	No studies in the modern literature
Urtica dioica, stinging nettle	Alleviates BPH, LUTS	1 RCT with negative results
Radix Multiflori Polygoni	Delays aging, improves erectile function	No studies in the Western literature
GABA, gamma-aminobutyric acid	Improves erectile function	May actually worsen ED [199]
Rehmannia glutinosa	Replenishes vitality	No studies in the modern literature
Caladium seguinum	Improves erectile function	No studies in the modern literature
Policosanol, Octacosanol, sugar cane wax	Improved erectile function, lowers cholesterol	No data regarding erectile function
Quercetin, Pteleopsis suberosa	Flavonoid used in BPH and prostate cancer prevention	Animal and cell culture data on prostate cancer

Curcumin, pumpkin seeds	Polyphenol used in BPH and prostate cancer	Stops growth of prostate cancer cells in vitro [200]
Paullinia cupana, guarana	Improves erectile function	In vitro data [201]
Catuama, ginger, zingiber	Improves erectile function	No studies in the Western literature
Urtica dioria, stinging nettle	Alleviates BPH, LUTS	1 promising crossover RCT [202], 2 successful RCTs in combination with sabal extract [203,204], 1 negative study in combination with Pygium africanum [205]
Pygium africanum, African plum, Tadenan	Alleviates BPH, LUTS	No rigorous human trials, but analysis of 18 small RCTs somewhat promising [206]
South African star grass, Hypoxis rooperi, beta-sitosterol, Azuprostat, Harzol	Alleviates BPH, LUTS	Encouraging RCTs [206–208], but no long-term safety data
Secale cerale, rye pollen, Cernilton	Alleviates BPH, LUTS	Review of 2 RCTS and 2 uncontrolled studies mildly encouraging [209]

[153,154]. Se is frequently administered with other antioxidants: The Su. Vi.Max trial found a combination of vitamins C, E, beta-carotene, Se, and Zn to reduce the incidence of prostate cancer risk in patients with low or normal PSA, but to increase it if the PSA was elevated [155]. A study with a combination of vitamins C, E, Se, and co-enzyme Q 10 found no effect compared with placebo in men with diagnosed prostate cancer and rising PSA levels [156]. A large National Cancer Institute (NCI)-funded trial with a combination product of selenium and vitamin E is currently ongoing [157,158]; however, the choice of selenium agent in that study has been criticized, and Se has also been described as a pro-oxidant [159].

Polyphenols and flavonoids are antioxidants found in fruit, vegetables, red wine, and tea, and are often marketed as extracts of grape seed or green tea. While one study showed that alcohol consumption in general does not appear to affect prostate cancer risk [160], others did find an inverse correlation [161] or even increased risk [161,162]. A highly publicized retrospective study found 6% reduction of relative risk for every glass of red wine consumed per week [163], but a Canadian study found better results with beer [164].

Tea, particularly green tea, has been noted to decrease the risk of prostate cancer [164–169] and contains significant amounts of catechins, a subgroup of polyphenols with particularly strong antioxidant properties [170]. However, other studies did not find benefits for prostate health [171–173], and a study of prostate cancer patients at the Mayo Clinic showed that 69% experienced green tea toxicity [174]. An excellent overview is given by Lee and colleagues [175], who doubted the generalizability of a Chinese study with unusually spectacular results [166], as prostate cancer is rare in the studied population.

Pomegranate juice, which contains polyphenols such as elagic acid, gallotannins, and anthocyanins, is known to inhibit prostate cancer growth in vitro [176]. In a recently published rigorous trial, PSA doubling time in patients after radiation or surgery who drank 8 oz of pomegranate juice daily increased from 15 months at baseline to 54 months with treatment [177].

Soy contains isoflavones, of which genistein is the best studied, and affects sex steroid synthesis and action [178]. An inverse relation between soy consumption and prostate cancer risk has been observed [167,179–181], but one study was equivocal [182] and one showed increased risk of prostate cancer [183]. One small trial suggested decreased T and PSA levels with soy isoflavone supplementation in men with early prostate cancer [151], but another study in healthy men only showed a mild decline in PSA [184]. A good overview over the estrogenic mechanism of action and therapeutic prospects of genistein is given by McCarty [185].

Zinc

The use of zinc for prostate health is rather controversial [102,186,187]. Zinc is preferably accumulated in healthy prostate tissue, whereas malignant cells have particularly low zinc levels [188]. While some observations reported decreased incidence of prostate cancer with higher zinc intake [189,190], others showed no effect [127,191,192], or even increased risk [193,194]. The fact that men in the Health Professionals' Follow-up study who were taking more than 100 mg of zinc per day doubled their risk of prostate cancer [193] is particularly disconcerting.

An overview of other herbal supplements, for which less data are available and which are commonly used in combination preparations is given in Table 1 [195–209].

Summary

Dietary supplements and nutraceuticals are commonly used by men with ED, decreased libido, BPH, and concerns about developing prostate cancer. Many preparations do not contain the advertised dosages of the active ingredient or are contaminated. There is some evidence for the efficacy of pharmaceutical-grade yohimbine for ED. In contrast to ginkgo, Panax ginseng and L-arginine, particularly when combined with pycnogenol or yohimbine, may also improve ED. ALC and PLC have been used successfully as adjuncts to PDE-5 inhibitors. DHEA increases estrogen more than it does testosterone, and plant formulations must undergo lab processing to take effect. Saw palmetto is widely prescribed for BPH, but probably is not as effective as once thought. Antioxidants like lycopene, vitamin E, selenium, polyphenols, and flavonoids show promise in reducing the incidence of prostate cancer, and the results of larger studies will shed further light on their applicability. In summary, dietary supplements and nutraceuticals, particularly those addressing erectile function and libido, need to undergo rigorous testing before they can be wholeheartedly recommended.

References

[1] Shah J. Erectile dysfunction through the ages. BJU Int 2002;90(4):433–41.
[2] Eisenberg DM, et al. Trends in alternative medicine use in the United States, 1990–1997: results of a follow-up national survey. JAMA 1998;280(18):1569–75.
[3] Scally MC, Hodge A. Health supplement regulations and consumer protection rights. South Med J 2000;93(12):1230–2.
[4] Scally MC, Hodge A, Street C. Prescription for change: health supplement regulations and protecting the public interest. J Natl Med Assoc 2001;93(6):230–2.
[5] Zeisel SH. Regulation of "nutraceuticals." Science 1999;285(5435):1853–5.
[6] Gunther S, et al. Demographic and health-related correlates of herbal and specialty supplement use. J Am Diet Assoc 2004;104(1):27–34.
[7] Barqawi A, et al. Herbal and vitamin supplement use in a prostate cancer screening population. Urology 2004;63(2):288–92.
[8] American Association of Clinical Endocrinologists medical guidelines for the clinical use of dietary supplements and nutraceuticals. Endocr Pract 2003;9(5):417–70.

[9] Betz JM, White KD, der Marderosian AH. Gas chromatographic determination of yohimbine in commercial yohimbe products. J AOAC Int 1995;78(5):1189–94.

[10] Parasrampuria J, Schwartz K, Petesch R. Quality control of dehydroepiandrosterone dietary supplement products. JAMA 1998;280(18):1565.

[11] Chua R, et al. Quality, labeling accuracy, and cost comparison of purified soy isoflavonoid products. J Altern Complement Med 2004;10(6):1053–60.

[12] Harkey MR, et al. Variability in commercial ginseng products: an analysis of 25 preparations. Am J Clin Nutr 2001;73(6):1101–6.

[13] Arlt VM, Schmeiser HH, Pfeifer GP. Sequence-specific detection of aristolochic acid-DNA adducts in the human p53 gene by terminal transferase-dependent PCR. Carcinogenesis 2001;22(1):133–40.

[14] Gratz SR, Gamble BM, Flurer RA. Accurate mass measurement using Fourier transform ion cyclotron resonance mass spectrometry for structure elucidation of designer drug analogs of tadalafil, vardenafil and sildenafil in herbal and pharmaceutical matrices. Rapid Commun Mass Spectrom 2006;20(15):2317–27.

[15] Fleshner N, et al. Evidence for contamination of herbal erectile dysfunction products with phosphodiesterase type 5 inhibitors. J Urol 2005;174(2):636–41 [discussion: 641];[quiz: 801].

[16] Centers R, et al. FDA cracks down on illegal sex drugs.

[17] D'Ovidio K, et al. Aflatoxins in ginseng roots. Food Addit Contam 2006;23(2):174–80.

[18] Trucksess M, et al. Determination of aflatoxins and ochratoxin A in ginseng and other botanical roots by immunoaffinity column cleanup and liquid chromatography with fluorescence detection. J AOAC Int 2006;89(3):624–30.

[19] Tournas VH, Katsoudas E, Miracco EJ. Moulds, yeasts and aerobic plate counts in ginseng supplements. Int J Food Microbiol 2006;108(2):178–81.

[20] Kudo K, et al. A case of poisoning in a man who drank a nutrition supplement containing methomyl, a carbamate pesticide. Fukuoka Igaku Zasshi 2005;96(7):305–10.

[21] Rogan WJ, et al. Recall of a lead-contaminated vitamin and mineral supplement in a clinical trial. Pharmacoepidemiol Drug Saf 1999;8(5):343–50.

[22] Tseng YL, Kuo FH, Sun KH. Quantification and profiling of 19-norandrosterone and 19-noretiocholanolone in human urine after consumption of a nutritional supplement and nor-steroids. J Anal Toxicol 2005;29(2):124–34.

[23] Baume N, et al. Research of stimulants and anabolic steroids in dietary supplements. Scand J Med Sci Sports 2006;16(1):41–8.

[24] Morris CA, Avorn J. Internet marketing of herbal products. Jama 2003;290(11):1505–9.

[25] Srinivasan VS. Challenges and scientific issues in the standardization of botanicals and their preparations. United States Pharmacopeia's dietary supplement verification program—a public health program. Life Sci 2006;78(18):2039–43.

[26] NIH Consensus Conference. Impotence. NIH Consensus Development Panel on Impotence. JAMA 1993;270(1):83–90.

[27] Benet AE, Melman A. The epidemiology of erectile dysfunction. Urol Clin North Am 1995; 22(4):699–709.

[28] Johannes CB, et al. Incidence of erectile dysfunction in men 40 to 69 years old: longitudinal results from the Massachusetts male aging study. J Urol 2000;163(2):460–3.

[29] Moyad MA. The placebo effect and randomized trials: analysis of alternative medicine. Urol Clin North Am 2002;29(1):135–55, x.

[30] Moyad MA, et al. Prevention and treatment of erectile dysfunction using lifestyle changes and dietary supplements: what works and what is worthless, part II. Urol Clin North Am 2004;31(2):259–73.

[31] Montorsi F, et al. Efficacy and safety of fixed-dose oral sildenafil in the treatment of erectile dysfunction of various etiologies. Urology 1999;53(5):1011–8.

[32] Dula E, et al. Efficacy and safety of fixed-dose and dose-optimization regimens of sublingual apomorphine versus placebo in men with erectile dysfunction. The Apomorphine Study Group. Urology 2000;56(1):130–5.

[33] Thompson IM, et al. Erectile dysfunction and subsequent cardiovascular disease. Jama 2005;294(23):2996–3002.
[34] Arlt W, et al. Biotransformation of oral dehydroepiandrosterone in elderly men: significant increase in circulating estrogens. J Clin Endocrinol Metab 1999;84(6):2170–6.
[35] Pawlikowski M. Adrenal cortex—the next biological clock? Neuro Endocrinol Lett 2005; 26(3):193–5.
[36] Olech E, Merrill JT. DHEA supplementation: the claims in perspective. Cleve Clin J Med 2005;72(11):965–6 968, 970-1 passim.
[37] Basar MM, et al. Relationship between serum sex steroids and Aging Male Symptoms score and International Index of Erectile Function. Urology 2005;66(3):597–601.
[38] Reiter WJ, et al. Serum dehydroepiandrosterone sulfate concentrations in men with erectile dysfunction. Urology 2000;55(5):755–8.
[39] Feldman HA, et al. Impotence and its medical and psychosocial correlates: results of the Massachusetts Male Aging Study. J Urol 1994;151(1):54–61.
[40] Reiter WJ, et al. Dehydroepiandrosterone in the treatment of erectile dysfunction: a prospective, double-blind, randomized, placebo-controlled study. Urology 1999;53(3):590–4 [discussion: 594–5].
[41] Reiter WJ, et al. Dehydroepiandrosterone in the treatment of erectile dysfunction in patients with different organic etiologies. Urol Res 2001;29(4):278–81.
[42] Genazzani AR, et al. Long-term low-dose dehydroepiandrosterone replacement therapy in aging males with partial androgen deficiency. Aging Male 2004;7(2):133–43.
[43] Jones JA, et al. Use of DHEA in a patient with advanced prostate cancer: a case report and review. Urology 1997;50(5):784–8.
[44] Morales AJ, et al. Effects of replacement dose of dehydroepiandrosterone in men and women of advancing age. J Clin Endocrinol Metab 1994;78(6):1360–7.
[45] Araghiniknam M, et al. Antioxidant activity of dioscorea and dehydroepiandrosterone (DHEA) in older humans. Life Sci 1996;59(11):PL147–57.
[46] Adimoelja A. Phytochemicals and the breakthrough of traditional herbs in the management of sexual dysfunctions. Int J Androl 2000;23(Suppl 2):82–4.
[47] Horton R, Tait JF. Androstenedione production and interconversion rates measured in peripheral blood and studies on the possible site of its conversion to testosterone. J Clin Invest 1966;45(3):301–13.
[48] Brown GA, et al. Effects of anabolic precursors on serum testosterone concentrations and adaptations to resistance training in young men. Int J Sport Nutr Exerc Metab 2000;10(3): 340–59.
[49] King DS, et al. Effect of oral androstenedione on serum testosterone and adaptations to resistance training in young men: a randomized controlled trial. Jama 1999;281(21):2020–8.
[50] Wallace MB, et al. Effects of dehydroepiandrosterone vs androstenedione supplementation in men. Med Sci Sports Exerc 1999;31(12):1788–92.
[51] Rasmussen BB, et al. Androstenedione does not stimulate muscle protein anabolism in young healthy men. J Clin Endocrinol Metab 2000;85(1):55–9.
[52] Leder BZ, et al. Metabolism of orally administered androstenedione in young men. J Clin Endocrinol Metab 2001;86(8) 3654–3568.
[53] Leder BZ, et al. Oral androstenedione administration and serum testosterone concentrations in young men. JAMA 2000;283(6):779–82.
[54] Brown GA, et al. Endocrine responses to chronic androstenedione intake in 30- to 56-year-old men. J Clin Endocrinol Metab 2000;85(11):4074–80.
[55] Brown GA, et al. Effects of androstenedione-herbal supplementation on serum sex hormone concentrations in 30- to 59-year-old men. Int J Vitam Nutr Res 2001;71(5): 293–301.
[56] Siegner AW Jr. The Food and Drug Administration's actions on ephedra and androstenedione: understanding their potential impacts on the protections of the Dietary Supplement Health and Education Act. Food Drug Law J 2004;59(4):617–28.

[57] Bahrke MS, Yesalis CE. Abuse of anabolic androgenic steroids and related substances in sport and exercise. Curr Opin Pharmacol 2004;4(6):614–20.

[58] DesJardins M. Supplement use in the adolescent athlete. Curr Sports Med Rep 2002;1(6): 369–73.

[59] Lue TF, Lee KL. Pharmacotherapy for erectile dysfunction. Chin Med J (Engl) 2000; 113(4):291–8.

[60] Toda N, Ayajiki K, Okamura T. Nitric oxide and penile erectile function. Pharmacol Ther 2005;106(2):233–66.

[61] Zorgniotti AW, Lizza EF. Effect of large doses of the nitric oxide precursor, L-arginine, on erectile dysfunction. Int J Impot Res 1994;6(1):33–5 [discussion: 36].

[62] Chen J, et al. Effect of oral administration of high-dose nitric oxide donor L-arginine in men with organic erectile dysfunction: results of a double-blind, randomized, placebo-controlled study. BJU Int 1999;83(3):269–73.

[63] Klotz T, et al. Effectiveness of oral L-arginine in first-line treatment of erectile dysfunction in a controlled crossover study. Urol Int 1999;63(4):220–3.

[64] Fitzpatrick DF, Bing B, Rohdewald P. Endothelium-dependent vascular effects of Pycnogenol. J Cardiovasc Pharmacol 1998;32(4):509–15.

[65] Stanislavov R, Nikolova V. Treatment of erectile dysfunction with pycnogenol and L-arginine. J Sex Marital Ther 2003;29(3):207–13.

[66] Tam SW, Worcel M, Wyllie M. Yohimbine: a clinical review. Pharmacol Ther 2001;91(3): 215–43.

[67] Ernst E, Pittler MH. Yohimbine for erectile dysfunction: a systematic review and meta-analysis of randomized clinical trials. J Urol 1998;159(2):433–6.

[68] Pittler MH, Ernst E. Trials have shown yohimbine is effective for erectile dysfunction. BMJ 1998;317(7156):478.

[69] Susset JG, et al. Effect of yohimbine hydrochloride on erectile impotence: a double-blind study. J Urol 1989;141(6):1360–3.

[70] Guay AT, et al. Clomiphene increases free testosterone levels in men with both secondary hypogonadism and erectile dysfunction: who does and does not benefit? Int J Impot Res 2003;15(3):156–65.

[71] Kernohan AF, et al. An oral yohimbine/L-arginine combination (NMI 861) for the treatment of male erectile dysfunction: a pharmacokinetic, pharmacodynamic and interaction study with intravenous nitroglycerine in healthy male subjects. Br J Clin Pharmacol 2005;59(1):85–93.

[72] Lebret T, et al. Efficacy and safety of a novel combination of L-arginine glutamate and yohimbine hydrochloride: a new oral therapy for erectile dysfunction. Eur Urol 2002;41(6): 608–13 [discussion: 613].

[73] Johnson S, Iazzetta J, Dewar C. Severe Raynaud's phenomenon with yohimbine therapy for erectile dysfunction. J Rheumatol 2003;30(11):2503–5.

[74] Cohen AJ, Bartlik B. Ginkgo biloba for antidepressant-induced sexual dysfunction. J Sex Marital Ther 1998;24(2):139–43.

[75] Balon R. Ginkgo biloba for antidepressant-induced sexual dysfunction? J Sex Marital Ther 1999;25(1):1–2.

[76] Kang BJ, et al. A placebo-controlled, double-blind trial of Ginkgo biloba for antidepressant-induced sexual dysfunction. Hum Psychopharmacol 2002;17(6):279–84.

[77] Wheatley D. Triple-blind, placebo-controlled trial of Ginkgo biloba in sexual dysfunction due to antidepressant drugs. Hum Psychopharmacol 2004;19(8):545–8.

[78] Williamson EM. Interactions between herbal and conventional medicines. Expert Opin Drug Saf 2005;4(2):355–78.

[79] Izzo AA, et al. Cardiovascular pharmacotherapy and herbal medicines: the risk of drug interaction. Int J Cardiol 2005;98(1):1–14.

[80] Kupiec T, Raj V. Fatal seizures due to potential herb-drug interactions with Ginkgo biloba. J Anal Toxicol 2005;29(7):755–8.

[81] Ramsay NA, et al. Complimentary and alternative medicine use among patients starting warfarin. Br J Haematol 2005;130(5):777–80.

[82] Kim JY, et al. Induction of nitric oxide synthase by saponins of heat-processed ginseng. Biosci Biotechnol Biochem 2005;69(5):891–5.

[83] Choi YD, Rha KH, Choi HK. In vitro and in vivo experimental effect of Korean red ginseng on erection. J Urol 1999;162(4):1508–11.

[84] Choi YD, Xin ZC, Choi HK. Effect of Korean red ginseng on the rabbit corpus cavernosal smooth muscle. Int J Impot Res 1998;10(1):37–43.

[85] Ryu JK, et al. Free radical-scavenging activity of Korean red ginseng for erectile dysfunction in non-insulin-dependent diabetes mellitus rats. Urology 2005;65(3):611–5.

[86] Kang KS, et al. Study on the nitric oxide scavenging effects of ginseng and its compounds. J Agric Food Chem 2006;54(7):2558–62.

[87] Choi HK, Seong DH, Rha KH. Clinical efficacy of Korean red ginseng for erectile dysfunction. Int J Impot Res 1995;7(3):181–6.

[88] Hong B, et al. A double-blind crossover study evaluating the efficacy of korean red ginseng in patients with erectile dysfunction: a preliminary report. J Urol 2002;168(5):2070–3.

[89] Price A, Gazewood J. Korean red ginseng effective for treatment of erectile dysfunction. J Fam Pract 2003;52(1):20–1.

[90] Cipolla MJ, et al. Propionyl-L-carnitine dilates human subcutaneous arteries through an endothelium-dependent mechanism. J Vasc Surg 1999;29(6):1097–103.

[91] Cavallini G, et al. Carnitine versus androgen administration in the treatment of sexual dysfunction, depressed mood, and fatigue associated with male aging. Urology 2004;63(4):641–6.

[92] Gentile V, et al. Preliminary observations on the use of propionyl-L-carnitine in combination with sildenafil in patients with erectile dysfunction and diabetes. Curr Med Res Opin 2004;20(9):1377–84.

[93] Cavallini G, et al. Acetyl-L-carnitine plus propionyl-L-carnitine improve efficacy of sildenafil in treatment of erectile dysfunction after bilateral nerve-sparing radical retropubic prostatectomy. Urology 2005;66(5):1080–5.

[94] Eng J, et al. A population-based survey of complementary and alternative medicine use in men recently diagnosed with prostate cancer. Integr Cancer Ther 2003;2(3):212–6.

[95] Chan JM, et al. Total and specific complementary and alternative medicine use in a large cohort of men with prostate cancer. Urology 2005;66(6):1223–8.

[96] Barnes PM, et al. Complementary and alternative medicine use among adults: United States, 2002. Adv Data 2004;(343):1–19.

[97] Carraro JC, et al. Comparison of phytotherapy (Permixon) with finasteride in the treatment of benign prostate hyperplasia: a randomized international study of 1,098 patients. Prostate 1996;29(4):231–40 [discussion: 241–2].

[98] Boyle P, et al. Updated meta-analysis of clinical trials of Serenoa repens extract in the treatment of symptomatic benign prostatic hyperplasia. BJU Int 2004;93(6):751–6.

[99] Gerber GS, et al. Randomized, double-blind, placebo-controlled trial of saw palmetto in men with lower urinary tract symptoms. Urology 2001;58(6):960–4 [discussion: 964–5].

[100] Beckman TJ, Mynderse LA. Evaluation and medical management of benign prostatic hyperplasia. Mayo Clin Proc 2005;80(10):1356–62.

[101] Bent S, et al. Saw palmetto for benign prostatic hyperplasia. N Engl J Med 2006;354(6):557–66.

[102] Chan JM, Gann PH, Giovannucci EL. Role of diet in prostate cancer development and progression. J Clin Oncol 2005;23(32):8152–60.

[103] Anlasik T, et al. Dietary habits are major determinants of the plasma antioxidant status in healthy elderly subjects. Br J Nutr 2005;94(5):639–42.

[104] Sies H, Stahl W, Sevanian A. Nutritional, dietary and postprandial oxidative stress. J Nutr 2005;135(5):969–72.

[105] Di Mascio P, et al. Carotenoids, tocopherols and thiols as biological singlet molecular oxygen quenchers. Biochem Soc Trans 1990;18(6):1054–6.

[106] Clinton SK, et al. cis-trans lycopene isomers, carotenoids, and retinol in the human prostate. Cancer Epidemiol Biomarkers Prev 1996;5(10):823–33.
[107] Giovannucci E. A review of epidemiologic studies of tomatoes, lycopene, and prostate cancer. Exp Biol Med (Maywood) 2002;227(10):852–9.
[108] Giovannucci E. Tomato products, lycopene, and prostate cancer: a review of the epidemiological literature. J Nutr 2005;135(8):2030S–1S.
[109] Giovannucci E, et al. Intake of carotenoids and retinol in relation to risk of prostate cancer. J Natl Cancer Inst 1995;87(23):1767–76.
[110] Giovannucci E, et al. A prospective study of tomato products, lycopene, and prostate cancer risk. J Natl Cancer Inst 2002;94(5):391–8.
[111] Wu K, et al. Plasma and dietary carotenoids, and the risk of prostate cancer: a nested case-control study. Cancer Epidemiol Biomarkers Prev 2004;13(2):260–9.
[112] Lu QY, et al. Inverse associations between plasma lycopene and other carotenoids and prostate cancer. Cancer Epidemiol Biomarkers Prev 2001;10(7):749–56.
[113] Vogt TM, et al. Serum lycopene, other serum carotenoids, and risk of prostate cancer in US Blacks and Whites. Am J Epidemiol 2002;155(11):1023–32.
[114] Etminan M, Takkouche B, Caamano-Isorna F. The role of tomato products and lycopene in the prevention of prostate cancer: a meta-analysis of observational studies. Cancer Epidemiol Biomarkers Prev 2004;13(3):340–5.
[115] Cohen JH, Kristal AR, Stanford JL. Fruit and vegetable intakes and prostate cancer risk. J Natl Cancer Inst 2000;92(1):61–8.
[116] Kolonel LN, et al. Vegetables, fruits, legumes and prostate cancer: a multiethnic case-control study. Cancer Epidemiol Biomarkers Prev 2000;9(8):795–804.
[117] Le Marchand L, et al. Vegetable and fruit consumption in relation to prostate cancer risk in Hawaii: a reevaluation of the effect of dietary beta-carotene. Am J Epidemiol 1991;133(3):215–9.
[118] Hayes RB, et al. Dietary factors and risks for prostate cancer among blacks and whites in the United States. Cancer Epidemiol Biomarkers Prev 1999;8(1):25–34.
[119] Kirsh VA, et al. A prospective study of lycopene and tomato product intake and risk of prostate cancer. Cancer Epidemiol Biomarkers Prev 2006;15(1):92–8.
[120] Cook NR, et al. Beta-carotene supplementation for patients with low baseline levels and decreased risks of total and prostate carcinoma. Cancer 1999;86(9):1783–92.
[121] Kirsh VA, et al. Supplemental and dietary vitamin E, beta-carotene, and vitamin C intakes and prostate cancer risk. J Natl Cancer Inst 2006;98(4):245–54.
[122] Heinonen OP, et al. Prostate cancer and supplementation with alpha-tocopherol and beta-carotene: incidence and mortality in a controlled trial. J Natl Cancer Inst 1998;90(6):440–6.
[123] Gann PH, et al. Lower prostate cancer risk in men with elevated plasma lycopene levels: results of a prospective analysis. Cancer Res 1999;59(6):1225–30.
[124] Goodman GE, et al. The association between lung and prostate cancer risk, and serum micronutrients: results and lessons learned from beta-carotene and retinol efficacy trial. Cancer Epidemiol Biomarkers Prev 2003;12(6):518–26.
[125] Eichholzer M, et al. Smoking, plasma vitamins C, E, retinol, and carotene, and fatal prostate cancer: seventeen-year follow-up of the prospective basel study. Prostate 1999;38(3):189–98.
[126] Stahelin HB, et al. Plasma antioxidant vitamins and subsequent cancer mortality in the 12-year follow-up of the prospective Basel Study. Am J Epidemiol 1991;133(8):766–75.
[127] Vlajinac HD, et al. Diet and prostate cancer: a case-control study. Eur J Cancer 1997;33(1):101–7.
[128] Tzonou A, et al. Diet and cancer of the prostate: a case-control study in Greece. Int J Cancer 1999;80(5):704–8.
[129] Deneo-Pellegrini H, et al. Foods, nutrients and prostate cancer: a case-control study in Uruguay. Br J Cancer 1999;80(3–4):591–7.
[130] Chan JM, et al. Supplemental vitamin E intake and prostate cancer risk in a large cohort of men in the United States. Cancer Epidemiol Biomarkers Prev 1999;8(10):893–9.

[131] Hartman TJ, et al. The association between baseline vitamin E, selenium, and prostate cancer in the alpha-tocopherol, beta-carotene cancer prevention study. Cancer Epidemiol Biomarkers Prev 1998;7(4):335–40.
[132] Rodriguez C, et al. Vitamin E supplements and risk of prostate cancer in U.S. men. Cancer Epidemiol Biomarkers Prev 2004;13(3):378–82.
[133] Hsing AW, et al. Serologic precursors of cancer. Retinol, carotenoids, and tocopherol and risk of prostate cancer. J Natl Cancer Inst 1990;82(11):941–6.
[134] Hayes RB, et al. Serum retinol and prostate cancer. Cancer 1988;62(9):2021–6.
[135] Hernaandez J, et al. The modulation of prostate cancer risk with alpha-tocopherol: a pilot randomized, controlled clinical trial. J Urol 2005;174(2):519–22.
[136] Huang HY, et al. Prospective study of antioxidant micronutrients in the blood and the risk of developing prostate cancer. Am J Epidemiol 2003;157(4):335–44.
[137] Giovannucci E. Gamma-tocopherol: a new player in prostate cancer prevention? J Natl Cancer Inst 2000;92(24):1966–7.
[138] Redman C, et al. Involvement of polyamines in selenomethionine induced apoptosis and mitotic alterations in human tumor cells. Carcinogenesis 1997;18(6):1195–202.
[139] Griffin AC. Role of selenium in the chemoprevention of cancer. Adv Cancer Res 1979;29: 419–42.
[140] Waters DJ, et al. Effects of dietary selenium supplementation on DNA damage and apoptosis in canine prostate. J Natl Cancer Inst 2003;95(3):237–41.
[141] Chun JY, et al. Mechanisms of selenium down-regulation of androgen receptor signaling in prostate cancer. Mol Cancer Ther 2006;5(4):913–8.
[142] Lee SO, et al. Selenium disrupts estrogen signaling by altering estrogen receptor expression and ligand binding in human breast cancer cells. Cancer Res 2005;65(8):3487–92.
[143] Dong Y, et al. Prostate specific antigen expression is down-regulated by selenium through disruption of androgen receptor signaling. Cancer Res 2004;64(1):19–22.
[144] van den Brandt PA, et al. Toenail selenium levels and the subsequent risk of prostate cancer: a prospective cohort study. Cancer Epidemiol Biomarkers Prev 2003;12(9):866–71.
[145] Ozmen H, et al. Comparison of the concentration of trace metals (Ni, Zn, Co, Cu and Se), Fe, vitamins A, C and E, and lipid peroxidation in patients with prostate cancer. Clin Chem Lab Med 2006;44(2):175–9.
[146] Li H, et al. A prospective study of plasma selenium levels and prostate cancer risk. J Natl Cancer Inst 2004;96(9):696–703.
[147] Nomura AM, et al. Serum selenium and subsequent risk of prostate cancer. Cancer Epidemiol Biomarkers Prev 2000;9(9):883–7.
[148] Yoshizawa K, et al. Study of prediagnostic selenium level in toenails and the risk of advanced prostate cancer. J Natl Cancer Inst 1998;90(16):1219–24.
[149] Lipsky K, et al. Selenium levels of patients with newly diagnosed prostate cancer compared with control group. Urology 2004;63(5):912–6.
[150] Nyman DW, et al. Selenium and selenomethionine levels in prostate cancer patients. Cancer Detect Prev 2004;28(1):8–16.
[151] Kumar NB, et al. The specific role of isoflavones in reducing prostate cancer risk. Prostate 2004;59(2):141–7.
[152] Ghadirian P, et al. A case-control study of toenail selenium and cancer of the breast, colon, and prostate. Cancer Detect Prev 2000;24(4):305–13.
[153] Duffield-Lillico AJ, et al. Selenium supplementation, baseline plasma selenium status and incidence of prostate cancer: an analysis of the complete treatment period of the Nutritional Prevention of Cancer Trial. BJU Int 2003;91(7):608–12.
[154] Duffield-Lillico AJ, et al. Baseline characteristics and the effect of selenium supplementation on cancer incidence in a randomized clinical trial: a summary report of the Nutritional Prevention of Cancer Trial. Cancer Epidemiol Biomarkers Prev 2002;11(7):630–9.
[155] Meyer F, et al. Antioxidant vitamin and mineral supplementation and prostate cancer prevention in the SU.VI.MAX trial. Int J Cancer 2005;116(2):182–6.

[156] Hoenjet KM, et al. Effect of a nutritional supplement containing vitamin E, selenium, vitamin C and coenzyme Q10 on serum PSA in patients with hormonally untreated carcinoma of the prostate: a randomised placebo-controlled study. Eur Urol 2005;47(4):433–9 [discussion: 439–40].

[157] Klein EA. Selenium and vitamin E cancer prevention trial. Ann N Y Acad Sci 2004;1031: 234–41.

[158] Lippman SM, et al. Designing the Selenium and Vitamin E Cancer Prevention Trial (SELECT). J Natl Cancer Inst 2005;97(2):94–102.

[159] Drake EN. Cancer chemoprevention: selenium as a prooxidant, not an antioxidant. Med Hypotheses 2006;67(2):318–22.

[160] Platz EA, et al. Alcohol intake, drinking patterns, and risk of prostate cancer in a large prospective cohort study. Am J Epidemiol 2004;159(5):444–53.

[161] Barba M, et al. Lifetime total and beverage specific–alcohol intake and prostate cancer risk: a case-control study. Nutr J 2004;3:23.

[162] Sharpe CR, Siemiatycki J. Case-control study of alcohol consumption and prostate cancer risk in Montreal, Canada. Cancer Causes Control 2001;12(7):589–98.

[163] Schoonen WM, et al. Alcohol consumption and risk of prostate cancer in middle-aged men. Int J Cancer 2005;113(1):133–40.

[164] Jain MG, et al. Alcohol and other beverage use and prostate cancer risk among Canadian men. Int J Cancer 1998;78(6):707–11.

[165] Heilbrun LK, Nomura A, Stemmermann GN. Black tea consumption and cancer risk: a prospective study. Br J Cancer 1986;54(4):677–83.

[166] Jian L, et al. Protective effect of green tea against prostate cancer: a case-control study in southeast China. Int J Cancer 2004;108(1):130–5.

[167] Sonoda T, et al. A case-control study of diet and prostate cancer in Japan: possible protective effect of traditional Japanese diet. Cancer Sci 2004;95(3):238–42.

[168] Kinlen LJ, et al. Tea consumption and cancer. Br J Cancer 1988;58(3):397–401.

[169] Bettuzzi S, et al. Chemoprevention of human prostate cancer by oral administration of green tea catechins in volunteers with high-grade prostate intraepithelial neoplasia: a preliminary report from a one-year proof-of-principle study. Cancer Res 2006;66(2):1234–40.

[170] Graham HN. Green tea composition, consumption, and polyphenol chemistry. Prev Med 1992;21(3):334–50.

[171] Sharpe CR, Siemiatycki J. Consumption of non-alcoholic beverages and prostate cancer risk. Eur J Cancer Prev 2002;11(5):497–501.

[172] Slattery ML, West DW. Smoking, alcohol, coffee, tea, caffeine, and theobromine: risk of prostate cancer in Utah (United States). Cancer Causes Control 1993;4(6):559–63.

[173] Ellison LF. Tea and other beverage consumption and prostate cancer risk: a Canadian retrospective cohort study. Eur J Cancer Prev 2000;9(2):125–30.

[174] Jatoi A, et al. A phase II trial of green tea in the treatment of patients with androgen independent metastatic prostate carcinoma. Cancer 2003;97(6):1442–6.

[175] Lee AH, et al. Protective effects of green tea against prostate cancer. Expert Rev Anticancer Ther 2006;6(4):507–13.

[176] Albrecht M, et al. Pomegranate extracts potently suppress proliferation, xenograft growth, and invasion of human prostate cancer cells. J Med Food 2004;7(3):274–83.

[177] Pantuck AJ, et al. Phase II study of pomegranate juice for men with rising prostate-specific antigen following surgery or radiation for prostate cancer. Clin Cancer Res 2006;12(13):4018–26.

[178] Holzbeierlein JM, McIntosh J, Thrasher JB. The role of soy phytoestrogens in prostate cancer. Curr Opin Urol 2005;15(1):17–22.

[179] Lee MM, et al. Soy and isoflavone consumption in relation to prostate cancer risk in China. Cancer Epidemiol Biomarkers Prev 2003;12(7):665–8.

[180] Jacobsen BK, Knutsen SF, Fraser GE. Does high soy milk intake reduce prostate cancer incidence? The Adventist Health Study (United States). Cancer Causes Control 1998; 9(6):553–7.

[181] Hebert JR, et al. Nutritional and socioeconomic factors in relation to prostate cancer mortality: a cross-national study. J Natl Cancer Inst 1998;90(21):1637–47.
[182] Nomura AM, et al. Cohort study of tofu intake and prostate cancer: no apparent association. Cancer Epidemiol Biomarkers Prev 2004;13(12):2277–9.
[183] Strom SS, et al. Phytoestrogen intake and prostate cancer: a case-control study using a new database. Nutr Cancer 1999;33(1):20–5.
[184] Maskarinec G, et al. Serum prostate-specific antigen but not testosterone levels decrease in a randomized soy intervention among men. Eur J Clin Nutr 2006.
[185] McCarty MF. Isoflavones made simple—genistein's agonist activity for the beta-type estrogen receptor mediates their health benefits. Med Hypotheses 2006;66(6):1093–114.
[186] Costello LC, et al. Zinc and prostate cancer: a critical scientific, medical, and public interest issue (United States). Cancer Causes Control 2005;16(8):901–15.
[187] Moyad MA. Lifestyle/dietary supplement partial androgen suppression and/or estrogen manipulation. A novel PSA reducer and preventive/treatment option for prostate cancer? Urol Clin North Am 2002;29(1):115–24, ix.
[188] Dhar NK, et al. Distribution and concentration of zinc in the subcellular fractions of benign hyperplastic and malignant neoplastic human prostate. Exp Mol Pathol 1973;19(2):139–42.
[189] Kristal AR, et al. Vitamin and mineral supplement use is associated with reduced risk of prostate cancer. Cancer Epidemiol Biomarkers Prev 1999;8(10):887–92.
[190] Key TJ, et al. A case-control study of diet and prostate cancer. Br J Cancer 1997;76(5): 678–87.
[191] West DW, et al. Adult dietary intake and prostate cancer risk in Utah: a case-control study with special emphasis on aggressive tumors. Cancer Causes Control 1991;2(2):85–94.
[192] Andersson SO, et al. Energy, nutrient intake and prostate cancer risk: a population-based case-control study in Sweden. Int J Cancer 1996;68(6):716–22.
[193] Leitzmann MF, et al. Zinc supplement use and risk of prostate cancer. J Natl Cancer Inst 2003;95(13):1004–7.
[194] Kolonel LN, Yoshizawa CN, Hankin JH. Diet and prostatic cancer: a case-control study in Hawaii. Am J Epidemiol 1988;127(5):999–1012.
[195] Sperling H, et al. An extract from the bark of Aspidosperma quebracho blanco binds to human penile alpha-adrenoceptors. J Urol 2002;168(1):160–3.
[196] Choi J, et al. Antinociceptive anti-inflammatory effect of Monotropein isolated from the root of *Morinda officinalis*. Biol Pharm Bull 2005;28(10):1915–8.
[197] Di Rocco A, et al. A pilot study of L-methionine for the treatment of AIDS-associated myelopathy. Neurology 1998;51(1):266–8.
[198] James JS. Frequent urination, leg cramps, leg weakness, erection difficulties: HIV myelopathy amino acid study. AIDS Treat News 2000;(344):3–4.
[199] Hitiris N, Barrett JA, Brodie MJ. Erectile dysfunction associated with pregabalin add-on treatment in patients with partial seizures: five case reports. Epilepsy Behav 2006;8(2): 418–21.
[200] Hong JH, et al. The effects of curcumin on the invasiveness of prostate cancer in vitro and in vivo. Prostate Cancer Prostatic Dis 2006;9(2):147–52.
[201] Zamble A, et al. Paullinia pinnata extracts rich in polyphenols promote vascular relaxation via endothelium-dependent mechanisms. J Cardiovasc Pharmacol 2006;47(4):599–608.
[202] Safarinejad MR. Urtica dioica for treatment of benign prostatic hyperplasia: a prospective, randomized, double-blind, placebo-controlled, crossover study. J Herb Pharmacother 2005;5(4):1–11.
[203] Sokeland J. Combined sabal and urtica extract compared with finasteride in men with benign prostatic hyperplasia: analysis of prostate volume and therapeutic outcome. BJU Int 2000;86(4):439–42.
[204] Lopatkin NA, et al. [Combined extract of Sabal palm and nettle in the treatment of patients with lower urinary tract symptoms in double blind, placebo-controlled trial]. Urologiia 2006;(2):12, 14–9 [in Russian].

[205] Melo EA, et al. Evaluating the efficiency of a combination of *Pygeum africanum* and sting-
ing nettle (*Urtica dioica*) extracts in treating benign prostatic hyperplasia (BPH): double-
blind, randomized, placebo controlled trial. Int Braz J Urol 2002;28(5):418–25.

[206] Wilt T, et al. Pygeum africanum for benign prostatic hyperplasia. Cochrane Database Syst
Rev 2002;1:CD001044.

[207] Klippel KF, Hiltl DM, Schipp B. A multicentric, placebo-controlled, double-blind clinical
trial of beta-sitosterol (phytosterol) for the treatment of benign prostatic hyperplasia. German BPH-Phyto Study group. Br J Urol 1997;80(3):427–32.

[208] Berges RR, Kassen A, Senge T. Treatment of symptomatic benign prostatic hyperplasia
with beta-sitosterol: an 18-month follow-up. BJU Int 2000;85(7):842–6.

[209] MacDonald R, et al. A systematic review of Cernilton for the treatment of benign prostatic
hyperplasia. BJU Int 2000;85(7):836–41.

ELSEVIER
SAUNDERS

Endocrinol Metab Clin N Am
36 (2007) 553–578

ENDOCRINOLOGY
AND METABOLISM
CLINICS
OF NORTH AMERICA

Index

Note: Page numbers of article titles are in **boldface** type.

A

Abdominal obesity, CPAP effects on, 354
  diabetes mellitus related to, 351
  in metabolic syndrome, 351–352
  testosterone relationship to, 350

Absolute estrogen excess, gynecomastia
  from, 499, 501

Acetyl-L-carnitine (ALC), for erectile
  dysfunction, 537–538

Acetylcysteine, for male infertility, 319

Acne, androgen excess causing, 445

Active-confronting coping, in infertility,
  524, 528

Acute illness, male hypogonadism and,
  335–337
    testosterone treatment efficacy
      studies in, 337–338

Addiction, to anabolic steroids, 485–486

Adipokines, in obstructive sleep apnea, 354

Adiponectin, testosterone therapy impact
  on, 353

Adipose tissue, estrogen production in, 369

Adolescents, ergogenic aids use by, 483–485

Adrenal gland, excess estrogen production
  by, gynecomastia from, 502–503

Adrenarche, 283

Adrenocortical tumors, feminizing, 502, 513

Adrenoleukodystrophy, X-linked recessive,
  387

Adult-onset hypogonadotropic
  hypogonadism, 293

Age/aging, erectile dysfunction and,
  androgen insufficiency with, 436, 439
    endothelial dysfunction in, 453
  gynecomastia related to, 498, 505
  osteoporosis related to, 402–403, 405,
    407

Aging Male Scale, 439

AIDS wasting syndrome, 334, 340–341

Alcohol abuse, osteoporosis related to,
  402–403

Alendronate, for osteoporosis, 410–411

Alexithymia, 525

Alkaline phosphatase, in osteoporosis,
  408–409

Alopecia, androgen insufficiency causing,
  436, 439, 441
  androgenetic, **379–398**
    classification of, 380–381
    clinical features of, 380
    diagnosis of, 382–383
    disease associations with, 387
    histology of, 383
    historical versus modern research
      on, 379
    overview of, 379, 392–393
    pathogenesis of, 383–387
    prevalence of, 380–381
    risk factors for, 387
    treatment of, 387–393
  psychosocial aspects of, 527–528

5-Alpha reductase enzyme, in androgen
  insufficiency and erectile dysfunction,
  441–442
    as first-line therapy, 444–445
  in androgenetic alopecia, 384–386
  prostate development role, 421, 423

5-Alpha reductase inhibitors, for androgen
  insufficiency and erectile dysfunction,
  442, 444–445
  for prostate cancer, 423

α-Blockers, erectile dysfunction treatment
  and, 468–469, 471

Alpha-Tocopherol Beta-Carotene (ATBC)
  trial, 539

Alprostadil, for erectile dysfunction,
  intracavernosal, 470–472

0889-8529/07/$ - see front matter © 2007 Elsevier Inc. All rights reserved.
doi:10.1016/S0889-8529(07)00051-5   *endo.theclinics.com*

histology of, 383
historical versus modern research on, 379
overview of, 379, 392–393
pathogenesis of, 383–387
    androgens role, 384–386
    genetics in, 386–387
    hair cycle changes in, 383–384
prevalence of, 380–381
risk factors for, 387
treatment of, 387–393

Androgenic pathway, prostate cancer and, 422–423
    as risk factor, 422–423
    preventive inhibition of, 423–424

Androgen-to-estrogen ratio, in gynecomastia, 504–507

Andrologic disease/disorders, deficiencies as. See *Androgen insufficiency*.
    hypogonadal. See *Hypogonadism*.
    reproductive. See *Infertility*.
    dietary supplements and nutraceuticals for, **533–552**
        common problems with, 534
        decrease libido indications, 534–538
        erectile dysfunction indications, 534–538
        herbal preparations, 536–537, 540–543
        infertility indications, 319–320
        overview of, 533–534, 543
        prostate indications, 538–539, 542–543
        survey on use of, 533–534
    erectile, **435–452**. See also *Erectile dysfunction (ED)*.
    genetics of. See *Gene mutations; Genetics*.
    gynecomastia as, **497–519**. See also *Gynecomastia*.
    hair loss as. See *Alopecia*.
    obesity and, **349–363**. See also *Obesity*.
    psychosocial aspects of, **521–531**
        counseling in, 527
        erectile dysfunction and, 526–527
        hypospadias and, 525–526
        infertility and, 522–525
        psychologic treatment in, 527
        research discussion on, 521, 527–529
        stress and coping in, 521–522
    pubertal. See *Puberty*.

Androstenedione, as sport performance-enhancing drug, 483, 487–488

for erectile dysfunction, 535–536
gynecomastia and, 502–503
prostate cancer risk and, 422
puberty role, 283
skin metabolism of, 384–385

ANDROTEST, 439

Anger, infertility and, 523

Angina, as phosphodiesterase type 5 inhibitor contraindication, 467–468

Anomalies, delayed puberty related to, 285
    in idiopathic hypogonadotropic hypogonadism, 289–292

Anosmia, 288, 291

Antiandrogen monotherapy, for prostate cancer, 426–428

Antiandrogens, for gynecomastia, 507
    for prostate cancer, 425
        combination therapies, 426
        controversies with, 426–428
        monotherapy, 426–428

Antiarrhythmics, as phosphodiesterase type 5 inhibitor contraindication, 467

Antibalding lotions, gynecomastia and, 503

Antibiotics, for male infertility, 315–316

Antibodies, antisperm, 306

Anticholinergics, for male infertility, 316

Antidepressants, erectile dysfunction and, 527

Anti-Doping Agencies, US, 485, 489
    World, 485, 489

Anti-Drug Abuse Act (1988), 482

Antiestrogens, for gynecomastia, 505, 513–514
    for male infertility, 316–317

Anti-müllerian hormone (AMH), neonatal role, 284

Antioxidants, for male infertility, 319–320
    for prostate health, 538–539, 542

Antiplatelet therapy, for testosterone therapy in CAD, 371

Antisperm antibodies, 306

Apomorphine, for erectile dysfunction, 469–470
    sublingual, 470
    with androgen insufficiency, 446

Appraisal-oriented coping, in infertility, 524

Lipid level, elevated. See *Dyslipidemia.*

Lipid uptake, testosterone impact on, 350, 371

Liver disease, aromatase inhibitors caution with, 318
  cirrhosis as, gynecomastia and, 506–507
  hypogonadism associated with, acute, 334–336
    chronic, 334, 342

Longitudinal bone growth, androgen role, 405

Lower urinary tract symptoms (LUTS), dietary supplements/nutraceuticals for, 534, 540–541

Lubricants, vaginal, infertility and, 298

Luteinizing hormone (LH), childhood physiology of, 284, 286
  for male infertility, 313–314
  in androgen insufficiency, and erectile dysfunction, 443, 447
    measurement of, 335
  in gynecomastia, 499, 501–502
  in hypogonadism diagnosis, hypogonadotropic, 287–289
    systemic disease and, 335–336
  in infertility evaluation, 302–303
  in obstructive sleep apnea, 353

Luteinizing hormone releasing-hormone (LHRH), for gynecomastia, 507

Lycopene, for prostate health, 539

M

Magnetic resonance imaging (MRI), in hypogonadotropic hypogonadism diagnosis, 287
  in infertility evaluation, 308

Male breast cancer, gynecomastia and, 503, 509

Male breast tissue, enlargement of. See *Gynecomastia.*
  fatty, 511
  sex hormone receptors in, 498–499

Male hypogonadism, general symptoms of, 333–334
  gynecomastia related to, primary, 503–504
    secondary, 504
  infertility related to, 302
  systemic disease in, **333–348**
    laboratory diagnosis of, 334–344

mechanism of action, 333–335, 344
  symptoms significance, 333–334
  testosterone treatment efficacy studies in, 337–338

Male infertility, delayed puberty and, 286
  diagnostic approach to, **297–311**
    differential, 303–306
    initial evaluation, 298–303
    purpose of, 297–298, 309
    pyospermia and, 306
    radiologic, 306–309
  environmental factors of, 525, 528
  genetics in, 504
  management of, **313–331**
    algorithm for, 324–325
    medical therapies for, 313–320
      empiric agents in, 316–320
      specific agents in, 313–316
    microsurgical procedures for, 325
    overview of, 313, 325
    surgical procedures for, 320–325
  obesity epidemic and, 350
  psychosocial aspects of, 522–525, 528
  reactive oxygen species and, 319

Male osteoporosis, **399–419**
  age-related, 402–403
  androgen insufficiency causing, 436
  causes of, 401–404
  clinical approach to, 408–409
  epidemiology of, 399–401
  estrogen deficiency causing, 318, 405–406
  idiopathic, 402–403, 407
  importance of, 399
  pathophysiology of, 401–402, 404–408
  secondary, 402–404
  treatment of, 409–412

Male reproductive function, deficiency of. See *Male infertility.*
  obesity epidemic and, 349–351

Mammography, for gynecomastia, 511, 513

Marital benefit, infertility and, 523

Masculinity, infertility and, 523, 528

Massachusetts Male Aging Study, 453, 458

Mastopathy, diabetic, gynecomastia and, 508–509

Meaning-based coping, in infertility, 524

Mechanical devices/therapies, for erectile dysfunction, penile prostheses as, 473–474
    vacuum erection devices as, 470–472
  for hirsutism, 445

Reproductive history, in infertility
evaluation, 297–298

Respiratory disease, chronic obstructive,
hypogonadism associated with, 334,
341–342
osteoporosis related to, 403

Respiratory illness, hypogonadism
associated with, 334–336

Retinitis pigmentosa, as phosphodiesterase
type 5 inhibitor contraindication, 467

Rheumatoid arthritis (RA), hypogonadism
associated with, 334, 343–344

Rhinitis, phosphodiesterase type 5
inhibitors causing, 467

Rigiscan measurements, of erectile
dysfunction treatment duration, 466

Risedronate, for osteoporosis, 410

Rotterdam Study, of osteoporosis, 400

S

Saw palmetto, for prostate health, 538

Scalp biopsy, for androgenetic alopecia,
382–383

Scalp reduction surgery, for androgenetic
alopecia, 390

Screening, for androgen insufficiency, 439
for sport ergogenic aid use, 485,
487–490

Secondary hypogonadism, gynecomastia
related to, 504
in critically ill patients, 336
in HIV-positive patients, 340–341

Secondary osteoporosis, in men, 402–404

Secondary sex characteristics, development
during puberty, 283, 499
in infertility evaluation, 299–300

Secrecy, infertility and, 523–524

Selective estrogen receptor modulators
(SERMs), for erectile dysfunction, 537
for gynecomastia, 505, 514
for osteoporosis, 411–412

Selenium, for prostate health, 539

Self-efficacy, infertility and, 522, 528

Semen. See also *Sperm concentration.*
mental stress impact on, 286

Semen analyses, for infertility diagnosis,
297, 300–301

differential, 305–306
normal parameters for, 301, 305–306

Seminal vesicle defects, infertility related to,
300, 305
radiographic imaging of, 307–308

Sepsis, hypogonadism associated with,
334–336

Sertoli cell failure, infertility related to, 302

Sertoli cell proteins, neonatal role, 284

Sertoli cell tumors, gynecomastia related to,
501–502

Severity of illness, systemic, hypogonadism
related to, 336–337

Sex hormone-binding globulin (SHBG),
androgen insufficiency and, diagnostic
level of, 440–441
follow-up monitoring of, 447
coronary artery disease and, 366–367
gynecomastia and, 501, 503, 505, 507
male hypogonadism and, in systemic
disease, 334, 336
metabolic syndrome and, 351

Sex steroid receptors, in male breast tissue,
498–499

Sex steroids. See also *specific hormone,*
e.g.,Testosterone.
cardiovascular effects of, **365–377**
coagulation and, 372–373
endothelial function in, 371–372
hypogonadism impact, 365–368
inflammation and, 372–373
myocardium in, 370
obesity and, 368–370
overview of, 365
testosterone in, 370–371
exogenous, 371–373
thrombosis in, 370–371
midlife loss of production of, 401
osteoporosis related to, 404–408
prostate cancer and, **421–434**. See also
Prostate cancer.

Sexual history, in androgen insufficiency
with erectile dysfunction, 436
in infertility evaluation, 298–299

Sexual relations, timing with ovulation, 298

Sexuality, hypospadias effect on, 525–526

Sexually transmitted diseases, in infertility
evaluation, 299

Shame, infertility and, 523

Short stature, diagnostic approach to, 285,
288

Moving?

Make sure your subscription moves with you!

To notify us of your new address, find your **Clinics Account Number** (located on your mailing label above your name), and contact customer service at:

E-mail: elspcs@elsevier.com

800-654-2452 (subscribers in the U.S. & Canada)
407-345-4000 (subscribers outside of the U.S. & Canada)

Fax number: 407-363-9661

Elsevier Periodicals Customer Service
6277 Sea Harbor Drive
Orlando, FL 32887-4800

*To ensure uninterrupted delivery of your subscription, please notify us at least 4 weeks in advance of move.